COMPUTATIONAL GENETICS AND GENOMICS

COMPUTATIONAL GENETICS AND GENOMICS

Tools for Understanding Disease

Edited by

GARY PELTZ, MD, PhD

*Department of Genetics and Genomics, Roche Palo Alto,
Palo Alto, CA*

HUMANA PRESS ✳ TOTOWA, NEW JERSEY

© 2005 Humana Press Inc.
999 Riverview Drive, Suite 208
Totowa, New Jersey 07512

www.humanapress.com

Production Editor: Amy Thau

Cover design by Patricia F. Cleary

Cover Illustration: A haplotype block emerging from a DNA double helix. Image by Myriam Kirkman-Oh, KO Studios, courtesy of Roche.

For additional copies, pricing for bulk purchases, and/or information about other Humana titles, contact Humana at the above address or at any of the following numbers: Tel.: 973-256-1699; Fax: 973-256-8341; E-mail: orders@humanapr.com or visit our website at www.humanapress.com

The opinions expressed herein are the views of the authors and may not necessarily reflect the official policy of the National Institute on Drug Abuse or any other parts of the US Department of Health and Human Services. The US Government does not endorse or favor any specific commercial product or company. Trade, proprietary, or company names appearing in this publication are used only because they are considered essential in the context of the studies reported herein.

This publication is printed on acid-free paper. ∞
ANSI Z39.48-1984 (American National Standards Institute) Permanence of Paper for Printed Library Materials.

Printed in the United States of America. 10 9 8 7 6 5 4 3 2 1
eISBN: 1-59259-930-3
Library of Congress Cataloging-in-Publication Data
Computational genetics and genomics : tools for understanding
    disease / edited by Gary Peltz. p. ; cm.
    Includes bibliographical references and index.
    ISBN 1-58829-187-1 (alk. paper)
    1. Medical genetics--Mathematical models. 2. Genomics
--Mathematical models.   I. Peltz, Gary, 1956-   .
    [DNLM: 1. Genomics--methods. 2. Computational Biology.
3. Disease Models, Animal. 4. Mice, Transgenic--genetics.
QU 58.5 C738 2005]
RB155.C595 2005
616'.042'0151--dc22
                                    2004022878

PREFACE

Ultimately, the quality of the tools available for genetic analysis and experimental disease models will be assessed on the basis of whether they provide new information that generates novel treatments for human disease. In addition, the time frame in which genetic discoveries impact clinical practice is also an important dimension of how society assesses the results of the significant public financial investment in genetic research. Because of the investment and the increased expectation that new treatments will be found for common diseases, allowing decades to pass before basic discoveries are made and translated into new therapies is no longer acceptable.

Computational Genetics and Genomics: Tools for Understanding Disease provides an overview and assessment of currently available and developing tools for genetic analysis. It is hoped that these new tools can be used to identify the genetic basis for susceptibility to disease. Although this very broad topic is addressed in many other books and journal articles, *Computational Genetics and Genomics: Tools for Understanding Disease* focuses on methods used for analyzing mouse genetic models of biomedically important traits. This volume aims to demonstrate that commonly used inbred mouse strains can be used to model virtually all human disease-related traits. Importantly, recently developed computational tools will enable the genetic basis for differences in disease-related traits to be rapidly identified using these inbred mouse strains.

On average, a decade is required to carry out the development process required to demonstrate that a new disease treatment is beneficial. However, the analysis of mouse genetic models and the application of the approaches described in this text will enable genetic discoveries to be made much more quickly. Providing insight into the genes and pathways regulating the disease-related traits among the inbred strains. The results can direct subsequent biological experimentation, clinical research, and human genetic analysis.

The book is organized into three parts: Part I: Theory and Technical Concepts, Part II: Selected Examples: Murine Models of Human Disease, and Part III: Selected Examples: The Genetic Basis for Human Disease. The chapters in the first section provide theoretical and practical overviews of the methodology used for analysis of murine genetic models of human

v

disease. Chapter 1 describes how new computational methods and analysis of biomedical traits among inbred mouse strains can accelerate the rate of genetic discovery. The statistical methods used for genetic analysis of murine experimental intercross progeny, which are referred to as quantitative trait locus mapping, are described in Chapter 2. Chapter 3 provides the first detailed overview of a recently developed haplotype-based computational genetic analysis method. If used by experimental mouse geneticists, this method can exponentially accelerate the rate of genetic discoveries made using murine disease models. The methods for organizing the pattern of genetic polymorphisms in the genome of inbred strains into haplotype blocks, which can be computationally analyzed, is described in Chapter 4. This chapter also compares the different methods used for generating haplotype blocks for mouse and man, and indicates how they can be used for very different applications. The section concludes with a description of the methods for discovering and characterizing genetic polymorphisms found among the commonly used inbred mouse strains in Chapter 5.

The second section provides an overview of murine models of asthma and lung disease, osteoporosis, and substance abuse. Although there are a multitude of available mouse models for many different human disease-related traits, these chapters were written by investigators who have developed the models that are used in the disease area they investigate. More importantly, they provide an overview of available mouse models and what has been learned from analysis of these models. In addition, they also indicate what models need to be developed in order to advance our understanding of these diseases. Because many disease-related processes can only be studied in vivo, it is important to examine the quality of the available disease models.

In the third section, two chapters describe how genetic analysis of human populations has provided information about the genetic basis for susceptibility to asthma and other inflammatory diseases. Hopefully, we will be able to write additional chapters about the genetic basis for many more diseases within the next few years.

Gary Peltz, MD, PhD

CONTENTS

PART III. SELECTED EXAMPLES:
THE GENETIC BASIS FOR HUMAN DISEASE

CONTRIBUTORS

JOHN ALLARD • *Department of Genetics and Genomics, Roche Palo Alto, Palo Alto, CA*

DEE AUD • *Department of Genetics and Genomics, Roche Palo Alto, Palo Alto, CA*

BETH BENNETT • *Institute for Behavioral Genetics, University of Colorado, Boulder, CO*

JANET CHENG • *Department of Genetics and Genomics, Roche Palo Alto, Palo Alto, CA*

CHRISTOPHER CHOU • *Department of Genetics and Genomics, Roche Palo Alto, Palo Alto, CA*

WILLIAM COOKSON • *Wellcome Trust Centre for Human Genetics, University of Oxford, Oxford, UK*

JOHN C. CRABBE • *Department of Behavioral Neuroscience, Oregon Health & Science University and Portland VA Medical Center, Portland, OR*

KIM CRONISE • *Departments of Psychology and Neuroscience, Middlebury College, Middlebury, VT*

ARIEL DARVASI • *The Institute of Life Sciences, The Hebrew University, Jerusalem, Israel*

CHRIS DOWNING • *Institute for Behavioral Genetics, University of Colorado, Boulder, CO*

HENRY A. ERLICH • *Human Genetics Department, Roche Molecular Systems Inc., Alameda, CA*

DOROTHEE FOERNZLER • *Roche Center for Medical Genomics, F. Hoffmann-La Roche Ltd., Basel, Switzerland*

SOREN GERMER • *Human Genetics Department, Roche Molecular Systems Inc., Alameda, CA*

JINGSHU GUO • *Department of Genetics and Genomics, Roche Palo Alto, Palo Alto, CA*

RUSSELL HIGUCHI • *Human Genetics Department, Roche Molecular Systems Inc., Alameda, CA*

MICHAEL J. HOLTZMAN • *Division of Pulmonary and Critical Care Medicine, Washington University School of Medicine, St. Louis, MO*

STEVEN HU • *Department of Genetics and Genomics, Roche Palo Alto, Palo Alto, CA*

SHARON JIANG • *Department of Genetics and Genomics, Roche Palo Alto, Palo Alto, CA*

THOMAS E. JOHNSON • *Institute for Behavioral Genetics, University of Colorado, Boulder, CO*

EDY Y. KIM • *Division of Pulmonary and Critical Care Medicine, Washington University School of Medicine, St. Louis, MO*

ROBERT F. KLEIN • *Bone and Mineral Research Unit, Oregon Health & Science University and Portland VA Medical Center, Portland, OR*

GUOCHUN LIAO • *Department of Genetics and Genomics, Roche Palo Alto, Palo Alto, CA*

JOHN D. MCPHERSON • *Department of Molecular and Human Genetics and Human Genome Sequencing Center, Baylor College of Medicine, Houston, TX*

JEFFREY D. MORTON • *Division of Pulmonary and Critical Care Medicine, Washington University School of Medicine, St. Louis, MO*

ANH NGUYEN • *Department of Genetics and Genomics, Roche Palo Alto, Palo Alto, CA*

GARY PELTZ • *Department of Genetics and Genomics, Roche Palo Alto, Palo Alto, CA*

ANNE PISANTÉ • *The Institute of Life Sciences, The Hebrew University, Jerusalem, Israel*

ANNE PUECH • *Centre National de Genotypage, Evry, France*

STEVE SHAFER • *Department of Anesthesia, Stanford University Medical Center, Stanford, CA*

JONATHAN USUKA • *Department of Genetics and Genomics, Roche Palo Alto, Palo Alto, CA*

JIANMEI WANG • *Department of Genetics and Genomics, Roche Palo Alto, Palo Alto, CA*

JUN WANG • *Human Genetics Department, Roche Molecular Systems Inc., Alameda, CA*

BENJAMIN YAKIR • *The Institute of Life Sciences, The Hebrew University, Jerusalem, Israel*

I

THEORY AND TECHNICAL CONCEPT

1
Computational Biology

Are We There Yet?

Gary Peltz

1. INTRODUCTION

Any parent who has taken young children on a car trip will understand the question in the title and its implied impatience with the duration of the journey. The same question can be put to the research community's journey toward understanding the genetic basis of complex disease. Recently developed genomic technologies, such as oligonucleotide microarrays and achievements including whole genome sequencing, have suggested that scientists can now analyze complex genetic diseases at a much more rapid pace. The analytic speed is further increased by the large amount of genetic and genomic information that is available in public databases, which enables several analytic steps to be computationally performed. However, it is clear that we have not yet arrived at our desired destination, that of knowing the genetic basis for complex disease susceptibility *(1)*. Therefore, it is an appropriate time to ask if complex disease research is moving in the right direction and if it is using the best road map and the appropriate type of transportation.

A significant percentage of research in academic and industrial laboratories is now directed toward understanding the pathogenesis of complex human diseases. In simple terms, a complex disease does not result from an alteration at a single genetic locus; but multiple, distinct genetic susceptibility loci contribute to its pathogenesis. Environmental factors may also have a large impact on susceptibility. The clinical phenotypes that are part of the spectrum of complex human diseases can be analyzed in the same manner as any complex genetic trait; they result from summation of effects from all contributing loci. This is fundamentally different from qualitative traits, such as the presence or absence of a disease diagnosis, in which individual

From: *Computational Genetics and Genomics*
Edited by: G. Peltz © Humana Press Inc., Totowa, NJ

phenotypes fall into discrete categories *(2)*. Complex disease-associated traits often show quantitative variation and exhibit an approximately normal distribution in the population. Quantitative variation is that which is measured on a numerical scale. A quantitative trait locus (QTL) is a genetic locus that contributes to a quantitative trait. It is the quantitative aspect of the disease-associated traits that facilitates genetic analysis *(2)*.

Complex diseases have been the focus of academic and industrial research efforts because they are common in the general population and have a large impact on human health. Rheumatoid arthritis provides one example of the impact a complex disease has on society. It has an overall prevalence of 1% among adults and affects approx 2.1 million people in the United States *(3)*. Its estimated annual cost (direct and indirect) was $8.7 billion in 1994 *(4)*, and this is expected to increase dramatically in the first two decades of the 21st century *(5)*. It is known that rheumatoid arthritis susceptibility is controlled by several different genetic loci, including those within and outside the HLA region. Family studies have clearly demonstrated a heritable predisposition to rheumatoid arthritis and many other common diseases, such as asthma, autism, schizophrenia, multiple sclerosis, systemic lupus erythematosus (SLE), and type 1 and type 2 diabetes mellitus (reviewed in ref. *1*). It is anticipated that identification of the genetic factors regulating susceptibility to complex disease will lead to a better understanding of the cause of these diseases, improved therapeutics, and even strategies for disease prevention.

In contrast, Mendelian (simple) genetic diseases result from alterations at a single genetic locus. For a Mendelian trait, the genetic alteration has a large phenotypic effect, and there is a one-to-one correspondence between the genotype and phenotype. Although these diseases may severely impact affected individuals, they appear in a relatively small number of individuals. For example, cystic fibrosis, the most common Mendelian-like genetic disease, has an incidence of 1 in 3300 Caucasians. The incidence is less in African Americans (1 in 15,300) and Asian-Americans (1 in 32,000), and is a very rare disease (less than 1 in 50,000) in Africa and Asia *(6)*. Linkage analysis and positional cloning are very powerful methods that have been used over the last 20 yr to identify the genetic loci responsible for cystic fibrosis and for more than 100 other monogenic human diseases *(7)*. The same approaches also identified genes responsible for a subset of some common disorders, such as breast cancer (BRCA-1, -2), colon cancer (familial adenomatous polyposis and hereditary nonpolyposis colon cancer), Alzheimer's disease (β-amyloid precursor protein, presenilin-1 and -2), and diabetes (maturity onset diabetes of youth -1, -2, and -3) (reviewed in ref. *1*).

However, the identified mutations account for only a small percentage of individuals with these diseases. For example, the identification of BRCA-1 and -2 mutations that are associated with susceptibility to breast cancer was a major accomplishment. They were identified by analysis of cohorts of individuals with an early onset and high familial incidence of breast cancer. However, only about 3% of all primary breast cancer in the general population (diagnosed at age <70 yr) is caused by the highly penetrant mutations *(8)*. Conventional linkage and positional cloning methods have had only limited success in identifying the genetic loci that underlie the most common traits and diseases in humans. Despite considerable effort, genetic variants accounting for susceptibility to most common disorders in the general population have not been identified.

It is clear that a new playbook and new rules must be developed to accelerate the rate at which complex disease-related traits can be successfully analyzed in humans. The thesis underlying this book is that an integrative approach, beginning with genetic analysis of complex disease-associated traits in experimental model organisms, provides an efficient and productive process for analysis of complex traits (Fig. 1). Most human disease-related traits can be modeled in experimental organisms, such as the mouse or rat. The experimental genetic models of complex disease-related traits can then be genetically analyzed using standard linkage and positional cloning methods. Identification of genetic loci within the linked regions can be accelerated by using an integrated approach employing currently available genetic and

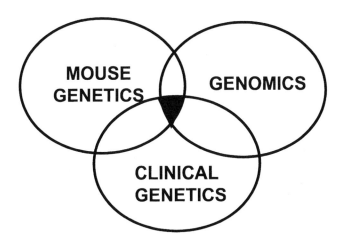

Fig. 1. Diagrammatic representation of an integrative approach used for analysis of complex disease-related traits.

genomic tools. In addition, the pace at which genetic discoveries can be made using mouse genetic models can be greatly accelerated by the use of recently developed computational tools. These will be described in this and other chapters in this book. The results of this analysis can direct subsequent biological experimentation, clinical research, and human genetic analysis. This type of analysis will provide insight into the genes and pathways regulating the complex disease-related traits in model organisms. The human homologs of the identified gene, as well as other elements in the pathway, can then be analyzed using human genetic analysis.

The conceptual basis for, and practical application of, genetic methods to investigate human disease biology are described in this book. The reasons for analyzing mouse models of human disease-related traits are presented in this chapter, along with an overview of how integrative and computational methods accelerate genetic analysis. A set of "rules" is discussed in the next section. These "rules" should not be viewed as absolutes. Rather, they are devices used to describe the rationale for the proposed methods for studying disease biology. Following this, three examples are provided. Each indicates how an integrated genetic and genomic approach enabled the genetic basis for disease-related phenotypic differences in experimental mouse genetic models to be identified. Lastly, an overview of how recently developed computational methods can accelerate the process of genetic discovery is provided. Subsequent chapters provide more detailed information on this computational method and specific applications.

2. SOME "RULES" FOR UNDERSTANDING THE DISEASE BIOLOGY

1. Complex traits are not simple. As discussed in the Introduction, the analysis of human cohorts using conventional linkage and positional cloning has enabled genetic mutations responsible for a number of monogenic diseases and a subset of monogenic-like diseases to be identified. The mutations identified by this method have a very large effect on susceptibility and exhibit a strong genotype–phenotype correlation. The mutations were identified in clinical cohorts with unusual presentations and account for an uncommon subset of individuals with a common disease. In contrast, positional cloning and linkage approaches have had only limited success in identifying the genetic loci that underlie the most common traits and diseases in humans. Despite considerable effort, genetic variants accounting for susceptibility to many common disorders in the general population have not been identified. Because multiple genetic loci are involved, and each individual locus makes a small contribution to

overall disease susceptibility, it has been quite difficult to identify common disease-susceptibility loci by applying conventional linkage and positional cloning methods to human populations. Furthermore, a genetic alteration at a single locus that is responsible for a major phenotypic effect in a small subset of the population may not bear any relationship to the genetic changes underlying subtle (quantitative) differences in the general population. Because of these factors, new tools and approaches must be developed to identify genetic factors underlying common human diseases.
2. We have to better utilize gene expression information and improve our understanding of the biological impact of alterations in gene expression patterns. The importance of global gene expression patterns as a tool for understanding genetic variation and genetic susceptibility to disease has not been fully appreciated. Cataloging changes in gene expression patterns and understanding its regulation are required and fundamental steps for understanding complex biological processes. The fact that 5% of genes in the genome are predicted to encode transcription factors *(9)* indicates how important this process is to cellular biology. The pattern of gene expression is precisely connected to the functioning of cells and tissues. When correlated with phenotype, it provides a rich source of information about the function of genes, cells, and tissues. Alterations in this pattern can be used to understand disease processes and susceptibility points. From a genetic perspective, the combinatorial effect of *cis-* and *trans-* sequence polymorphisms on the level of expression of a single gene allows for more possible phenotypic diversity than a quantitative estimate of the amount of genotypic variation within a population would predict. The expression level(s) of a given gene (or genes) within a pathway can be very finely modulated. This provides a genetic control mechanism that can be modulated in a much finer manner than could be achieved through alterations in the coding sequence of a protein. Consistent with this, promoter-specific transcription activators are quite abundant in the human genome. One analysis suggested that the human genome may contain over 2000 promoter-specific transcription activators in the human genome *(9)*.

Ribonucleic acid (RNA) splicing provides another mechanism for directly modifying information contained in the genome and provides another source for genetic regulation of complex traits. The biological importance of RNA splicing is supported by a recent experimental observation that at least 74% of human multiexon genes are alternatively spliced *(10)*. Others have estimated that 40–60% of human genes produce alternatively spliced gene products *(11)*. Premessenger (m)RNA splicing involves the removal of introns and joining exons to form mature mRNAs

with intact translation reading frames (for review *see* refs. *12* and *13*). This complex process is regulated by both intronic and exonic nucleotide sequences (reviewed in ref. *14*). In addition to the invariant GT and AG intronic dinucleotide sequences at the 5′ (donor) and 3′ (acceptor) exon–intron junctions, there are other less-conserved sequence motifs that regulate pre-mRNA splicing. Enhancer and silencer sequences that promote or inhibit the splicing process have been identified in both exonic and intronic sequences. Genetic variation in these sequences can produce a complete absence of correctly spliced transcripts or the presence of aberrantly spliced transcripts. As demonstrated in yeast, a genetic change in RNA-processing proteins can have a genome-wide effect on transcription *(15)*. Similarly, a genetic polymorphism in a pre-mRNA-splicing protein could affect isoform-specific gene expression patterns, biological processes, phenotype, or disease susceptibility *(14,16)*. For example, analysis of the regulation of CD44 cell surface glycoprotein isoform expression demonstrates that an alteration in pre-mRNA splicing plays a role in a disease process. Because it has 10 alternatively spliced exons, the *CD44* gene is transcribed into a variety of isoforms, which are expressed in a developmental stage and tissue-specific pattern *(17)*. In several human malignancies, certain CD44 splice variants are predominantly expressed. In a mouse model, changes in the relative level of CD44 isoform transcripts were accompanied by a significant change in the expression of several (SR family) splicing factors expressed during tumorigenesis in the mammary gland *(18)*. Mutations in a 5′ splice site in exon 10 of the microtubule-associated protein *tau* gene, which regulate alternative splicing and tau protein isoform expression, were associated with frontotemporal dementia and Parkinsonism linked to chromosome 17 *(19)*. Interestingly, these mutations disrupted a stem-loop structure in tau RNA, and the stability of this secondary structure affected the ratio of tau isoform expression in vitro. A significant fraction (10–15%) of disease-causing mutations in human genes affects pre-mRNA splicing (*see* Human Gene Mutation Database, http://archive.uwcm.ac.uk and ref. *14*).
3. Patterns of polymorphism within a chromosomal region—not an individual single nucleotide polymorphism (SNP) or a restricted subset of SNPs within the coding sequences of a single gene—is the unit for evaluating the effect of genotypic changes on phenotype.

The central dogma of molecular biology indicated that individual genes are transcribed into RNA, which is then translated into protein. Because of the importance of the central dogma to scientific research, geneticists have focused on sequence variation within a gene as the unit for studying the consequences of genetic variation. Often, polymorphism scanning has been confined to genomic sequences within or near exons *(20)*. However, genetic variation is not introduced into the genome by processes that respect boundaries between genes, nor does it select for coding sequences. Furthermore, the effect of a sequence change may not be confined to a single gene. Therefore, it is likely to be more efficient and productive to evaluate sequence variation over a chromosomal region when assessing the effect of genotype on phenotype.

Although SNPs at different sites within a chromosomal region can be identified and characterized individually, alleles at different positions along a chromosome can be associated. The presence or absence of an allele at one site can provide information about alleles at other sites; this association between alleles is called *linkage disequilibrium.* A haplotype can be defined as the relationship between deoxyribonucleic acid (DNA) sequence variants in the same gene, region, or chromosome. Analysis of polymorphisms over large genomic segments of the human genome has indicated that polymorphic variation at multiple sites within a chromosomal region can be grouped into patterns ("haplotypes") with high linkage disequilibrium *(20–23)*. Regions with low linkage disequilibrium separate the haplotypic blocks. The size of the genomic sequence contained within a haplotypic block can range from a few to over 100 kb. Analysis of human chromosome 21 indicated that about half the haplotypic blocks identified, each with an average size of 7.8 kb, could be defined by less than three SNPs, and less than three different haplotypes within a block encompassed most of the population (80%) *(23)*. Unfortunately, the structure of the haplotypic blocks cannot be determined empirically. A large amount of detailed sequence information must be available to identify the haplotype-defining SNPs and the conserved blocks. It is also likely that the size and structure of the haplotypic blocks will change as sequence information from more individuals is obtained and analyzed. However, analysis of the haplotypic patterns enables individuals within a population to be segmented into a finite number of small groups sharing the same haplotype for a particular chromosomal region. Identification of haplotypes to segment the human population has great potential. This will decrease the amount of genotyping required to characterize a genomic region, and the haplotypic information will enable a human population to be segregated into a finite number of different groups. The frequency of disease or disease-associated traits can be compared among the groups with different genetic haplotypes within a chromosomal region. It is hoped that this will provide a more efficient method for identification of disease-susceptibility regions in human populations. One of the first examples of linkage disequilibrium mapping using haplotypes was the identification of a 250-kb region of human chromosome 5q31 associated with Crohn's disease susceptibility *(24)*. There were 11 SNPs with strong linkage disequilibrium in the 5q31 region associated with Crohn's disease susceptibility, and it was not possible to identify an individual disease-associated SNP. These results are consistent with the possibility that a set of polymorphisms within a chromosomal region, which may effect more than a single gene, contribute to the disease susceptibility.

Similarly, inbred mouse strains are particularly useful for genetic analysis because the entire genome of an inbred strain is effective in linkage disequilibrium. The parental origin of DNA segments in intercross progeny over entire chromosomes can be inferred by analysis of only a few polymorphic markers *(25)*. Furthermore, there is extensive linkage disequilibrium among polymorphisms in the genome of inbred strains. Analogous to the human population, SNPs among the inbred strains can be organized into haplotypic blocks *(26)*. Analysis of regions linked to susceptibility to complex disease-related traits in mouse models has also indicated that genetic changes across chromosomal regions affecting multiple genes, rather than within a particular gene, may contribute to susceptibility. For example, a region on chromosome 1 that controls autoantibody production in a mouse model of SLE was analyzed. Polymorphisms within a set of co-linear interferon-inducible genes in this region were responsible for differential autoantibody production in this model *(27)*. This result appears to be applicable to other mouse models of human disease-related traits. Fine-mapping analysis often identifies several distinct subloci within a linked chromosomal region that independently contribute to the phenotypic trait. Additional analysis of a linked chromosomal region regulating autoantibody production and nephritis in the murine model of systemic lupus demonstrated that the interval consisted of at least four distinct genetic loci *(28)*. Similarly, the ability of our "digital disease" computer program to identify chromosomal regions regulating complex traits in mice is likely to result from recognition of patterns of genetic variation over large (10 cm) regions within the mouse genome *(29)*. Analysis of the patterns of variation over larger regions is likely to be informative in situations when analysis of a single SNP does not reveal genotype–phenotype correlation.

4. Integrative approaches must be utilized to efficiently analyze complex biological processes. Only a limited amount of resolution can be achieved with the use of any single approach for analyzing a complex biological

system. However, two orthogonal approaches can be simultaneously applied to investigate a complex biological problem. Although each approach may have its own inherent limitations, the integrated use of data arising from each of the two separate approaches can provide a more efficient and precise analysis. The integrated use of gene expression data obtained with high-density oligonucleotide microarrays in conjunction with the SNP genotyping method has been shown to accelerate QTL analysis *(27,30,31)*. The identification of a genetic locus within a defined genetic interval is accelerated by analysis of differentially expressed genes within the region in selected tissues obtained from the parental strains. A computational method for performing genetic analysis will be described in this book. This computational method enables candidate chromosomal regions and specific genes to be identified very quickly for phenotypes that differ among inbred mouse strains. If so, databases with tissue-specific gene expression and phenotypic information across mouse strains could be used in conjunction with the murine SNP database to computationally identify candidate disease genes. In a hypothetical experiment, the expression of roughly 25,000 murine genes in an affected tissue obtained from different mouse strains can be profiled. In this hypothetical example, assume that 2% of these genes will be differentially expressed within tissues obtained from strains with a phenotypic difference. The resulting list of 500 gene candidates could be computationally reduced by 99% to about five genes, by identifying genes that are encoded within a 15-cm chromosomal region that is linked to the trait. This approach provides a reasonable starting point for analysis of complex disease biology and should reduce the frustrations and overcome the difficulties associated with QTL analysis in murine complex disease models. Complex trait analysis will be greatly accelerated by the development of other methods that can examine changes in all genes within an organism. Consistent with this, it has recently been demonstrated that gene expression levels can be analyzed as heritable traits in mice, plants, and humans *(32)*. Producing a catalog of gene expression differences among commonly used inbred mouse strains would accelerate analysis of identified chromosomal regions controlling genetic traits. Although proteomic technologies are quite promising, they currently lack the bandwidth needed for genome-wide analysis. Hopefully, improved proteomic technologies will soon be developed, which can be utilized for genetic analysis in the very near future.

5. The problem with experimental mouse or rat models of human disease is not with the models themselves, but with the way they have been inappropriately utilized and interpreted. As one example, the pathogenesis

of human immune-mediated diseases has been studied in many different rodent models. An organ-specific inflammatory response is induced in rodent experimental models by sensitization and subsequent re-exposure to an experimental antigen. There are mouse and rat models of allergen-induced experimental asthma *(33,34)*, collagen-induced arthritis *(35–37)*, and experimental allergic encephalitis *(38,39)*, in which antigen-triggered inflammation is induced in the lungs, joints, and brain, respectively. The organ-specific inflammation developing in these experimental models has characteristics that resemble human asthma, rheumatoid arthritis, or multiple sclerosis. The pharmaceutical industry has used these models for preclinical testing of potential therapeutic agents. The effect of an exogenous agent on the antigen-induced organ-specific inflammatory process in these experimental models is characterized to assess whether a potential therapeutic will have efficacy in a human disease. However, utilization of available rodent experimental models for this purpose has been fraught with problems. A tested compound can ameliorate inflammation in these models by inhibiting the immune-mediated response to the inciting antigen. Unfortunately, the clinical manifestations of a human immune-mediated disease often appear years to decades after an individual has been sensitized to an antigen. In contrast, the rodent models are analyzed within days to 1 mo after initial antigen exposure. Although initiated by an immune response to antigen, the human immune-mediated diseases become clinically apparent when the underlying pathogenic processes no longer involve the initial response to the disease-inciting antigen. Therefore, efficacy in human clinical cohorts is likely to be unrelated to efficacy in the preclinical mouse models.

The differences observed in the innate and adaptive immune responses of mouse and man have recently been reviewed *(40)*. These differences can affect different components of the immune response and can be the basis for differences in the observed response to experimental interventions. Because there are 65–75 million years of evolutionary distance between mouse and man, it should not be a surprise that there are differences between these two species. However, overemphasizing the catalog of differences between the immune response of murine and man can lead to neglect of the key point. The vast majority of the fundamental mechanisms and processes regulating the murine and human immune responses are very similar. Therefore, the mechanisms underlying immune-mediated phenotypic differences of biomedical importance are quite likely to be shared by mouse and man. Although the exact site at which the genetic change is introduced is quite likely to differ between the two species, the controlling pathways are likely to be similar.

Although the murine models have limited utility for predicting the efficacy of human therapeutics in clinical trials, they have been quite useful for identifying genetic susceptibility elements for human disease. As in the human population, inbred mouse strains are differentially susceptible to developing organ-specific inflammation in response to experimental antigen exposure protocols. Therefore, these experimental mouse models of human inflammatory disease have been genetically analyzed to identify genetic elements contributing to susceptibility or resistance to the disease-related process. It is striking that different investigators have identified similar genetic loci regulating susceptibility in different experimental rodent models of human disease-related traits *(38,41)*. Most importantly, the genetic regions identified in some rodent experimental models are syntenic to the regions identified by analysis of human cohorts with immune-mediated diseases. Analysis of 21 previously published genome-wide scans indicated that several clinically distinct human autoimmune diseases—including asthma, rheumatoid arthritis, and multiple sclerosis—may be controlled by a common set of susceptibility loci, and the loci were syntenic to those found through analysis of experimental mouse models *(42)*. The similarities in genetic loci identified in human and rodent models extend beyond inflammatory disease. Six chromosomal regions regulating hypertension were identified in a murine genetic model. There was a high degree of concordance between the chromosomal regions identified in the mouse model and those found in human populations (four of six) and rat experimental models (five of six) *(43)*. It is not known how often the genetic loci regulating complex traits in murine models will directly translate into human susceptibility elements. However, it is very likely that the genes and pathways identified in the experimental rodent models will provide key insight into how complex disease-associated traits are genetically controlled in human populations. Most human disease genes isolated by positional cloning have highly similar homologs in rodents *(44)*.

6. Understanding the biological impact of the genetic changes underlying complex traits will require the development of new methods for biological analysis. Most biological experimentation examines pathways that have a major effect on cell and tissue function. This is similar to the rather profound phenotypic changes associated with genetic changes underlying Mendelian traits. In contrast, the biological impact of genetic changes underlying complex traits will be much more subtle, more difficult to dissect in isolation, and will be sensitive to the overall genetic background and the environment. It will not be possible to confirm the

identity of many complex trait loci by functional complementation or with gene knockouts *(2)*. This makes it much more difficult to identify and understand the biological impact of genetic variation at complex trait loci. It is likely that the criteria and methods currently used for biological analysis will have to be altered for complex traits. Phenotypic effects in gene knockout mice or changes caused by exogenous gene complementation are unlikely to be seen in these complex systems. The supporting evidence for the biological effect of an individual genetic alteration underlying a complex trait is likely to be indirect. A preponderance of supporting evidence and the absence of negative evidence will often be the determining criteria. Gene or protein expression differences, response to environmental factors, effects of other components in the pathway, and the involvement of orthologs in other species will be analyzed for subtle biological effects produced by genetic alterations underlying complex traits. The plethora of information generated by genetic analysis of complex traits will spur advances in cell biology and organ physiology. It is likely that QTL affect cellular differentiation and organ development. Therefore, more sensitive and efficient methods for studying cellular differentiation process and tissue development will have to be developed. Small molecules will be more extensively used to analyze the biological pathways impacted by genetic variation. Small molecules have provided key information about protein function in several areas of biology. Tetrodotoxin was used to analyze the action potential *(45)*, whereas prostaglandin J2 and peroxisome proliferator-activated receptor-γ (PPAR-γ) agonists enabled a pathway regulating adipogenesis to be analyzed *(46,47)*. However, a large amount of time and cost is required to produce a highly specific chemical inhibitor for a desired gene product. Therefore, small interfering RNAs (siRNAs), which decrease the expression of a selected mRNA by gene silencing, provide a powerful new tool for biological analysis (reviewed in ref. *48*). Although there are limitations that are because of the limited extent and time of siRNA-mediated RNA knockdown, siRNAs can be used to assess the biological importance of many different types of candidate genes in vitro. Furthermore, the availability of siRNA libraries targeting a large number of specific mouse and human genes *(49)* further increases the utility of this tool. Once the current limitations resulting from off-target and temporally limited effects are overcome, siRNAs will be the first of a number of new tools that enable a more efficient process of biological characterization of genetically identified gene candidates.

3. THREE EXAMPLES: INTEGRATIVE APPROACH
TO COMPLEX TRAIT ANALYSIS IN MICE

Commonly used genetic mapping tools identify chromosomal regions affecting complex traits in rodent models of human disease-related traits. However, identification of the causative genetic factor within a linked chromosomal region is essential for obtaining new information about a disease or biological process. The process of identifying genetic loci within linked chromosomal regions is difficult and often unproductive, which has been a source of frustration for many *(50)*. However, the following three examples demonstrate how the combined use of whole genome gene expression profiling and QTL analysis of mouse genetic models enables the efficient identification of causative genetic variants within linked regions.

3.1. Murine Experimental Model of Asthma

An integrative approach was utilized to analyze a well-characterized murine genetic model that mimics the pathophysiology of human allergic asthma (Fig. 2). In this model, allergen exposure results in airway hyperresponsiveness,

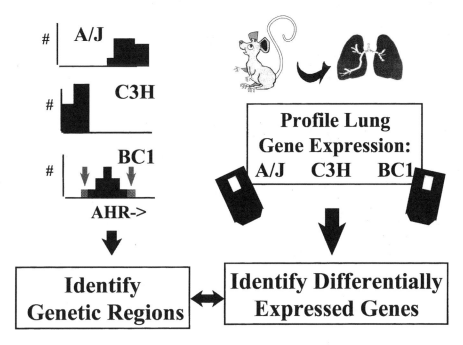

Fig. 2. Diagrammatic representation of an integrated genetic and genomic approach for analyzing a murine experimental genetic model of allergic asthma.

increased airway epithelial mucus content, antigen-specific IgE in serum, and pulmonary eosinophilia *(51,52)*. Inbred mouse strains vary markedly in their susceptibility to disease induction in this model. Two strains with markedly different susceptibilities to experimental allergen-induced asthma were used: the A/J strain is highly susceptible to allergen-induced airway hyperresponsiveness and the C3H/HeJ strain is highly resistant. Analysis of the inheritance pattern of the asthmatic response in intercross progeny led to the identification of regions on chromosomes 2 and 7 that regulated asthma susceptibility in this experimental model. To identify gene candidates, pulmonary gene expression was profiled using oligonucleotide microarrays. After phenotypical assessment, lungs were harvested from parental (A/J, C3H/HeJ) and F1 mice and from eight first-generation backcross progeny (BC1) that exhibited phenotypically extreme allergen-induced airway responsiveness. As indicated in Fig. 3, 2718 of the 7350 genes on the microarray were expressed in the lungs of the parental strains. A total of 739 genes were differentially expressed in the lungs

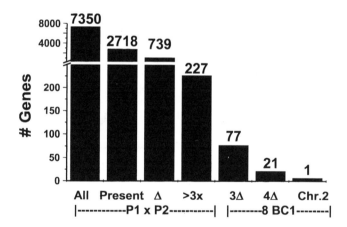

Fig. 3. Identification of a gene regulating susceptibility in an experimental murine genetic model of allergic asthma. The number of differentially expressed genes after comparison of gene expression profiles was determined after examining the number of genes: on the oligonucleotide array (all); expressed in the lungs of the two parental mouse strains (present); differentially expressed between the two strains according to the criteria provided by the manufacturer (Δ); computationally determined to be over threefold different (3×) between the two strains; or differentially expressed among the eight BC1 intercross progeny examined. The gene expression profile of five pairs of phenotypically extreme BC1 progeny was compared as described in the text. The number of differentially expressed genes when three (3Δ) or four (4Δ) of the five comparisons indicated that the gene was differentially expressed is shown.

of A/J and C3H/HeJ mice (Δ), and 227 genes exhibited a more than threefold change in expression when these two parental strains were compared (>3x).

Differential gene expression was also assessed within groups of high-responder (A/J and 4 BC1-high) and low-responder (C3H and 4 BC1-low) mice. The expression data were filtered for differential expression using five intragroup pairwise comparisons. Only 77 genes were differentially expressed if three of the five comparisons were different (3Δ), and 21 genes were differentially expressed when four of the five comparisons were different (4Δ). The initial expression data set was confirmed by expression profiling additional high-responder and low-responder intercross progeny to yield a total of 18 data points. This analysis revealed that only a single differentially expressed gene was located within one of the identified QTL intervals. Complement factor 5 (*C5*), located at 23.5 cm on chromosome 2, was the only gene that met the differential expression criteria and was located in one of the defined QTL intervals.

The level of *C5* expression was significantly associated with genotype and correlated closely with the magnitude of allergen-induced asthmatic response (Fig. 4). This correlation was strengthened when genotyping of the lone BC1-low responder mouse with an aberrantly low level of pulmonary

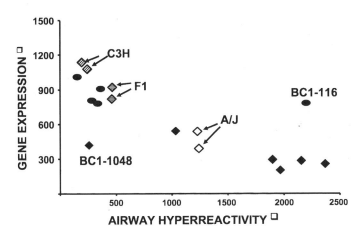

Fig. 4. Complement factor 5 (*C5*) gene expression and genotype correlates with allergen-induced airway hyperresponsiveness. *C5* transcript levels in whole lungs of ovalbumin-sensitized A/J, C3H, and F1 (A/J × C3H) mice are indicated; six high-responder BC1 and six low-responder BC1 mice are shown in comparison to their dynamic airway hyperresponsiveness. BC1 mice with *C5* deficiency are represented by diamonds and BC1 mice that are *C5* heterozygous are shown as circles. (Reproduced with permission from ref. *30*.)

C5 mRNA expression revealed that it was homozygous for the A/J allele at the *C5* locus. All of the other intercross progeny that were resistant to experimental asthma induction had a C3H-derived C5 allele. Subsequent analysis revealed that the presence of a deletion in the coding sequence of *C5* in susceptible mice leads to the absence of C5 protein and susceptibility to the asthmatic trait *(30)*. The mechanism by which a genetic deficiency in C5 could lead to susceptibility to an asthmatic trait could then be characterized. Subsequent experimental analysis revealed that C5 deficiency effected the production of cytokines regulating the asthmatic response. IL-12 is a cytokine with potent effects on T-cell differentiation. When produced in the airways, it can prevent or reverse allergic asthma. Inhibition of C5-mediated signaling by blockade of the C5a receptor rendered human monocytes unable to produce IL-12 in vitro. This provided a plausible mechanism for the regulation of susceptibility to asthma by alleles of *C5* in mice.

3.2. Analysis of an Experimental Murine Genetic Model of Osteoporosis

Osteoporosis is one of the most common bone and mineral disorders in all aging communities. It is characterized by low bone mass resulting in fractures from relatively minor trauma. Although lifestyle and environmental factors contribute to osteoporosis, genetic factors are also of great importance *(53)*. Bone mineral density achieved in early adulthood (peak bone mass) is a major determinant of osteoporotical fracture risk. Genetic segregation analyses in inbred mouse strains have identified linkage between peak bone mineral density and several chromosomal regions, but the identities of the underlying genes remain unknown. To identify genes that might regulate bone mineral density, we used a combined genetic and genomic approach. A region on mouse chromosome 11 that was shown to strongly influence peak bone mineral density in F2 (B6 × D2) intercross progeny was investigated *(29,54)*. A D2 background congenic mouse, with an 82-Mb region of chromosome 11 replaced by the corresponding region of the B6 genome, was used in these studies. Congenic mice had increased peak bone mineral density (whole body and femoral) and improved measures of femoral shaft strength (failure load and stiffness) relative to heterozygous or D2 littermates. Linkage analysis of intercross progeny generated using the chromosome 11 congenic mice further narrowed the interval regulating bone mineral density to a 31-Mb region between 54.7 and 85.4 Mb on chromosome 11. Microarray analysis of kidney and cartilage tissue obtained from parental and congenic mice indicated that *Alox15* was the only differentially expressed gene within the identified region on chromosome 11. *Alox15* expression in the kidney of D2 mice was nearly 20-fold greater than that observed in B6 kidney. Analysis of genomic DNA identified 15 polymorphisms in the *Alox15* gene that distinguished the D2 and B6 strains *(31)*.

The identification of *Alox15* as a candidate genetic locus regulating bone mass was quite intriguing. It codes for a murine 12/15 lipoxygenase that converts arachidonic and linoleic acids into endogenous ligands for PPAR-γ *(55)*. Activation of this pathway in marrow-derived mesenchymal progenitors stimulates adipogenesis and inhibits osteoblastogenesis *(56)*. Lipoxygenases had been implicated in the pathogenesis of several diseases, including atherosclerosis, asthma, cancer, and glomerulonephritis. However, the biological functions of murine or human *Alox15* had not yet been determined with certainty. In fact, an *Alox15* knockout mouse was reported not to have any detectable difference from wild-type littermates *(57)*.

An in vitro osteoblast differentiation system was used to demonstrate that transient overexpression of *Alox15* in murine bone marrow stromal cell cultures restricted osteoblast differentiation *(56)*. These in vitro observations led to the hypothesis that genetically determined, constitutively high *Alox15* expression limited peak bone mass attainment by suppressing osteogenesis through activation of PPAR-γ-dependent pathways. The effect of *Alox15* on skeletal development in vivo was then investigated. The skeletal phenotype of *Alox15* knockout mice was compared to that of age-matched B6 progenitors. Although body weight and whole-body bone mineral density were similar between the two strains, femoral bone mineral density and biomechanical indices of femoral shaft strength were increased in *Alox15* knockout mice. To limit the possible effects of background strain, the effect of crossbreeding D2 and *Alox15* knockout mice on bone mass acquisition was examined. Three hundred F2 offspring of this pairing with 0, 1, or 2 copies of the intact *Alox15* allele were characterized. F2 mice with no intact *Alox15* alleles exhibited significantly higher whole body bone mineral density and increased femoral bone strength than mice that were homozygous for the alleles mediating high-level *Alox15* expression. These experiments demonstrated that reduced expression of *Alox15* rescued mice from a low bone mass phenotype that was associated with high levels of *Alox15* expression. We also examined the skeletal effects of pharmacological inhibitors of 15-lipoxygenase in two rodent models of osteoporosis. Mice with severely reduced bone mass, owing to constitutive overexpression of an interleukin-4 (IL-4) transgene *(58)*, were treated with an *Alox15* inhibitor for 12 wk after weaning. Because IL-4 was known to upregulate *Alox15* expression in a number of tissues, we hypothesized that increased *Alox15* expression may contribute to the defective skeletal phenotype in this model. Treatment with the *Alox15* inhibitor resulted in increased whole body bone mineral density, femoral bone mineral density, and femoral shaft failure load. Treatment with another *Alox15* inhibitor also prevented bone loss in a rat model of estrogen deficiency (postmenopausal) osteoporosis *(56)*. These results indicated that pharmacological inhibition of 12/15-lipoxygenase in vivo can improve bone mass and strength during skeletal development, as well as offset the bone loss that accompanies estrogen deficiency.

3.3. Identification of a Genetic Locus for Autoantibody Production Using a Mouse Model

An integrated approach was also used to identify a genetic locus regulating autoantibody production in a murine model of a human autoimmune disease *(27)*. SLE affects a number of organ systems and is considered to be a prototypic systemic autoimmune disease. The common denominator among SLE patients is the production of autoantibodies reactive with multiple self-proteins. The hallmark of this disease is elevated serum levels of antinuclear antibodies. Hybrids of New Zealand black (NZB) and New Zealand white (NZW) mice develop a severe immune complex-mediated glomerulonephritis associated with high serum levels of IgG antinuclear autoantibodies, and these mice are considered to be an excellent model of human SLE *(59)*. Genetic analyses have demonstrated that the major histocompatibility complex (MHC) and multiple non-MHC loci from both New Zealand strains contribute to the lupus phenotype *(60–63)*. The region on distal chromosome 1, for which contributing genes from both NZB and NZW parental strains have been localized, is among the most interesting *(27,41,59,64–66)*. One NZB-derived lupus-susceptibility locus on distal chromosome 1 (named *Nba2* for *New Zealand black autoimmunity 2*) was identified in multiple different backcrosses and showed linkage as a QTL with nearly all of the lupus autoantibodies studied *(61)*. These findings suggested that this locus might act as an immune response gene that influences antigen-driven B-cell responses to self-antigens.

A congenic mouse was used to characterize the *Nba2* lupus-susceptibility locus. The B6.NZB-*Nba2* (or B6.*Nba2*) congenic mouse has the *Nba2*-containing distal chromosome 1 region (~79–109 cm) of NZB introgressed onto the nonautoimmune C57BL/6 (B6) strain. This congenic mouse produced all of the lupus-associated antibodies. To identify gene candidates within the *Nba2* region, gene expression in spleen cells obtained from 4-mo-old (pre-autoimmune) B6.*Nba2* congenic and B6 parental mice were profiled using oligonucleotide microarrays. Only two differentially expressed genes within the *Nba2* interval, interferon-inducible genes *Ifi202* and *Ifi203*, were identified by comparison of gene expression in congenic and parental NZB mice *(67)*. These two co-linear genes were differentially expressed when NZB and NZW spleen cells were compared. Analysis of different cell types within the spleen indicated that increased *Ifi202* expression was localized to splenic B cells and to non-T/non-B cells. The NZB-derived IFI202 allele was preferentially expressed in F1 mice relative to the NZW allele. These results, along with analyses of promoter region polymorphisms and differential *IFI202* protein expression implicated *Ifi202* as a candidate gene. B cells from NZB and B6.*Nba2* congenic mice were resistant to apoptosis induced by crosslinking surface IgM, which coincided with high expression of IFI202 in the apoptosis-resistant B cells. Increased expression of IFI202 has been shown to inhibit apoptosis *(68,69)*, and decreased expression led to increased susceptibility to apoptosis under certain physiological conditions *(70)*. Inhibition of B-cell apoptosis provides a mechanism by which increased IFI202 expression enhances lupus susceptibility. Apoptosis is critically involved in the maintenance of B-cell tolerance, and inhibition of B-cell apoptosis through mutations in another gene (Fas[*lpr*]) was shown to contribute to a lupus-related phenotype in another mouse strain *(71)*. The integrated approach to analysis of the NZB/W murine genetic model identified a novel genetic mechanism regulating autoantibody production.

4. NEW MOUSE STRAINS AND TOOLS TO ACCELERATE GENETIC ANALYSIS

The last two examples demonstrate the utility of congenic mice for identification of a genetic locus within a linked region. Congenic mouse strains are constructed by repeated backcrossing of a donor strain onto a background strain, with selection at each generation for the presence of a desired donor chromosomal region. Because this involves serial backcrossing and selection among progeny, construction of congenic mice is a process that is costly in both dollars and time. Therefore, the availability of a series of well-characterized congenic mouse strains, with different chromosomal regions from one strain placed onto the genetic background of a recipient strain, provides a valuable tool for genetic analysis. They will be useful for rapidly assessing the impact of genotypic changes within a defined chromosomal region on the phenotype and for identification of the genetic locus regulating the phenotype.

As one example, a set of congenic mice were produced, with each strain having a single A/J-derived chromosome placed on the C57BL/6 host background. Each of the 21 chromosome substitution strains had one of its

19 autosomes or one of two sex chromosomes derived from the A/J donor strain. The rest of the chromosomes were from the C57BL/6 mice *(72)*. Recently, this congenic strain set was used to analyze 53 different traits, and over 150 chromosomal regions regulating these traits were identified *(73)*. Two other groups have produced overlapping sets of congenic strains with smaller chromosomal regions from the donor strain introgressed into the genome of another recipient strain *(74,75)*. These sets of congenic substrains, in which a single identified segment of the genome of one mouse strain is replaced by that of another strain, provide a useful tool for analysis of the effect of genetic variation on phenotypic responses. Application of well-characterized experimental strategies for genetic mapping *(76)* to the genome-wide congenic strain sets will enable genetic regions regulating complex traits in experimental mouse models to be rapidly identified. This requires characterization of the phenotype in the parental strains and in each congenic substrain. In one example, this approach was used to identify a genetic locus for susceptibility to malaria using a set of A/J and C57BL/6 congenic strains *(77)*.

Chemical mutagenesis was used to introduce new genetic mutations into inbred mouse strains. There are several large efforts to dissect complex traits in the mouse using chemical mutagenesis to produce artificial mutants, which can be screened for phenotypes of interest *(78–80)*. This resulted from difficulties encountered by investigators using standard methods for QTL analysis (reviewed in ref. *50*). It was hoped that this approach would provide a powerful alternative method for complex trait analysis. This method is attractive because new mutations are introduced into the genetic background of an inbred mouse strain, and all genes in the genome are susceptible to mutagenesis. This approach has been, and will be, useful for identifying highly penetrant genes, particularly those having a profound effect on embryonic and organ development *(81)*. A clever strategy has been developed to enable screening for recessive mutations, but it does require several generations of intercrossing mutagenized mice *(81)*. However, it is unlikely that this approach will be generally useful for analysis of complex genetic traits. Identification of genes with a large phenotypic effect may not reveal how polygenic traits are regulated. Because most phenotypic screens performed on mutagenized progeny are not for quantitative traits, it is unlikely that genes of small effect will be identified. It is also statistically unlikely that an individual progeny will have mutations in multiple different loci that will produce quantitative trait variance. However, mutagenesis programs may produce a very useful collection of genetic variation on a known background. DNA and sperm from mutagenized male mice can be archived, and the archived DNA can be scanned for mutations in selected genes. The sperm can be recovered from mice with mutations in genes of interest and used to produce mice for phenotypic studies *(82)*.

The application of an SNP-based genotyping method for analysis of murine intercross progeny provides another tool that facilitates genetic analysis. An improved strategy for SNP scoring with allele-specific oligonucleotide primers and kinetic (real time) monitoring of polymerase chain reaction (PCR) amplification *(83)* was utilized for mouse genotyping *(65)*. Allele-specific amplification results from the use of oligonucleotide primers specific for one or the other SNP variant sequence. This approach provides an efficient and low-cost method for SNP-allele genotyping. The genotyping reaction is performed within a single microtiter well and does not require any post-PCR analytic steps. Most importantly, this method can determine allele frequencies in pooled DNA samples. A subset of phenotypically extreme progeny can be selected, and their DNA can be aggregated into pools. Allele frequency differences between the pooled samples can be used to identify linkage regions, which exponentially reduce the amount of genotyping required for analysis of experimental intercrosses. A web-accessible database, which enables computational selection of allele-specific primers for genotyping experimental mouse intercrosses, was established. The oligonucleotide primer sequences and conditions for performing over 750 allele-specific kinetic PCR genotyping assays *(83)* are provided in the mouse SNP database *(see* http:\\mouseSNP.roche.com and ref. *65)*.

5. COMPUTATIONAL APPROACHES
TO COMPLEX DISEASE BIOLOGY

Genetic analysis of murine models requires generation, phenotypic screening, and genotyping of a large number of intercross progeny. Even with improved genotyping tools, this laborious, expensive, and time-consuming process has greatly limited the rate at which genetic loci can be identified in experimental mouse or rat models. It usually requires at least 2 yr to generate and characterize the 200–1000 intercross progeny required for genetic analysis. To accelerate this process, a computational method that can predict linkage regions by analysis of phenotypic data generated from inbred mouse strains was developed *(65)*. The computational prediction method can be used in conjunction with databases of gene expression and phenotypic information to markedly accelerate complex trait analysis. Although it is at an early stage, the computational approach can eliminate many months to years of laboratory work and reduce the time required for QTL interval identification to milliseconds. Five years ago, at least five scientists working for a 5-yr period would be required to carry out the analysis of a complex trait in an experimental mouse model. Using the computational method described in this book, one scientist could complete the initial steps in analysis of a complex trait in an experimental mouse model in 1 d.

Experimental murine genetic models can be analyzed using currently available genetic and genomic tools. However, the rate can be exponentially accelerated through application of recently developed computational tools. Databases of gene expression information and DNA sequence polymorphisms among inbred mouse strains enable genetically controlled, disease-related traits to be computationally analyzed. Although computational methods may not generate a complete "solution to the riddle" posed by a complex trait, they can identify candidate genes and pathways that serve as starting points for subsequent biological and genetic analysis. If the databases and methods are sufficiently developed, the computationally identified gene candidates will have a reasonable probability of contributing to the disease-related phenotype.

Almost all human complex diseases and disease-related phenotypes can be experimentally modeled in rats and mice. Genetic and genomic tools that enable computational analysis of complex traits in mice are currently available (Fig. 5). Web-accessible databases of DNA sequence polymorphisms across 21 murine strains (*see* ref. *65* and http://mouseSNP.roche.com) and phenotypic information (http://www.jax.org) across inbred mouse strains are enabling tools for computational analysis of complex traits. Of course, an investigator can also experimentally obtain phenotypic information among inbred mouse strains for any trait of interest. One algorithm that utilizes information within the mouse SNP database to computationally identify

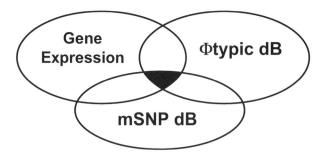

Fig. 5. Diagrammatic outline of the integrative approach used for computational analysis of complex disease-related traits in mouse models.

chromosomal regions regulating susceptibility or resistance to disease-related traits was described *(65)*. After entry of phenotypic information obtained from inbred mouse strains, the phenotypic and genotypic information is computationally analyzed by this method to predict the chromosomal regions regulating the phenotypic trait. The computational predictions were evaluated using 10 experimentally verified QTL intervals from seven phenotypic traits analyzed as true positives. There was a statistically highly significant level of concordance between the predicted and experimentally verified intervals *(65)*. Several factors contributed to the quality of the computational predictions. The use of inbred mouse strains housed under the same conditions minimizes environmental variability, and timed experimental intervention and multiple sampling limit the experimental error in phenotypic assessment. The inbred strains are homozygous at all loci, which eliminates confounding effects owing to heterozygosity found in human populations. We do not yet fully understand the limitations of the computational prediction method nor do we know the optimal inbred strains to use for generating the phenotypic data. Clearly, the method may not provide the correct predictions for all traits studied. However, it has the exciting potential of drastically reducing the time required for identifying chromosomal regions with genetic loci regulating complex disease-associated traits.

Recently, we have produced another computational genetic mapping method that utilizes a significantly different methodology *(84)*. This new method has increased statistical validity and makes predictions that are more precise. As discussed in subsequent chapters, there is a large amount of linkage disequilibrium among the polymorphisms found among the inbred mouse strains *(26)*. This linkage disequilibrium means that the pattern of genetic variation across regions of the genome can be characterized by knowing the alleles at a relatively few positions within each region. Among the inbred *Mus musculus* strains, each discrete region contains a relatively small number of distinct genetic patterns. This drastically reduces the number of comparisons required for computational genetic analysis. Instead of comparing a phenotypic pattern with individual SNP alleles, we have developed a new method that compares the observed phenotypic data with different haplotypes that extend across larger genomic regions. Once the haplotypic structure of the mouse genome is understood, it facilitates computational mapping of genetic traits. The haplotype-based method utilizes the same principle of finding patterns of genetic variation that correlate with phenotypic differences among the strains as was used by the digital disease method. However, the haplotype-based computational mapping method is radically different; it is based on a highly quantitative model. As described, this method has been successfully utilized to map the genetic loci for previously known traits, as well as for discovering a novel functional genomic element in mouse *(84)*.

After the genetic regions controlling complex traits have been computationally identified, candidate genes can then be computationally identified. This requires the availability of a database of gene expression information generated from tissues obtained from a panel of inbred mice. The tissues related to the disease-related phenotypes can be obtained from a panel of inbred mouse strains and used for gene expression profiling using microarrays. The resulting strain and tissue-specific gene expression information can be stored in a database, which includes the chromosomal location for each gene. The database can be interrogated to identify differentially expressed genes within a target tissue for each disease-related phenotype that are contained within a predicted region. The correlation of the expression profile, genetic variation, and phenotypic information among the phenotypically extreme strains can be evaluated to assess the predicted candidates. Computational analysis of a mouse model of experimental allergic asthma can be used as an illustrative example of this process. A computational genome scan using phenotypic measurements for allergen-induced airway hyperresponsiveness obtained from four inbred strains was performed *(65)*. The strongest peaks identified were intervals on chromosomes 2, 7, 10, and 11. The next step in this analysis required the creation of a database containing the expression levels for 25,000 genes in the lungs of the four strains under basal conditions and after allergen stimulation. This database was computationally interrogated to identify differentially expressed genes in the lungs when high- (A/J) and low-responder (C3H/HeJ) strains were compared. Next, identifying those encoded within the computationally predicted chromosomal regions reduced the list of differentially expressed genes. In this case, *C5* would be among the differentially expressed genes encoded within the computationally predicted region on mouse chromosome 2. The mouse SNP database indicates that a 2-bp deletion is present in the 5′ end of the *C5* gene in the high-responder strain, and the low-responder strain does not have this deletion. Therefore, analysis of the gene expression, computational prediction, and SNP data identified *C5* as a candidate gene. An investigator could then analyze the possible role of this computationally identified candidate gene in the pathogenesis of experimental allergic asthma. A computationally derived list of gene candidates can be produced for each complex disease-related trait analyzed in this manner.

Even in the absence of full genomic information, the power of the approach outlined here for discovery of genetic susceptibility loci is evident. With the full sequence of mouse, rat, and human genomes currently in sight, these methods should find broad usage in the search for genetic susceptibility loci underlying complex human diseases. The recent sequencing of the human genome has generated a great deal of excitement. However, we do not yet understand all of the information contained within this sequence nor do we understand how sequence variation within the human population affects human traits. It is rather ironic that analysis of rodent experimental models, many developed decades earlier, will provide the key to interpreting the information contained within the human genome.

ACKNOWLEDGMENT

The work described in this chapter was partially supported by a grant from the National Human Genome Research Institute (1 RO1 HG022162-01) awarded to the author. I would like to also thank the many collaborators who have developed the interesting mouse experimental genetic models of human disease-related traits with whom I have had the pleasure of working.

REFERENCES

1. Risch NJ. Searching for genetic determinants in the new millennium [Review]. Nature 2000;405:847–856.
2. Mackay TFC. The genetic architecture of quantitative traits. Annu Rev Gen 2001;35:303–339.
3. Lawrence RC, Helmick CG, Arnett FC, et al. Estimates of the prevalence of arthritis and selected musculoskeletal disorders in the United States [see comments]. Arthritis Rheum 1998;41:778–799.
4. Yelin E. The costs of rheumatoid arthritis: absolute, incremental, and marginal estimates [Review]. J Rheumatol Suppl 1996;44:47–51.
5. Helmick CG, Lawrence RC, Pollard RA, Lloyd E, Heyse SP. Arthritis and other rheumatic conditions: who is affected now, who will be affected later? National Arthritis Data Workgroup. Arthritis Care Res 1995;8:203–211.
6. Genetic testing for cystic fibrosis. NIH Consens Statement Online 1997 Apr 14–16 1997;15:1–37.
7. Collins FS. Positional cloning moves from perditional to traditional [erratum appears in Nat Genet 1995 Sep;11:104]. Nat Genet 1995;9:347–350.
8. Peto J, Collins N, Barfoot R, et al. Prevalence of BRCA1 and BRCA2 gene mutations in patients with early-onset breast cancer [see comments]. J Natl Cancer Inst 1999;91:943–949.
9. Tupler R, Perini G, Green MR. Expressing the human genome. Nature 2001;409:832, 833.
10. Johnson JM, Castle J, Garrett EP, et al. Genome-wide survey of human alternative pre-mRNA splicing with exon junction microarrays. Science 2003;302: 2141–2144.

11. Modrek B, Lee C. A genomic view of alternative splicing. Nat Genet 2002; 30:13–19.

12. Keene JD. Ribonucleoprotein infrastructure regulating the flow of genetic information between the genome and the proteome [Review]. Proc Natl Acad Sci USA 2001;98:7018–7024.

13. Kramer A. The structure and function of proteins involved in mammalian pre-mRNA splicing [Review]. Ann Rev Biochem 1996;65:367–409.

14. Nissim-Rafinia M, Karem B. Splicing regulation as a potential genetic modifier. Trends Genet 2002;18:123–127.

15. Clark TA, Sugnet CW, Ares M. Genomewide analysis of mRNA processing in yeast using splicing-specific microarrays. Science 2002;296:907–910.

16. Mendell JT, Dietz HC. When the message goes awry: disease-producing mutations that influence mRNA content and performance [Review]. Cell 2001;107: 411–414.

17. Bajorath J. Molecular organization, structural features, and ligand binding characteristics of CD44, a highly variable cell surface glycoprotein with multiple functions [Review]. Proteins 2000;39:103–111.

18. Stickeler E, Kittrell F, Medina D, Berget SM. Stage-specific changes in SR splicing factors and alternative splicing in mammary tumorigenesis. Oncogene 1999;18:3574–3582.

19. Grover A, Houlden H, Baker M, et al. 5′ splice site mutations in tau associated with the inherited dementia FTDP-17 affect a stem-loop structure that regulates alternative splicing of exon 10. J Biol Chem 1999;274: 15,134–15,143.

20. Johnson GC, Esposito L, Barratt BJ, et al. Haplotype tagging for the identification of common disease genes. Nat Genet 2001;29:233–237.

21. Daly MJ, Rioux JD, Schaffner SF, Hudson TJ, Lander ES. High-resolution haplotype structure in the human genome. Nat Genet 2001;29:229–232.

22. Reich DE, Cargill M, Bolk S, et al. Linkage disequilibrium in the human genome. Nature 2001;411:199–204.

23. Patil N, Berno AJ, Hinds DA, et al. Blocks of limited haplotype diversity revealed by high-resolution scanning of human chromosome 21 [see comments]. Science 2001;294:1719–1723.

24. Sun B, Rizzo LV, Sun SH, et al. Genetic susceptibility to experimental autoimmune uveitis involves more than a predisposition to generate a T helper-1-like or a T helper-2-like response. J Immunol 1997;159:1004–1011.

25. Neuhaus IM, Beier D. Efficient localization of mutations by interval haplotype analysis. Mamm Genome 1998;9:150–154.

26. Wade CM, Kulbokas EJ, Kirby AW, et al. The mosaic structure of variation in the laboratory mouse genome. Nature 2002;420:574–578.

27. Rozzo SJ, Allard J, Choubey D, et al. Evidence for an interferon-inducible gene, Ifi202, in the susceptibility to systemic lupus. Immunity 2001; 15:435–443.

28. Morel L, Blenman KR, Croker BP, Wakeland EK. The major murine systemic lupus erythematosus susceptibility locus, Sle1, is a cluster of functionally related genes. Proc Natl Acad Sci USA 2001;98:1787–1792.

29. Grupe A, Germer S, Usuka J, et al. In silico mapping of complex disease-related traits in mice [see comments]. Science 2001;292:1915–1918.
30. Karp CL, Grupe A, Schadt E, et al. Identification of complement factor 5 (C5) as a susceptibility locus for experimental allergic asthma. Nat Immunol 2000;1:221–226.
31. Klein RF, Alard J, Avnur Z, et al. Regulation of bone mass in mice by the lipoxygenase gene Alox15. Science 2004;303:229–232.
32. Schadt E, Monks SA, Drake TA, et al. Genetics of gene expression surveyed in maize, mouse and man. Nature 2003;422:297–302.
33. Drazen JM, Takebayashi T, Long NC, De S, Shore SA. Animal models of asthma and chronic bronchitis [Review]. Clin Exp Allergy 1999;29 (Suppl 2):37–47.
34. Wills-Karp M, Ewart S. The genetics of allergen-induced airway hyperresponsiveness in mice. Am J Crit Care Med 1997;156:S89–S96.
35. Joe B, Wilder RL. Animal models of rheumatoid arthritis [Review]. Mol Med Today 1999;5:367–369.
36. Yang HT, Jirholt J, Svensson L, et al. Identification of genes controlling collagen-induced arthritis in mice: striking homology with susceptibility loci previously identified in the rat. J Immunol 1999;163:2916–2921.
37. McIndoe RA, Bohlman B, Chi E, Schuster E, Lindhardt M, Hood L. Localization of non-Mhc collagen-induced arthritis susceptibility loci in DBA/1j mice. Proc Natl Acad Sci USA 1999;96:2210–2214.
38. Bergsteinsdottir K, Yang HT, Pettersson U, Holmdahl R. Evidence for common autoimmune disease genes controlling onset, severity, and chronicity based on experimental models for multiple sclerosis and rheumatoid arthritis. J Immunol 2000;164:1564–1568.
39. Steinman L. Assessment of animal models for MS and demyelinating disease in the design of rational therapy [Review]. Neuron 1999;24:511–514.
40. Mestas J, Hughes-Christopher CW. Of mice and not men: differences between mouse and human immunology. J Immunol 2004;172:2731–2738.
41. Vyse TJ, Todd JA. Genetic analysis of autoimmune disease [Review]. Cell 1996;85:311–318.
42. Becker KG, Simon RM, Bailey-Wilson JE, Freidlin B, Biddison WE, McFarland HF, et al. Clustering of non-major histocompatibility complex susceptibility candidate loci in human autoimmune diseases. Proc Natl Acad Sci USA 1998;95:9979–9984.
43. Sugiyama F, Churchill GA, Higgins DC, et al. Concordance of murine quantitative trait loci for salt-induced hypertension with rat and human loci. Genomics 2001;71:70–77.
44. Mushegian AR, Bassett DE, Boguski MS, Bork P, Koonin EV. Positionally cloned human disease genes: patterns of evolutionary conservation and functional motifs. Proc Natl Acad Sci USA 1997;94:5831–5836.
45. Narahashi T, Moore JW, Scott WR. Tetrodotoxin blockage of sodium conductance increase in lobster giant axons. J Gen Physiol 1964;47:965–974.

46. Kliewer SA, Lenhard JM, Willson TM, Patel I, Morris DC, Lehmann JM. A prostaglandin J2 metabolite binds peroxisome proliferator-activated receptor gamma and promotes adipocyte differentiation. Cell 1995;83:813–819.

47. Lehmann JM, Moore LB, Smith-Oliver TA, Wilkison WO, Willson TM, Kliewer SA. An antidiabetic thiazolidinedione is a high affinity ligand for peroxisome proliferator-activated receptor gamma (PPAR gamma). J Biol Chem 1995;270:12,953–12,956.

48. Novina CD, Sharp PA. The RNAi revolution. Nature 2004;430:161–164.

49. Paddison PJ, Silva JM, Conklin DS, et al. A resource for large-scale RNA-interference-based screens in mammals. Nature 2004;428:427–431.

50. Nadeau JH, Frankel WN. The roads from phenotypic variation to gene discovery: mutagenesis versus QTLs. Nat Genet 2000;25:381–384.

51. Wills-Karp M, Luyimbazi J, Xu X, Schofield B, Neben TY, Karp CL, et al. Interleukin-13: central mediator of allergic asthma [see comments]. Science 1900;282:2258–2261.

52. Gavett SH, Wills-Karp M. Elevated lung G protein levels and muscarinic receptor affinity in a mouse model of airway hyperractivity. Am J Physiol 1993;265:L493–L500.

53. Peacock M, Turner CH, Econs MJ, Foroud T. Genetics of osteoporosis. Endocr Rev 2002;23:303–326.

54. Klein OF, Carlos AS, Vartanian KA, et al. Confirmation and fine mapping of chromosomal regions influencing peak bone mass in mice. J Bone Miner Res 2001;16:1953–1961.

55. Huang JT, Welch JS, Ricote M, et al. Interleukin-4-dependent production of PPAR-gamma ligands in macrophages by 12/15-lipoxygenase. Nature 1999; 400:378–382.

56. Lecka CB, Moerman EJ, Grant DF, Lehmann JM, Manolagas SC, Jilka RL. Divergent effects of selective peroxisome proliferator-activated receptor-gamma 2 ligands on adipocyte versus osteoblast differentiation. Endocrinology 2002;143:2376–2384.

57. Sun D, Funk CD. Disruption of 12/15-lipoxygenase expression in peritoneal macrophages. J Biol Chem 1996;271:24,055–24,062.

58. Lewis DB, Liggitt HD, Effmann EL, et al. Osteoporosis induced in mice by overproduction of interleukin 4. Proc Natl Acad Sci USA 1993;90: 11,618–11,622.

59. Vyse T, Kotzin B. Genetic basis of systemic lupus erythematosus. Curr Opin Immunol 1996;8:843–851.

60. Vyse TJ, Kotzin BL. Genetic susceptibility to systemic lupus erythematosus [Review]. Annu Rev Immunol 1998;16:261–292.

61. Vyse TJ, Todd JA. Genetic analysis of autoimmune disease [Review]. Cell 1996;85:311–318.

62. Kono DH, Theofilopoulos AN. Genetic susceptibility to spontaneous lupus in mice [Review]. Curr Dir Autoimmun 1999;1:72–98.

63. Wakeland EK, Liu K, Graham RR, Behrens TW. Delineating the genetic basis of systemic lupus erythematosus [Review]. Immunity 2001;15:397–408.

64. Morel L, Rudofsky UH, Longmate JA, Schiffenbauer J, Wakeland EK. Polygenic control of susceptibility to murine systemic lupus erythematosus. Immunity 1994;1:219–229.

65. Grupe A, Germer S, Usuka J, Aud D, Belknap JK, Klein RF, et al. In silico mapping of complex traits in mice. Science 2001;292:1915–1918.

66. Drake CG, Rozzo SJ, Vyse TJ, Kotzin BL. Absence of coding sequence polymorphism in the serum amyloid P component gene (Sap) in autoimmune New Zealand black mice. Mamm Genome 1996;7:466, 467.

67. Walley AJ, Cookson WO. Investigation of an interleukin-4 promoter polymorphism for associations with asthma and atopy. J Med Genet 1996;33:689–92.

68. Wang H, Liu C, Lu Y, et al. The interferon- and differentiation-inducible p202a protein inhibits the transcriptional activity of c-Myc by blocking its association with Max. J Biol Chem 2000;275:27,377–27,385.

69. D'Souza S, Xin H, Walter S, Choubey D. The gene encoding p202, an interferon-inducible negative regulator of the p53 tumor suppressor, is a target of p53-mediated transcriptional repression. J Biol Chem 2001;276:298–305.

70. Koul D, Lapushin R, Xu HJ, Mills GB, Gutterman JU, Choubey D. p202 prevents apoptosis in murine AKR-2B fibroblasts. Biochem Biophys Res Commun 1998;247:379–382.

71. Sobel ES, Katagiri T, Katagiri K, Morris SC, Cohen PL, Eisenberg RA. An intrinsic B cell defect is required for the production of autoantibodies in the lpr model of murine systemic autoimmunity. J Exp Med 1991;173: 1441–1449.

72. Nadeau JH, Singer JB, Matin A, Lander ES. Analysing complex genetic traits with chromosome substitution strains [published erratum appears in Nat Genet 2000;25:125] [Review]. Nat Genet 2000;24:221–225.

73. Singer JB, Hill AE, Burrage LC, et al. Genetic dissection of complex traits with chromosome substitution strains of mice. Science 2004;304:445–448.

74. Iakoubova OA, Olsson CL, Dains KM, et al. Genome-tagged mice (GTM): two sets of genome-wide congenic strains. Genomics 2001;74:89–104.

75. Fortin A, Diez E, Rochefort D, et al. Recombinant congenic strains derived from A/J and C57BL/6J: a tool for genetic dissection of complex traits. Genomics 2001;74:21–35.

76. Darvasi A. Experimental strategies for the genetic dissection of complex traits in animal models. Nat Genet 1998;18:19–24.

77. Fortin A, Cardon LR, Tam M, Skamene E, Stevenson MM, Gros P. Identification of a new malaria susceptibility locus (Char4) in recombinant congenic strains of mice. Proc Natl Acad Sci USA 2001;98:10,793–10,798.

78. Nolan PM, Peters J, Strivens M, et al. A systematic, genome-wide, phenotype-driven mutagenesis programme for gene function studies in the mouse. Nat Genet 2000;25:440–443.

79. Hrabe de Angelis MH, Flaswinkel H, Fuchs H, et al. Genome-wide, large-scale production of mutant mice by ENU mutagenesis. Nat Genet 2000;25:444–447.

80. Vinuesa CG, Goodnow CC. Illuminating autoimmune regulators through controlled variation of the mouse genome sequence. Immunity 2004;20:669–679.

81. Herron BJ, Lu W, Rao C, et al. Efficient generation and mapping of recessive developmental mutations using ENU mutagenesis. Nat Genet 2002;30: 185–189.

82. Coghill EL, Hugill A, Parkinson N, et al. A gene-driven approach to the indentification of ENU mutants in the mouse. Nature Genet 2002;30:255–256.

83. Germer S, Holland MJ, Higuchi R. High-throughput SNP allele-frequency determination in pooled DNA samples by kinetic PCR. Genome Res 2000;10:258–266.

84. Liao G, Wang J, Guo J, et al. In silico genetics: identification of a novel functional element regulating H2-Eα gene expression. Science 2004;306:690–695.

2

Statistical Theory in QTL Mapping

Benjamin Yakir, Anne Pisanté, and Ariel Darvasi

1. INTRODUCTION

Variability may be introduced in an observed phenotype by a range of elements. Inherited genetic factors, as well as environmental and behavioral conditions, may affect the phenotype. The blend of all these interactions gives rise to the unique being every living creature is. Experimental genetics has traditionally been, and still is, a very powerful tool for dissecting the genetic factors out of the blend that results in the observed phenotype complexity.

Unlike human genetics, a major advantage of experimental genetics is the ability to control the genetic background through inbred strain crosses, whereas nongenetic factors are kept relatively constant under controlled laboratory conditions. In reality, the ideal experiment is almost never feasible, and uncontrolled sources of variation and complex interactions may still obscure the underlying genetic effect.

Even under the best conditions, mapping quantitative trait loci (QTL) is a demanding endeavor. Any given QTL or genomic polymorphism contributes only a limited fraction of the phenotypical variation. This complex inheritance may involve partial penetrance, heterogeneity, the joint action of several genes, environmental effects, and more. The genetic dissection of complex traits is unavoidably based on a statistical approach. The aim in this chapter is to describe our view of the fundamental principles on which the statistical approach is based.

In a nutshell, the theory we will discuss involves the attempt to detect and locate weak signals in a noisy environment. This calls for the usage of large samples. Thereby, our probabilistical framework involves the distribution of statistics computed from large samples in the context of what is known as *local alternatives*. In statistical language, this theory is called *large sample theory*. Modern technology puts at our disposal the ability to genotype these

From: *Computational Genetics and Genomics*
Edited by: G. Peltz © Humana Press Inc., Totowa, NJ

samples over a practically unlimited collection of molecular genetic markers. The statistical investigation should make full use of this data. Stochastical processes are more appropriate as a model in this context than the separate investigation of individual markers. The statistical tools that were developed in the context of stochastical processes, in particular scanning statistics, are applicable also in the context of QTL mapping.

One should realize that QTL mapping is a multistage process that proceeds through several steps. The first step typically involves detection of chromosomes, or very large segments of chromosomes, which are likely to contain a QTL. In the next steps an attempt is made to narrow down the region containing the QTL. Finally, after a reduction to a small enough chromosomal segment, the gene associated with the variability in the investigated phenotype may be cloned, and its specific alleles may be identified. Several factors determine which tool is most appropriate at which stage. By the word tool we mainly mean here the selection of the cross and/or genetic resource. Phenotyping and genotyping methods may also be included in this context. A major factor, which determines to a large extent the advantages and disadvantages of a given tool for a given stage of the process, is the expected number of recombination events. This factor is directly determined by the breeding protocol. Statistically, recombination is reflected in the correlation among markers that reside on the same chromosome and between the markers and the QTL. In principle, an increase in the number of recombination events reduces the correlation. Reduction in the correlation is usually a blessing in the stages of fine-mapping but an obstacle in the first stage of detection. Another important factor is the strength of the statistic signal. The strength is usually summarized in the form of a noncentrality parameter; it is affected both by biological mechanisms by which the genetic variability is reflected as a phenotypic variability and by the breeding protocol. Other factors to be considered include, of course, the availability of the different resources and their respective costs.

Many attributes make the mouse an ideal mammalian model organism, especially for genetic investigations for which a wealth of resources have been established over the years. The relatively short generation time of the mouse, their easy breeding, and well-documented biological properties have led to the development of well-characterized, genetically designed specific strains *(13,14)*. These privileged circumstances have been exploited in both gene-to-phenotype and phenotype-to-gene studies. With the advent of molecular genetics, the use of DNA polymorphisms *(11)* has allowed for a refined identification of interstrains genetic divergence *(4)*. Correlation of the human and mouse genetic maps *(6,15)*, finally, makes the genetic analyses carried out in mice applicable to human diseases by means of comparative mapping *(15)*. Mouse inbred strains are invaluable models for many complex diseases (for review *see* ref. *12*). The use of more specialized genetic resources, such as congenics, chromosome substitution strains, recombinant inbred (RI), along with various statistical packages *(12)* has already led to a primary dissection of a few complex, multigenic traits. A detailed description of the mouse strains and their use in genetics can be found in Lee Silver (*see* ref. *17* and http://www.princeton.edu/lsilver/book/MGcontents.html).

In the present chapter we examine the statistical aspects of QTL mapping, with special emphasis on the relevant parameters, their impact on the genetic design to be chosen, and reciprocally, their adjustment under the various genetic models.

2. DESIGN OF GENETIC EXPERIMENTS IN MICE

A genetic mapping program in mice is typically initiated by the selection of two pure inbred strains that exhibit a substantial difference in terms of the observed phenotype. An inbred strain lacks genetic variation. All mice within the strain carry two identical copies of each autosome and are thus genetically identical for all practical purposes. Conversely, genetic variation is present between strains, leading presumably to the between-strains average phenotypical difference. Crossing the two strains gives rise to offspring that are a genetic combination of the two parental strains. The process of recombination then blends the genomes further in subsequent crosses, generating mice with chromosomes that are a mosaic of segments from the two parental genomes. Correlating the parental origin of the genetic material at various loci with the measured level of the trait is the major statistical tool for identifying the genetic factors associated with the phenotype.

Several experimental designs have been developed in the context of QTL analysis. The most widely used designs are the backcross (BC), the intercross (F2) designs, and to some extent RI strains (*see* Fig. 1). The statistical theory we present here is given primarily in the context of those three designs.

3. THE STATISTICAL MODEL

Denote by Y the phenotype measurement for a random mouse. This measurement may vary both within and between lines of pure inbred mice. Some of this variability may be attributed to genetic and some to nongenetic factors. For a given locus showing polymorphism between two given lines of inbred strains, denote by A_1 the allele originating from one strain and by A_2 the allele originating from the other. Intercrossing the two inbred strains may give rise

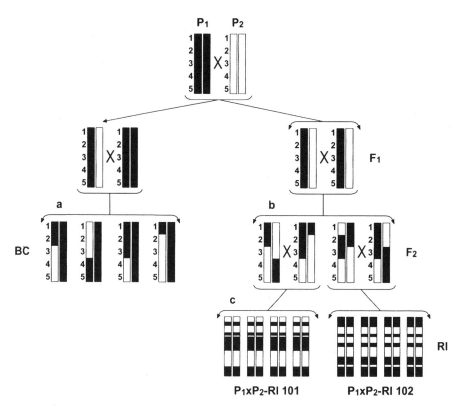

Fig. 1. The three cross designs: (a) backcross (BC), (b) intercross (F_2), and (c) recombinant inbred (RI). An outcross between two inbred lines (P_1 and P_2) produces the F_1 generation, with all the mice heterozygous over the whole genome; (a) the F_1 can be crossed back to one of the parental strain (P_1) to produce the BC; (b) an intercross within the F_1 will result in F_2 offspring; (c) strict inbreeding between F_2 pairs, for many generations, and following a single pair of chromosomes, will generate RI strains. All the individuals within a given RI strain carry the same homozygous, recombinant genotype.

to three genotypes. If X represents the copy number of allele A_2 in a genotype, then the variable X can take the values 0, 1, or 2. The model potentially assigns a different average level of Y for each genotype. At the same time, the variance of Y, or other characteristics of its distribution, is assumed to be independent of the genotype. The relation between the genotype and the phenotype is given in the regression formula:

$$Y = \mu + \alpha \cdot X + \delta \cdot I_{\{X=1\}} + e, \tag{1}$$

where e is a zero mean random deviate and I_A is the indicator function of an event A. (Specifically, $I_{\{X=1\}}$ is equal to 1 if the mouse is heterozygous and 0 if it is homozygous.) The coefficient α represents the *additive effect*, the coefficient δ represents the *dominant effect*, and the term μ is the intercept. μ is the expected level of Y for an (A_1A_1) homozygote. The expected level for an (A_2A_2) homozygote is 2α, and the expected level for a heterozygote is $\alpha + \delta$.

The deviate e incorporates all remaining factors that contribute to the variability. Such factors can include the genetic contribution from loci other than the one investigated, as well as environmental factors. We assume that this deviate is normally distributed and is uncorrelated with the genotype variable X.

The chosen cross design between the two inbred strains (BC, F2, RI, etc.) affects the distribution of the random variable X, as well as the distribution of the deviate e. For example, if the BC is formed by crossing back the F1 mice to the (A_1A_1) inbred strain, then X may take either the value 1 or the value 0, both with 0.5 probability. On the other hand, if the F1 mice are crossed one with another in order to form the intercross (F2), then X may take the values 0 or 2 with 0.25 probability and the value 1 with 0.5 probability. Finally, the RI mice are inbred strains, hence homozygous; X may take the value 0 or 2 with 0.5 probability each.

The phenotypical variance, the variance of Y, is a combination of variances that arises from several sources. The genetic variance is the part of the variance that is associated with the specific QTL. The source of the genetic variance is the variability of X. For the BC design, X may take only two values, the contribution of X to equation (1) simplifies to $(\alpha + \delta) \cdot X$. The variance of this component is $(\alpha + \delta)^2/4$, because the variance of X, a binomial $(1, 1/2)$ random variable, is $1/4$. For the F2 design, the genetic variance is the variance of $\alpha \cdot X + \delta \cdot I_{\{X = 1\}}$. Because X and $I_{\{X=1\}}$ are statistically uncorrelated, this variance is the sum of the variances of its components. The variance of $\alpha \cdot X$ is $\alpha^2/2$, because X has a binomial $(2, 1/2)$ distribution for the F2. The variance of $\delta \cdot I_{\{X = 1\}}$ is $\delta^2/4$, because the variance of the indicator is $1/4$. Overall, the genetic variance in the F2 is $\alpha^2/2 + \delta^2/4$. For the RI design, the relevant term is $\alpha \cdot X$ because RI lines are by definition homozygous. The variance here is α^2, because X equals 0 or 2 with 0.5 probability each.

Which of these three terms for the genetic variances is larger depends on the genetic model of the trait. For an additive model ($\delta = 0$) the genetic variance of an RI is twice as large as the genetic variance of the F2 and four times larger than that of the BC. However, for a dominant model ($\alpha = \delta$) the genetic variance of the RI is equal to the genetic variance of the BC. The genetic variance of the intercross is 25% smaller.

The heritability coefficient (H^2) is a preliminary approach for assessing the efficiency of a design. This coefficient is the ratio between the variance of the genetic term—the term involving X—and the overall variability of Y. It may take values between 0 and 1. The closer the coefficient is to 1, the more informative the design is. In the opposite case, values of H^2 closer to 0 make the statistical inference more difficult.

The H^2 may give a rough idea regarding the statistical merits of a design. A much better insight is provided when considering two additional parameters—the parameter of noncentrality at the QTL and the between-markers correlation coefficient. We devote the rest of this section to the definition of these quantities and the computation of their values for the three designs. In the subsequent sections we illustrate the role of these terms in the assessment of the properties of various statistical inferential tools.

3.1. The Parameter of Noncentrality

Statistical inference is based on correlating the genetic information at given polymorphical loci (genetic markers) with the phenotypical expression Y. A given collection of mice can be subdivided according to their genotype at a given locus (the levels of the variable X). This leads to the formation of up to three subclasses. The statistical analysis proceeds by comparing the differences in the levels of phenotypical expression (Y) between the subclasses.

Consider the BC design, and let us assume initially that we know the genetic configuration at the functional polymorphism that affects the quantitative trait. The variable X may have here only two values. A natural summary statistic (Z) computes the difference between the average expression levels in each group.[*] For convenience, this statistic is standardized to have a standard deviation of 1. We define the parameter of noncentrality to be the expected value of this Z:

$$\mathbb{E}(Z) \approx \frac{\sqrt{n}(\alpha + \delta)}{2\sigma}, \tag{2}$$

where n is the number of BC mice that were genotyped and σ is the standard deviation of the deviate e from the regression model (1). The ($\alpha + \delta$) arises as the expectation of the difference between the average phenotypes of the heterozygote and of the homozygote. The expectation in (2) is obtained by

---

[*]A slightly better statistic is the standardized sample regression coefficient. However, the statistic based on the difference of the averages is asymptotically equivalent and, in our view, is easier to interpret. Consequently, we will analyze this statistic.

dividing the expectation of the difference by its standard deviation, namely $(2\sigma / \sqrt{n})$.[*] (As a matter of fact, one can justify using the statistic Z as an approximate score statistic for testing the null hypothesis that the locus is not associated with the trait, i.e., $\alpha + \delta = 0$. We will not follow this more formal route. The interested reader is referred to ref. 5).

For the RI design also, X can take only two values. The standardized difference between the two types of homozygotes, which we call again Z, has the noncentrality parameter[**]:

$$\mathbb{E}(Z) \approx \frac{\sqrt{n}\alpha}{\sigma}. \tag{3}$$

In the F2 design, all three subBclasses can be realized. This leaves more flexibility in constructing statistics. For example, we shall use the statistic Z_α in order to make inference on the additive effect. Z_α is based on estimating the slope α in model (1). It essentially reflects the differences in phenotype average levels between the two homozygote types (standardized to have a standard deviation of 1). Likewise, we shall use the statistic $Z\delta$ (the difference in phenotypical average levels between the heterozygotes and homozygotes) in order to investigate deviations from the additive model. The expectations of these two types of statistics are[***]:

$$\mathbb{E}(Z_\alpha) \approx \frac{\sqrt{n}\alpha}{\sqrt{2}\sigma}, \quad \mathbb{E}(Z_\delta) \approx \frac{\sqrt{n}\delta}{2\sigma} \tag{4}$$

One can use a $2°$ of freedom χ^2 statistic in order to simultaneously test both the additive and dominance effects *(5)*. This statistic has the form: $Z_\alpha^2 + Z_\delta^2$.

Although this is not reflected in the above formulae, the σ value depends on the adopted breeding protocol and may vary between the BC, F2, and RI designs.

---

[*]About half the mice are heterozygotes. The variance of the phenotype across heterozygotes, as well as across homozygotes, is σ^2 (because X is given in each case). Therefore, the variance of the averages is $\sigma^2/(n/2)$. The variance of the difference is the sum of the variances, which leads to the expression of the standard deviation.

[**]About half the mice are homozygous for the alternative alleles. The expected difference between the two types of homozygotes is 2α. The variance of the averages for each homozygote type is $\sigma^2/(n/2)$. Hence, the expectation of Z is $(2\alpha)/\sqrt{2\sigma^2/(n/2)} = \sqrt{n}\alpha/\sigma$.

[***] The expectation of the difference between the two homozygote types is 2α. The frequency of each homozygote type is about $n/4$. This leads to a variance of the average difference of $8\sigma^2/n$, which gives the expression of the expectation of Z is (2_α).

The contribution of an (A_1A_1) homozygote to the expectation is μ. The contribution of an (A_2A_2) homozygote to the expectation is $\mu + 2\alpha$. The relative frequency of (A_1A_1) among homozygotes is about $1/2$. Consequently, the expectation of the average of the homozygotes is $\mu + \alpha$. The expectation among heterozygotes is $\mu + \alpha + \delta$. Therefore, the expectation of the difference is δ.

3.2. The Correlation Coefficient

The second parameter of interest is the intermarkers correlation coefficient. Given a pair of markers, consider the pair of computed Z statistics, one for each marker. The intermarkers correlation coefficient is the statistical correlation between these two statistics. This correlation is computed under the null assumption of both markers not being linked to a QTL ($\alpha = \delta = 0$). The value of this parameter is determined only by the recombination fraction between the two loci. It is independent of the additive and dominant coefficients of the trait (the parameters that determine the noncentrality parameter).

Consider a pair of markers on a random BC mouse, located at locus s and locus t on the same autosome denoted by $X(s)$ and by $X(t)$, the genotypes at both loci, respectively. Each may take either the value 0 or the value 1. Let θ be the recombination fraction between these two loci. The probability of the event $\{X(t) = 1\}$, given $\{X(s) = 1\}$, is $1-\theta$, because this event occurs if, and only if, the gamete inherited from the F1 parent is not recombinant. One can use the above conditional probability in order to show that the correlation between $X(t)$ and $X(s)$ is equal to $1-2\theta$. The associated test statistics $Z(t)$ and $Z(s)$ are (approximately) linear combinations, over a sample of mice, of the $X(t)$ and $X(s)$ variables. Consequently, for a large sample size,

$$\text{corr}(Z(t), Z(s)) \approx \text{corr}(X(t), X(s)) = 1-2\theta. \tag{5}$$

Consider next a random F2 mouse. Now, $X(s)$ and $X(t)$ may take three values each and two types of statistics are computed: Z and Z_δ. The probability transition matrix of going from $X(s)$ to $X(t)$ is given by:

$$\mathbb{P}(X(t) = i \mid X(s) = 2) = [(1-\theta)^2, 2\theta(1-\theta), \theta^2)],$$
$$\mathbb{P}(X(t) = i \mid X(s) = 1) = [\theta(1-\theta), \theta^2 + (1-\theta)^2, \theta(1-\theta)],$$
$$\mathbb{P}(X(t) = i \mid X(s) = 0) = [\theta^2, 2\theta(1-\theta), (1-\theta)^2)].$$

(As an example, observe that because in this case both gametes from the F1 parents should not be recombinant. Similar considerations provide the other entries in the above matrix.) Direct calculations give that here again the correlation between $X(t)$ and $X(s)$ is equal to $1-2\theta$. Consequently, because Z_α is approximately a linear combination of X:

$$\text{corr}(Z\alpha(t), Z\alpha(s)) \approx 1-2\theta. \tag{6}$$

In a similar way, the correlation coefficient between $I_{\{X(t) = 1\}}$ and $I_{\{X(s) = 1\}}$ is equal to $(1-2\theta)^2$. Z_δ is approximately a linear combination of $I_{\{X = 1\}}$. Hence,

$$\text{corr}(Z_\delta(t), Z_\delta(s)) \approx (1-2\theta)^2. \tag{7}$$

The Z_α variables are not correlated with any of the Z_δ variables.

An RI mouse has two identical copies of each autosome. The parental origin at two loci is the same ($X(t) = X(s)$) if that chromosome is not recombinant and vice versa. Denote by θ_{RI} the recombination fraction for a random gamete in the RI sample. The classical result of Haldane and Waddington (8) can be used in order to attain the approximation:

$$\theta_{RI} \approx 4\theta/(1 + 6\theta) \qquad (8)$$

(*See* ref. *9* for a general derivation of this and other results by a presentation of the problem in terms of finite population dynamics.) Considerations similar to those used for the BC give the following for the RI result:

$$\text{corr}(Z(t), Z(s)) \approx 1-2\theta_{RI} \approx 1-8\theta/(1 + 6\theta). \qquad (9)$$

This completes the computation of the intermarkers correlations for the three designs.

4. LARGE SAMPLE THEORY AND GAUSSIAN PROCESSES

The selection of inferential statistics should not be taken lightly. The choice may substantially affect the efficiency of the statistical analysis. This selection is typically guided by the prior assumption of the way genetic and nongenetic factors interact with the measured phenotype. This prior assumption is reflected in the statistical model that formulates the interaction. The model presented in equation (1) is an example of such a statistical model. This model is consistent with a prior assumption that a single major locus is responsible for a substantial part of the phenotypical variation, with other genetic factors, if any, adding only a small contribution each to that variation. Moreover, this model disables some forms of nonadditive epistasis and some forms of gene/environmental interaction.

In the sequel we will consider separately the statistical properties of inferential statistics for each of the three experimental designs. These statistics are computed based on the phenotypical and genotypical data collected over a collection of markers. Model (1) of a single major gene and dense genotyping is consistent with the approach of computing an inferential statistic for each marker at a time. (If the markers are not so densely spaced, interval mapping may be preferred *(11,5)*.) The inferential statistic will be of the form Z in the BC and RI designs and of the form in the F2 design. Other models may propose the use of other types of test statistics. (i.e., in order to detect interacting genes, one may consider inferential statistics, computed from the phenotypical and genetic data for a pair of markers, for all such possible pairs; *see* ref. *10*.)

The first step in the investigation of the properties of statistical procedures involves the determination of the distribution of the inferential statistics.

Let us focus on a given autosome. Markers are genotyped at loci t_1, t_2, ..., t_m (a total of m markers). For the BC and RI we denote the summary statistics by $Z(t_1)$, $Z(t_2)$, ..., $Z(t_m)$. For the F2 we denote them by $Z_\alpha(t_1)$, $Z_\alpha(t_2)$, ..., $Z_\alpha(t_m)$ and $Z_\alpha(t_1)$, $Z_\delta(t_2)$, ..., $Z_\delta(t_m)$. According to the large sample theory, the joint distribution of these statistics is approximately multinormal. Multinormal distributions are fully determined by the means and variances of the components and by the correlations between components. The components were standardized to have a variance of 1. The correlations were computed in (5) for the BC, in (6) and (7) for the F2, and in (9) for the RI. Thus, we are left only with the task of determining the means of the components.

The key concept in the determination of the means of the components (and a useful concept in general in statistics) is the concept of *sufficiency*. A statistic is called sufficient if it contains all the relevant information for making statistical inference (i.e., more formally, if conditioning on the statistic eliminates the dependency between parameters of the model and the distribution of the data). Assume a QTL is present at locus s. Let us figure that this locus is also genotyped and that an appropriate test statistic is computed (where the test statistic is $Z(s)$ in the BC and RI cases or $(Z_\alpha(s), Z_\delta(s))$ in the F2 case). Because, by assumption of model (1), the given QTL is the only genetic factor on the chromosome that contributes to the phenotypic variability, the particulars of these imaginary statistics, had we had them, would have been sufficient for determining the association with the trait. Therefore, the information at the other loci is no longer relevant, whether it is available or not.

This sufficiency assumption forces a given relation between the mean of a statistic computed at a marker ($Z(t)$) and the mean of the statistic ($Z(s)$) at the QTL, namely:

$$\mathbb{E}[Z(t)] = \mathrm{corr}(Z(t), Z(s)) \times \mathbb{E}[Z(s)]. \tag{10}$$

The right-hand side of (10) is the outcome of the noncentrality parameter, given in (2) for the BC, in (4) for the F2, and in (3) for the RI. The correlation coefficient between loci is computed in (5), (6), (7), and (9) for the three designs. In summary, the means of the components can be determined by identifying the parameter of noncentrality at the QTL and the correlation between the QTL and the various markers.

The Haldane model of crossovers is a popular model that leads to a simple relation between the genetic distance and the recombination fraction. Applying this function yields a correlation coefficient of the general form: $\exp\{-\beta|t - s|\}$ with β varying between the BC and the F2 designs (the correlation coefficient for the RI design does not have this form). Multinormal vectors with such correlation structure are denoted Orenstein–Uhlenbeck processes. Yet, as we shall see in the following sections, the statistical properties of the inferential procedures based on the multinormal process do not depend on the exact form of the correlation function but on a rather weaker property.

5. DETECTING A QTL

Mapping a QTL is a multistage process. The first step, following the phenotypical and genotypical data collection, is the determination of the reflection in the collected data of the presence of a QTL. It should be noted that even when a genetic influence on the trait is undisputable, its effect may be too weak, and our data may not be sufficient, in order to distinguish it from random fluctuations. Therefore, the first question to be addressed is: Can we detect a strong enough signal for the presence of a QTL? If the answer for this question is affirmative then we can proceed in the process of mapping the QTL. If, however, the answer is negative, then we ought to revise our strategy. Such a revision may include an increase in the sample size within the framework of the current design, using a different cross design, and so on.

The field in statistics theory that deals with the issue of determining the presence of a signal in a noisy environment is called *hypothesis testing*. According to this theory, one should select a test statistic with a distribution that best reflects the presence of a signal, and base the conclusion on the computed value of that statistic. In the case of QTL mapping we identified such statistics—the statistics of the form Z in the BC and RI designs and the statistics $Z_\alpha^2 + Z_\delta^2$. in the F2 design. Large values of the statistics in the latter case or large absolute values of the statistics in the former cases are an indication of the presence of a QTL in the vicinity of the marker: a strong effect of the QTL will be reflected by a nonzero noncentrality parameter of the statistics, which will tend to deviate its value away from 0.

The simple theory of hypothesis testing, which is based on normal distribution, would have been applicable had we looked at a single marker, and a single marker only. However, in our case we examine a sequence of test statistics, one for each marker. An extreme value in *any* of the test statistics is an indication of the presence of a QTL. Thus, in reality, our test statistic is $\max_{ti} |Z_\alpha^2 (t_i)|$ in the case of the BC and RI designs and $\max_{ti} [Z_\alpha^2 (t_i) + Z_\delta^2. (t_i)]$ in the case of the F2 design, when the maximization is taken across all markers. It turns out that the distribution of these statistics is no longer normal, even though each component has a normal distribution. The determination of the threshold, which will assure a given significance level for the experiment, is based on the distribution of the maximal test statistic in the absence of a QTL. This distribution, as we shall see in equations (11) and (12), depends on the form of the test statistics, the number of markers used for scanning, and on the correlation between the inferential statistics. This correlation is a function of the distance between markers and the design of the cross.

The probability of reaching the threshold is less than the product of the number of markers examined by the probability of reaching the threshold with a single marker. This last probability is easily computed using the normal distribution in the case of the BC and RI, or the χ^2 distribution on 2° of freedom in the case of the F2. This upper bound, also known as the *Bonferroni upper bound*, is actually a reasonable approximation of the true probability when the correlation between markers is not too high. However, when the correlation between markers is high, a better approximation of the probability takes the form:

$$\mathbb{P}(\max_{t_i} | Z(t_i) | \geq z) \approx [C + (\beta L z^2) \cdot v(2z^2 \beta \Delta)] \cdot \mathbb{P}(| Z | \geq z), \tag{11}$$

when the basic test statistic is a single normal variable Z, and the form:

$$\mathbb{P}(\max_{t_i}[Z_\alpha^2(t_i) + Z_\delta^2(t_i)] \geq u) \approx [C + (\beta L u) \cdot v(2u\beta\Delta)] \cdot \mathbb{P} \quad (Z_\alpha^2 + Z_\delta^2 \geq u), \tag{12}$$

when the basic test statistic is a χ^2 statistic. Here, the number of markers, used for the Bonferroni upper bound, is replaced by the term in the square brackets. The components that determine the value of these approximations are the number of chromosomes scanned (C); the sum of lengths between the first and the last marker in each chromosome, across all those chromosomes (L, measured in cM); the threshold (z in the first formula and u in the second); the probability of reaching the threshold with a single marker ($\mathbb{P}(| Z | \geq z)$ in the first formula and $\mathbb{P}(Z_\alpha^2 + Z_\delta^2 \geq u)$ in the second); and the components that reflect the correlation between markers. These components are the average distance between consecutive markers (Δ, measured in cM) and the rate with which the correlation between two markers approaches 1 as the markers get closer to each other (β). This last term is equal to 0.02 in the BC design, 0.08 in the RI design, and it turns out to be $(0.02 + 0.04)/2 = 0.03$ in the F2 design.

The function $v(\cdot)$ appearing in these formulae was originally developed in the context of random walks and renewal theory. It appears in other fields of statistics as well, including change-point detection and scanning statistics. It takes the form:

$$v(y) = \frac{2}{y} \exp\left\{-2\sum_{n=1}^{\infty} \Phi(-\sqrt{ny}\,/\,2)\right\}, \tag{13}$$

where $\Phi(\cdot)$ is the cumulative probability function of the normal distribution. It turns out that the function $\upsilon(\cdot)$ approaches the value of 1 as y approaches 0. The function can be approximated by $\exp\left\{-0.583\sqrt{y}\right\}$ for small values of y *(16)*. When markers become denser and denser, the distance between them, Δ, becomes smaller. This makes the arguments of the function $\upsilon(\cdot)$ in (11) and (12) approach 0. In the asymptotic case, the formula represents the probability of false detection with a continuum of markers. This formula is obtained by removing the function $\upsilon(\cdot)$ from the expressions in (11) and (12). At the other extreme, the function can be approximated by $2/y$ for large values of y. Substituting the function with this approximation reproduces the Bonferroni upper bound, because $\Delta = L / (m - C)$. Therefore, one can view the function $\upsilon(\cdot)$ as a correction term, which takes into account both the discreteness of the markers and the correlation between them.

Computing the power is an essential requirement for designing the experiment. The power is the probability of detecting the QTL, i.e., the probability of reaching the given threshold when a QTL is present. This probability depends on the expectations of the statistics computed at the markers. These expectations are tilted to have a nonzero value on the chromosome carrying the QTL. As we saw in (10), the expectations depend on the noncentrality parameter and on the correlations between the markers and the QTL. A simple lower bound for the power can be obtained by considering the probability of reaching the threshold in either of the two markers flanking the QTL. A refined approximation will take into account the possibility of reaching the threshold for markers that are further away from the QTL. We will not present these approximations here. The interested reader is referred to ref. *5*.

6. ESTIMATING MAP LOCATION

In the first stage of mapping a QTL the issue is to evaluate the reflection in the data of the presence of a QTL. If the answer to this evaluation is affirmative, then the continuation of the process of mapping involves narrowing down the candidate region likely to contain a QTL as much as possible. In its initial stage, this process involves the construction of a confidence interval (CI) for the QTL based on the data used for detection.

One procedure for constructing confidence intervals is by examining tests for the presence of a QTL at various loci. A QTL is assumed to exist somewhere along the chromosome. However, its exact location is unknown. According to this procedure, a locus s is included in the confidence interval if the hypothesis that s is the exact location of a QTL is *not* rejected. It follows that if the significance level for that test is 10%, then the confidence level of the resulting CI is 90%. Likewise, if the significance level of the tests is 5%, then the confidence level is 95%.

One approach for constructing such location tests makes the simplifying assumption that the QTL is completely linked to one of the markers, or in other words, the correlation coefficient between the QTL and one of the markers is 1. Yet, the marker that is completely linked to the QTL remains unknown. The problem of constructing a CI reduces, through this assumption, to the problem of testing each of the markers for being completely linked to the QTL. In the CI, all the markers that were not rejected by the test are included. Naturally, this approach may produce better results when markers are densely spaced, in which case the simplification made does not introduce much error. It may be less satisfactory when the number of markers is limited. In the latter case one may try other approaches of constructing confidence intervals. We will not refer to such approaches. The reader may find an evaluation of several of these approaches in ref. *(5)*.

The decision to exclude a marker s from the CI (reject the hypothesis that s is the QTL) may be based on the relation:

$$\max_t Z^2(t) - Z^2(s) > x, \tag{14}$$

when a single degree of freedom statistic is used (BC, RI) or on the relation:

$$\max_t [Z_\alpha^2(t) + Z_\delta^2(t)] - [Z_\alpha^2(s) + Z_\delta^2(s)] > x, \tag{15}$$

when a 2° of freedom statistic is used (F2).

The selection of x to assure the desired confidence level may depend, however, on the unknown parameter of noncentrality, because the distribution of the statistics in (14) and (15) depends on that parameter. Still, a remedy to this problem may be provided by the notion of sufficiency. As was claimed before, the statistic $Z(s)$ in case (14) and the statistic $(Z_\alpha(s), Z_\delta(s))$ in case (15) are sufficient statistics for the parameters of model (1), including the noncentrality parameter. Consequently, the conditional probability of the events (14) or (15), given the value of the sufficient statistic, is independent of that unknown parameter. The threshold x can be selected based on this conditioned computation. The result is a confidence interval with the prescribed confidence level, regardless of what the true value of the noncentrality parameter is.

It should be noted that technically the problem of constructing a confidence interval for the QTL location is not like the problem of constructing a confidence interval for the population expectation. In the latter case, one typically takes an interval of about two standard deviations in each direction of the sample average in order to get a CI with a confidence level of 95%. This construction relies on the fact that the distribution of the sample average is normal. The length of this interval decreases at a rate that is proportional $1/\sqrt{n}$, where n is the sample size (because the variance of the sample average is equal to the variance of a single observation, divided by the sample size). In QTL mapping, on the other hand, the estimate of the location of the QTL does not have a normal distribution, even when the sample size is large. Therefore, taking two standard deviations about its value will not result in a proper CI.

The difference between the normal case and QTL mapping is reflected also in the expression for the expected length of the CI. An approximation for this length for the case of a one degree of freedom statistic Z is provided in *(5)*:

$$\frac{x}{\beta\mu^2} + \frac{x^2}{2\beta\mu^4} + \frac{2(1 - v(2\mu^2\beta\Delta))^{1/2}}{\beta\mu^2} + \frac{v^2(2\mu^2\beta\Delta)}{2\beta}. \qquad (16)$$

Again, Δ is the average distance between markers, β is the rate of convergence to 1 of the covariance between markers as the distance between decreases, and $v(y)$ is the function presented in (13). The term μ is the noncentrality parameter. x is the threshold for the test. This threshold is essentially independent of the sample size. The noncentrality parameter, on the other hand, increases at a rate proportional to $\sqrt{n}$. It turns out, since the approximation is roughly proportional to $1/\mu^2$, that the expected length of the confidence interval decreases at a rate proportional to $1/n$ (compared to the $1/\sqrt{n}$, in the normal case).

7. FINE-MAPPING STRATEGIES

After detecting a QTL, a confidence interval for its location is computed. This confidence interval tends to be quite wide, perhaps 20 or 30 cM wide. Such wide intervals most likely contain dozens of genes that are good candidates to be the QTL. However, direct techniques of cloning, which may be used in order to verify that a given polymorphic sequence is the QTL, are lengthy and expensive. Therefore, it is critical to narrow down the search region, to below 1 cM, before the more direct measures can be applied. The process of narrowing down the interval containing the QTL is often called *fine-mapping*.

There is a major difference between fine-mapping of a Mendelian trait and fine-mapping of a QTL. In the former case there is a 1:1 relation between the presence or absence of the trait and the genetic composition at the functional composition. Thereby, one can barricade the functional polymorphism precisely by the identification of recombinant chromosomes and relating them to the phenotypical expression. In the latter case, on the other hand, there is no such 1:1 relation, only statistical correlations between the genetic composition and the phenotypic expression. Consequently, one must revert to statistical procedures in order to carry out the task. These statistical procedures may be based on hypothesis testing, parallel in spirit to the task of QTL detection, or on the construction of a CI, similar to problem of estimating map location. The main concern in fine-mapping, however, is that the resulting region will be narrow enough.

Examining (16) we see that the two main parameters that determine its width are the parameter of noncentrality (μ) and the parameter that captures the rate of recombination in a close proximity to the QTL (β). The larger these parameters are, the shorter the confidence interval is expected to be. Fine-mapping is most efficiently conducted by selecting an experimental design that maximizes these parameters. An example of such design is to use an advanced intercross design, or F_i, as proposed in *(3)*. F_i stands for the ith generation of intercrossing. The rate of recombination (β) increases approximately linearly in i. This leads to a reduction in the width of the CI.

An alternative experimental design is the recombinant inbred segregation test (RIST). According to this design, RI strains are selectively crossed with their parental lines in such a way that ensures recombination in the investigated region. The simple chromosomes identification, which is used in Mendelian traits, is replaced by a statistical test to determine on which side of the recombination point the QTL is located. Choosing the appropriate RIST design, either the RIST-BC or the RIST-F2 design, will maximize the noncentrality parameter and improve the performance of the procedure. For a comprehensive review on fine-mapping strategies *see* ref. *(2)*.

8. DISCUSSION

In this chapter we have presented the statistical framework for QTL analysis in its various stages. Because any QTL will usually explain only a small fraction of the phenotypical variation, large samples cannot be avoided. We have emphasized on the two parameters that have the largest effect on this theory. The first is the noncentrality parameter, which reflects the proportion of variance explained by the QTL being studied, and the second is the extent of correlation between the functional polymorphism and the genetic marker tested and between pairs of markers. Different designs can be implemented for QTL analysis, and in this chapter we have described how the relevant parameters affect the use of each of the main experimental designs, namely, F2, BC, and RI strains.

QTL analysis consists of a number of steps as described throughout the chapter. The general theory presented here can serve as a basis for the analysis of any such stages. For example, although both the first and the second stages, QTL detection and map location, are affected by the same two parameters, their effect might be of opposite direction: the detection stage requires as little recombination as possible, whereas extensive recombination is preferred for localization.

The difficulty in QTL analysis lies in the large samples required for detection and the limited breakdown of the correlation in adjacent chromosomal regions. The sample sizes may reach unattainable numbers if the genetic architecture of the trait consists of many genes with small effect each. This has caused very few success stories in QTL analysis. Nevertheless, some have indeed succeeded in taking a QTL project all the way to the identification of the relevant genes. One such example is the *Mom1* gene affecting multiplicity and size of tumor induced by the Apc^Min mutation in mice *(1)*. In tomato, the *ORFX* gene was found to have an effect on fruit weight *(7)*. More recently, a complex genetic architecture influencing high-temperature growth could be resolved in yeast, using an elegant genetic approach *(18)*. With the advances of the postgenomic era other examples will undoubtedly follow. Multidisciplinary approaches, including comparative genetics, expression analysis, bioinformatics, proteomics, and so on, will undoubtedly help in this difficult endeavor.

REFERENCES

1. Cormier RT, Hong KH, Halberg RB, et al. Secretory phospholipase Pla2g2a confers resistance to intestinal tumorigenesis. Nat Genet 1997;17:88–91.
2. Darvasi A. Experimental strategies for the genetic dissection of complex traits in animal models. Nat Genet 1998;18:19–23.
3. Darvasi A, Soller M. Advanced intercross lines, an experimental population for fine genetic mapping. Genetics 1995;141:943–951.
4. Dietrich W, Katz H, Lincoln SE, et al. A genetic map of the mouse suitable for typing intraspecific crosses. Genetics 1992;131:423–447.
5. Dupuis J, Siegmund D. Statistical methods for mapping quantitative trait loci from a dense set of markers. Genetics 1999;151:373–386.
6. Eppig JT, Nadeau JH. Comparative maps: the mammalian jigsaw puzzle. Curr Opin Genet Dev 1995;5:709–716.
7. Frary A, Nesbitt TC, Grandillo S, et al. fw2.2: a quantitative trait locus key to the evolution of tomato fruit size. Science 2000;289:85–88.
8. Haldane JBS, Waddington CH. Inbreeding and linkage. Genetics 1931; 16:357–374.
9. Kimura M. A probability method for treating inbreeding systems, especially with linked genes. Biometrics 1963;19:1–17.

10. Korol AB, Ronin YI, Kirzhner VM. Interval mapping of quantitative trait loci employing correlated trait complexes. Genetics 1995;140:1137–1147.
11. Lander ES, Botstein D. Mapping Mendelian factors underlying quantitative traits using RFLP linkage maps [published erratum appears in Genetics 1994;136:705]. Genetics 1989;121:185–199.
12. Manly KF, Olson JM. Overview of QTL mapping software and introduction to map manager QT. Mamm Genome 1999;10:327–334.
13. Moore KJ, Nagle DL. Complex trait analysis in the mouse: the strengths, the limitations and the promise yet to come. Annu Rev Genet 2000;34:653–686.
14. Morse HC, III. The laboratory mouse: a historical perspective. In: Foster HL, Small JD, Fox JG, eds. The mouse in biomedical research. vol. 1. History, genetics, and wildmice. New York: Academic, 1981.
15. O'Brien SJ, Menotti-Raymond M, Murphy WJ, et al. The promise of comparative genomics in mammals. Science 1999;286:458–462, 479–481.
16. Siegmund D. Sequential analysis: tests and confidence intervals. New York: Springer, 1985.
17. Silver LM. Mouse genetics: concepts and applications. New York, Oxford: Oxford University Press, 1995. http://www.princeton.edu/lsilver/book/MGcontents.html.
18. Steinmetz LM, Sinha H, Richards DR, et al. Dissecting the architecture of a quantitative trait locus in yeast. Nature 2002;416:326–330.

3

Haplotype-Based Computational Genetic Analysis In Mice

Jianmei Wang and Gary Peltz

1. INTRODUCTION

A number of significant discoveries have resulted from genetic analysis of model experimental organisms. Improved methods for quantitative trait analysis, a process referred to as quantitative trait locus (QTL) mapping, have enabled investigators to make genetic discoveries. This mapping method requires the experimental generation of intercross progeny derived from two selected parental strains, chosen because they differ in a trait of interest. Through correlative analysis of the measured phenotype and geno-type at multiple positions in the genome for each intercross progeny, regions of the genome responsible for the differences in the trait are identified. The genomic regions that quantitatively contribute to the trait are referred to as QTL. QTL analysis has been successfully used to map important traits in crop plants, cattle, fruit flies, mice, and many other model organisms. The statistical basis for QTL mapping has been thoroughly investigated (reviewed in ref. *1*). Based on this statistical underpinning, experimental crosses using model organisms can be designed to reliably detect QTLs, even when the involved regions make a relatively small contribution to the trait being studied.

Many traits of biomedical importance are now routinely studied by genetic analysis of mammalian experimental models, primarily using inbred mouse or rat strains. However, there are significant liabilities associated with QTL analysis, especially when applied to mammalian organisms. First, the resolution of QTL mapping is limited. An implicated region identified by QTL analysis typically ranges from 10 to 100 Mb in size.

Because of inherent limitations within QTL mapping methods, the resolution does not increase significantly as the density of the markers and the

From: *Computational Genetics and Genomics*
Edited by: G. Peltz © Humana Press Inc., Totowa, NJ

number of intercross progeny analyzed are increased *(2)*. The 95% confidence interval is often greater than half a chromosome for a genetic locus of moderate effect, even when identified by analysis of 500 or more intercross progeny *(3)*. Second, a significant amount of time and cost is required for generating and analyzing mouse or rat intercross progeny. The process of generating, genotyping, and phenotyping 200–1000 mice or rats required for analysis of a selected trait usually requires a 2-yr period. The genetic interval can be further narrowed by analysis of an experimentally produced congenic strain. The congenic mouse is produced by introgressing the involved segment of the genome from one strain onto the genetic background of the other strain. Generation of congenic strains requires an additional 2 yr, adding more time onto an already long process. Other independent methods of analysis are then used to identify the genetic variant(s) within the QTL interval causing the trait difference.

To overcome the cost, time, and resolution issues associated with QTL analysis, we have developed a computational method for genetic mapping that correlates phenotypic differences among a set of inbred mouse strains with genotypic differences *(4)*. Although this method was developed for analysis of genetic traits in mice, it can be applied to any experimental organism. However, to use an organism other than the mouse, there must be well-maintained inbred strains, a physical map of the genome, and a database characterizing the pattern of genetic variation among the strains analyzed. The set of genetic markers must be dense enough to cover all genes of interest and should characterize all polymorphic patterns for all the inbred strains selected for analysis. Most importantly, computational mapping by this method does not require generation of intercross progeny. Phenotypic analysis is performed on only a selected set of available parental strains. Although establishing the genotypic database for the inbred strain panel is costly, the cost is well justified, because it is amortized across all subsequently performed experiments. The computational method maps traits at high resolution using a relatively small number of inbred strains, usually to an interval that is below the size of a single gene. This increased precision is possible because the density of genotypic markers is very high, and the computational mapping method does not depend on recombinations occurring over two generations, which are relatively rare events. Furthermore, homozygosity of the genome of the inbred strains eliminates confounding effects because of allelic heterogeneity at a locus, and modeling the effects of dominance and additivity is not required. In addition to its low cost and precision, the computational mapping method has one other significant advantage. Because genetically identical and widely available inbred strains are analyzed, it enables the results to be repeated and widely replicated. The ability to analyze complex genetic traits remains an advantage for conventional QTL mapping approaches at this time. The computational mapping methods have relatively low power for analyzing genetic traits regulated by a large number of different genetic loci, each of small effect size (Table 1). However, as the number of strains that are genetically and phenotypically analyzed is increased, the complexity of the genetic traits that can be analyzed by the computational mapping method will increase. Although we are currently analyzing 20 or fewer inbred strains, it is not unlikely that the number of characterized inbred mouse strains will increase to nearly 100 within 3–5 yr.

Previously, a genome-wide computational mapping method was developed and referred to as digital disease *(5)*. This method utilized a relatively crude calculation of the correlation coefficient between trait values measured among inbred mouse strains and single nucleotide polymorphism (SNP) alleles within chromosome regions. It correctly mapped selected traits to 30-cM chromosomal regions. In this chapter, we outline a haplotype-based computational method for genetic analysis of phenotypic traits using inbred mouse strains. The haplotype-based method utilizes the same principle of finding patterns of genetic variation that correlate with phenotypic differences among the strains. However, the haplotype-based computational mapping method is radically different; it is based on a highly quantitative model. This method correctly identified known genetic loci for previously characterized traits and was used to discover a novel allele-specific enhancer element in the mouse genome *(4)*.

Table 1
Comparison: Quantitative Trait Locus (QTL) and Haplotype-Based Computational Genetic Analysis

Method	QTL analysis	Haplotype-based computational analysis
Process	Produce, genotype and phenotype 200–1000 F2 or BC1	Order and phenotype 10–20 strains
Reproducibility	Each F2 is unique	Can reorder strains
Resolution	10–100 Mb	Individual genes
Effort	3–5 scientists 3–10 yr	1 scientist < 1 d
Detection power	Handles high complexity	Handles limited complexity

BC, backcross.

The commonly used inbred mouse strains were developed from a limited number of founder mice. The genome of each inbred mouse strain resembles a patchwork of a small number of ancestral chromosomes *(6)*. The observed linkage disequilibrium among the inbred mouse strains is much greater than that in the population of mice in the wild. This strong linkage disequilibrium means that the pattern of genetic variation within a genomic region can be characterized by knowing the alleles at a relatively few positions. The genome of the inbred strains can be efficiently organized into semi-independent regions, and each region contains a relatively small number of distinct genetic patterns. This drastically reduces the number of comparisons required for computational genetic analysis. Instead of comparing a phenotypic pattern with individual SNP alleles, the haplotype-based method compares the phenotype with different haplotypes that extend across larger genomic regions *(4)*. We will describe how a map of the haplotypic structure of the mouse genome was constructed and how this enabled computational analysis of genetic traits to be performed. Following this, a quantitative model for haplotype-based computational mapping method is presented.

2. A HAPLOTYPE MAP FOR INBRED MOUSE STRAINS

As previously noted in the human genome, SNP alleles in close physical proximity in the genome of inbred mouse strains were often correlated, resulting in the presence of "SNP haplotypes" appearing within block-like structures *(7)*. Each haplotype within a block apparently originated from a common ancestral chromosome, whereas block size reflects other processes, including recombination and mutation. In general, the block structure and haplotype diversity depends on the genealogical history of the population used to construct the block structure and the local mutation and recombination rate. An appropriate haplotype map for QTL mapping purpose should be constructed using inbred strains with similar overall genetic background, yet display sufficient phenotypic differences. Because linkage disequilibrium decays as the distance between markers increase, it cannot be fully characterized by any simple block structure. When methods that produce very large blocks are used, the linkage disequilibrium among alleles within a large haplotype block is relatively weak. In this case, finer structures within the block are not identified, and distinct haplotypes within the block may be missed. However, when methods that produce very short blocks are used, then strong linkage disequilibrium between neighboring blocks will be missed. There are many different ways to define the block structure. All of these methods produce haplotype blocks that balance two desired proprieties. The size of the block should be as large as possible, but all distinct haplotypes within the block should be identified. In other words, if a group of inbred strains share alleles within a region, they should share a haplotype within the corresponding block. For the human population, there is the additional requirement that the number of "haplotype-tagging SNPs" (htSNPs) that must be genotyped to characterize the genetic pattern within a block should be as small as possible *(8)*.

Because there are differences in the way in which haplotype maps are utilized for analysis of human populations and inbred mouse strains, different algorithms should be utilized for construction of murine and human haplotype blocks. We developed a novel method, derived from the one previously used for human SNP analysis *(7)*, to analyze murine genetic variation and to define the structure of haplotypic blocks in the mouse genome. This new method was developed for construction of a haplotype map for inbred mouse strains and is presented in Chapter 4. In this section, we present the theory for this method and describe how it differs from other methods used for human haplotype map construction *(7–10)*. The allelic data in this mouse SNP database (*see* http://mouseSNP.roche.com) was used for haplotype map construction. It contains more than 2 million alleles that were assayed across 18 inbred mouse strains for the 134,500 SNPs. In the end, allelic data from 16 closely related mouse strains were used to construct the haplotype map.

To construct the mouse haplotype map, a set of all possible candidate blocks was constructed for each chromosome. A candidate block consists of two or more consecutive SNPs that are separated by less than 1 Mb, and at least 80% of the strains have a haplotype shared by at least one other strain. Each candidate block was then assigned a score, which was calculated as the number of SNPs within the block divided by two to the power of the number of haplotypes. The final block structure was constructed by selecting the block with the highest score from among the set of candidate blocks. Any blocks that overlapped the selected block were then discarded. This process was repeated until all SNPs were analyzed. Any SNP that was not included within the selected blocks was included as a single SNP block. The 80% coverage condition guarantees that there is extensive haplotype sharing among the strains within a haplotypic block. This condition also increases the computational efficiency, because it restricts the candidate blocks to those with three or fewer strains having a unique haplotype. When the coverage condition is changed to 70 or 90%, the block structures are relatively unchanged, except for only a few blocks. This algorithm generated longer blocks with fewer haplotypes. The block score definition implies that if a long block has a subblock within it, consisting of at least half of the SNPs and fewer haplotypes, then the shorter block would be selected in the final block structure instead of the longer one.

Although there are similarities between the methods for construction of mouse and human haplotypes, our mouse algorithm produces a very different type of haplotype map from the methods used for human haplotype construction. The advantage of the new method for computational mapping in inbred strains is illustrated by comparing the two algorithms. For human populations, it has been suggested that htSNPs can be used to define the structure of haplotype blocks *(7)*. The htSNPs are selected allelic markers that capture most of the variation within a selected region. They define the existing patterns of genetic variation within a region for the population studied and require a minimal amount of genotyping to characterize that pattern. A score function for a haplotype block generated by this method is the total number of SNPs divided by the number of htSNPs, which is approximately $(\#\text{SNPs})/\log_2(\#\text{haplotypes})$. Because $\log_2(\#\text{haplotypes}) << 2^{(\#\text{haplotypes})}$, the human algorithm strongly favors relatively longer blocks, and each block contains an increased number of haplotypes. To accommodate the large amount of genetic diversity in the human population, the selected htSNPs must identify the within-block haplotype of only 80% of the individuals analyzed *(7)*. The presence of up to 20% of other haplotypes within each block further increases the extent of haplotype diversity. Although these compromises are appropriate for extracting the pattern of genetic variation in a genetically diverse human population, it is neither necessary nor appropriate for haplotype analysis of the inbred strains. As the number of haplotypes within a block increases, the extent of linkage disequilibrium within the block decreases. Therefore, the block structure generated using our new algorithm, which is described in Chapter 4, captures the strong linkage groups within a murine block much better than the algorithms used for human populations. Our method for generating haplotype maps in the mouse is also more appropriate for high-resolution QTL mapping. When applied to mouse SNP allelic data, only approximately three haplotypes were found in most blocks among the 16 strains analyzed.

This algorithm uses an iterative method to identify blocks of SNPs. As a first step, larger blocks with fewer haplotypes were identified. There is a high degree of linkage disequilibrium among the SNPs within these blocks. The remaining SNPs form very small or even single SNP blocks. It is possible that very short blocks may be identified by chance rather than as a result of sharing of an ancestral chromosomal segment. Of note, any combination of two (or three) SNPs generates only four (or eight) different genotypic patterns. Because of this limited number of possible genotypes, allele sharing among strains within short haplotype blocks (less than four SNPs) may result from a random co-occurrence of the same genetic alteration. These blocks may not result from true linkage disequilibrium among the strains, and other sequence variation within these small blocks may not conform to the genotype of the flanking markers. For these small blocks, the trait values should be compared with individual allelic markers. In contrast, a haplotypic block constructed with four or more SNPs generated by this algorithm is highly likely to reflect the presence of true linkage disequilibrium within the block. Therefore, our computational mapping studies use haplotype blocks that contain four or more SNPs.

3. A METHOD FOR HAPLOTYPE-BASED COMPUTATIONAL GENETIC MAPPING

In traditional murine QTL mapping, genetic analysis is usually performed by analysis of genotypic data obtained from 50 to 200 markers used to analyze the genome of the intercross progeny. The chromosomal regions containing the genetic loci are identified using interval mapping, which models the recombination between the marker and the loci. On the other hand, computational mapping using inbred strains takes advantage of a dense set of markers characterizing all sequence variation in functional regions across the entire genome. Even though most individual SNPs are binary, many regions of strong linkage disequilibrium have more than two distinct alleles among the inbred strains. Some multiallelic sequence variation within a locus can result in more than two distinct phenotypes (*see* major histocompatibility complex [MHC] example in ref. *4*). The haplotypic blocks defined in Heading 2 represent natural grouping of SNPs into such multiallelic regions. When haplotypic blocks are used as markers instead of individual SNPs, the number of comparisons in association study is reduced by roughly 100-fold.

This computational analysis is performed under the assumption that the causative genetic locus has been analyzed and haplotypes for this locus that distinguish among the inbred strains have been identified. Additionally, the contribution of a single locus to the quantitative trait must be relatively large in order for the genetic effect to be detectable. The minimum effect size depends on the available number of strains. Although the assumptions and requirements may seem stringent, many traits, even complex traits, can be investigated. Mapping quantitative traits onto nonbinary markers requires new analytical methodology. We will describe how phenotypic traits can be computationally analyzed and specific candidate genetic loci can be identified. We will also provide quantitative statistical measures used to assess the results of a computational mapping experiment.

3.1. A Linear Model for Haplotype-Based Computational Mapping of Genetic Traits

Genetic researchers have traditionally applied a linear model to analyze a quantitative trait using the observed variance among a defined population. For a model in which an observed difference is caused by a single genetic locus, the total phenotypic variance is first partitioned into genetic and environmental variances. Following this, the genetic variance is further divided into a variance resulting from additive and dominance effects. The additive effect is half the measured trait value difference between the two strains with homozygous alleles. The dominance effect is quantified as the difference in measured trait values between strains with heterozygous alleles and the average of those with homozygous alleles. Experimental intercross progeny can be heterozygous at many genetic loci, but the parental inbred mouse strains are homozygous at all genetic loci. Therefore, the dominant effect does not contribute to genetic variance among the parental inbred strains. This greatly simplifies the analysis of genetically controlled trait differences among inbred strains, which provides a key advantage to our haplotype-based mapping method. Assuming that the genotypic differences within the gene controlling the selected trait of interest have been characterized, the linear model for the trait becomes

$$y_j = f(G_j) + \varepsilon_j \tag{1}$$

where y_j is the trait value for the jth inbred strain, $f(G_j)$ is the component of the phenotypic trait that is determined by the genotype controlling the trait, and ε_j is the residual variance in the jth strain that is independent of the genetic effect at the given locus. Assume that genetic heterogeneity within the gene is fully captured by known haplotypes with the haplotypic block constructed using allelic markers within the gene. Following this, the genotype contribution G_j takes value in $\{H_1, H_2, ..., H_k\}$, corresponding to the k distinct haplotypes within the gene found among the inbred strains analyzed. $k = 2$ or 3 for most of the haplotype blocks. The trait value determined by the genotype component is now:

$$f(H_i) = \mu_i, \quad i = 1, 2, ..., k.$$

For a trait whose value varies among the inbred strains, mapping the genetic locus becomes a process of finding the haplotype block whose genetic variance explains the largest amount of the total trait variance. In other words, the residual variance var(ε) is minimized, where

$$\text{var}(\varepsilon) = \frac{1}{n-1} \sum_{j=1}^{n} \varepsilon_j^2 = \frac{1}{n-1} \sum_{i=1}^{k} \sum_{l=1}^{n_i} (y_l - \mu_l)^2.$$

If the number of haplotypes within each haplotype block is fixed, the problem is further reduced to simple linear regression. Note that in general, the number of haplotype k varies among blocks, and $\mu_i = \frac{1}{n_i}\sum_{l=1}^{n_i} y_l$ is the estimated trait value determined by the genotype. Here n_l is the number of strains with haplotype H_l. Var(ε) is the "within-group sum of squares" divided by $n-1$. The within-group sum of squares

$$SSW(Y,\pi) = \sum_{i=1}^{k}\sum_{l=1}^{n_i}(y_l - \bar{y}_i)^2$$

is used as the criterion function for the k mean clustering algorithm *(11)*. It is the most commonly used measure of the clustering quality of the data set Y that partitions with fixed number of clusters. Let SST be the total sum of squares for the measured trait values. It is easy to see that SST for data set Y is: $SST(Y) = SSW(Y,\pi) + SSB(Y,\pi)$, where $SSB(Y,\pi) = \sum_{l=1}^{k} n_i(\bar{y}_i - \bar{y}^2)$ is the between-group sum of squares. Similarly, the total variance var(Y) consists of the genetic variance and the residual variance. The normalized sum of squares

$$\frac{SSW(Y,\pi)}{SST(Y)} = \frac{var(\varepsilon)}{var(Y)}$$

can be interpreted as the proportion of the total variance that is *not* explained by the genotype of the gene in question.

The normalized within-group sum of squares provides an objective measure to compare the genetic effect only for blocks with fixed number of haplotypes. It is not fair to compare the residual variance for different k, because different numbers of parameters (μ_1, μ_2, ..., μ_k) were fit. In order to appropriately compare the normalized within-group sum of squares for different k, it is necessary to use parametric statistics. We apply the analysis of variance (ANOVA) design to analyze genetic effect. In (1), assume that the residual term ε_j is independent and normally distributed with mean zero and constant variance σ^2. For each haplotype block, the F statistics are calculated as:

$$F = \frac{SSB(Y,\pi)/(k-1)}{SSW(Y,\pi)/(n-k)}.$$

The F statistics can then be used to test the null hypothesis

$$H_0 : \mu_1 = \mu_2 = \ldots = \mu_k.$$

For each block, a p value is calculated by comparing F with the theoretical F distribution of degree $k-1$ and $n-k$ (Fig. 1). The correlation between strain groupings within haplotypic blocks and phenotypic trait values is assessed by this calculated p value. Note that the p value calculated from

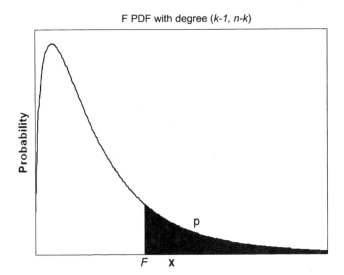

Fig. 1. Graph demonstrating how a p value for a computationally predicted haplotype block is calculated from the F statistic analysis. The calculated p value corresponds to the shaded area under the curve for the F probability density function of degree $(k-1, n-k)$.

F statistic analysis is an approximate p value. It cannot be interpreted as an exact estimate of the probability of a false-positive result. When the distribution of the residual terms ε_j deviates from normality or the sample size is small, the p value is not accurate. Furthermore, it is not corrected for multiple comparisons.

When allelic information is missing, the correct haplotype may not be available for all strains within a haplotypic block. For these blocks, the trait values can be compared with genotype for only reduced set of strains. When key strains are missing, the p values obtained after computational mapping using a reduced set of strains may be much smaller than would be obtained if the allelic data for all the strains were used. This does not indicate that the block is better correlated with the trait data. In order to rank blocks more appropriately, an adjustment factor is applied to the p values obtained using blocks with missing haplotypes. For a block with k haplotypes and some strain haplotype missing, let p_{min} be the minimum p value among all possible partitions of n strains into k haplotypes, and let p'_{min} be the minimum p value among all possible partitions of the subset of the strains into k haplotypes. The multiplicative factor $\min\{p_{min}/p'_{min}, 1\}$ is applied to the p value score. This crudely defined factor ensures that the p value for a block with missing alleles is not better than the best p value if the missing alleles were filled in.

Box 1: Number of Clusters

The problem of comparing the genetic effect of haplotype blocks with different number of haplotypes is related to the classical number-of-cluster problem, namely, what is the optimal number of clusters for a given data set. To date, there is no satisfying statistical theory or single best answer to this question. Milligan and Copper studied the problem by comparing 30 published methods and ranked them based on their performance on simulated data sets *(12)*. The best method for doing this was the Calinski and Harabasz index *(13)*. By this method, the variance ratio criterion (VRC) is calculated according to the following formula: VRC = $[SSB/(k-1)]/[SSW/(n-k)]$. It has exactly the same form as the F statistics used in our analysis. Instead of comparing how the p values correspond to the F statistics, the F statistics with different degrees of freedom are directly compared. Note that even though the VRC has the same form as the F statistics, it is only an empirical measure, not a parametric statistic. It is intended for multidimensional data without assumption on the distribution. The justification of VRC is partly based on its properties. In the special case of equal distance between all pairs of points, VRC = 1 for all cases. Although this property is desirable for general spatial cluster analysis, the quantitative phenotypic trait values are one dimensional. The case of equal distance between pairs of points is not possible. Instead, the p value of the F statistics gives a better measurement of the genetics effect for the null hypothesis. Table 2 shows the critical F statistics corresponding to the different significance level for $n = 16$ and $k = 2$, 3, and 4. The estimated genetic effect, represented by $\eta^2 = SSB - (k - 1) \times MSE/SSW + MSE$ is also shown. For larger values of k, a greater genetic effect is needed to achieve the same level of significance.

The p value calculated from the F statistics measures the extent of correlation between the recorded trait values and haplotype blocks. These uncorrected p values provide a rough estimate of the significance of the association. However, the true statistical significance of an association is difficult to determine for several reasons. First, the true distribution of the residuals (ε_j) is unlikely to be normal. Second, strong linkage disequilibrium exists between blocks in physical proximity. Because of this, there is no easy way to correct for multiple comparisons without being too conservative. Third, it is difficult to quantify the effect of missing data on a result. An appropriate approach to

Table 2
Critical Threshold $F_{k-1, n-k, \alpha}$ and Estimated Genetic Effect
Corresponding to the Critical Threshold as a Function of α for $n = 16$

α	$k = 2$		$k = 3$		$k = 4$	
	F_{crit}	η^2	F_{crit}	η^2	F_{crit}	η^2
0.1	3.10	0.18	2.76	0.30	2.61	0.39
0.01	8.86	0.39	6.70	0.51	5.95	0.60
1e-03	17.14	0.55	12.31	0.65	10.80	0.73
1e-04	28.75	0.67	20.31	0.76	17.90	0.82
1e-05	45.17	0.76	31.66	0.83	28.41	0.88
1e-06	67.06	0.83	48.43	0.88	44.70	0.92

estimate the significance threshold is by using a permutation test *(13,14)*. Assuming from the null hypothesis that there is no association between the trait values and the genotypes of any haplotype blocks in the genome, we can construct a distribution of the *p*-value scores that are generated by randomly shuffling the trait values. Each time, the trait values are rearranged according to a random permutation of 1, 2, ..., *n*. The best *p*-value score among all haplotype blocks in the genome is recorded. After the experiment is repeated *n* times, the recorded scores are ordered, and the $100(1-\alpha)\%$ critical value for the best genome-wide score is obtained by taking the $100(1-\alpha)$ percentile value of the ordered scores. Empirically, 1000 shuffles are needed in order to obtain a stable estimate of critical value for $\alpha = 0.05$. The critical value generated through this permutation test automatically accounts for multiple comparison, linkage disequilibrium and missing-data effect.

3.2. Categorical Trait Analysis

For phenotypic traits that have values in unordered categories, such as mouse coat color or the MHC phenotype *(15)*, the procedures described in Subheading 3.1. can be used to map genetic loci with a few modifications. The categorical data are first transformed into multidimensional data points, such that the distance between distinct categories is equal. The MHC-K phenotype in mice is a categorical phenotype represented by letters b, k, d, u, and v *(15)*. Each categorical phenotype was transformed into vectors (0,0,0,0,1), (0,0,0,1,0), (0,0,1,0,0), (0,1,0,0,0), and (1,0,0,0,0) in five-dimensional space. Using the standard Euclidean metric, the *F* statistics can be calculated. Because the statistics are scale invariant, any such transformation into metric space with equal distance between categories is equivalent. Because these points are in multidimensional space, it does not make sense to calculate the p values corresponding to the F statistics, which is based on the assumption of normal distribution of residuals in one dimension. Instead, the F statistic itself, or what is more appropriately called pseudo F statistics, can be used directly to evaluate the association. In fact, this is the Calinski–Harabasz index used in comparing clusters with different k *(16)* (Box 1).

3.3. Statistical Power for Computational Mapping

Given a set of measurements divided into k groups, ANOVA tests the null hypothesis that the k means from the different groups are equal. The total variance σ_T^2 consists of within-group variance and between-group variance.

$$\sigma_T^2 = \sigma_B^2 + \sigma_W^2.$$

For a power analysis using one-way ANOVA, one standard way to define the effect size is *(17)*:

$$\eta^2 = \frac{\sigma_B^2}{\sigma_T^2} = \frac{\text{SSB}}{\text{SST}}.$$

In our case, the groups are defined by haplotypes, and η^2 is the genetic effect of the haplotypes on the trait value. Let n be the total sample size and k be the number of groups. When the group sizes are equal, the F statistics for samples with effect size η^2 follows the noncentral F distribution $F(k-1, n-k, \lambda)$ with the noncentrality parameter

$$\lambda = \frac{n\sigma_B^2}{\sigma_W^2} = \frac{n\sigma_B^2}{\sigma_T^2 - \sigma_B^2} = \frac{n\eta^2}{1-\eta^2}.$$

Therefore, the power of the one-way ANOVA test with significance level α is given by:

$$\text{Power}(\alpha, \eta^2, n, k) = \text{Prob}(F(k-1, n-k, \lambda) < F_{\text{crit}}) \quad (2)$$

where $F_{\text{crit}} = F_{(1-\alpha, k-1, n-k)}$ is the $(1-\alpha)$ quantile of the F distribution with $k-1$ and $n-k$ degrees of freedom. Note that within a haplotype block, the number of strains with each different haplotype is usually not the same. Therefore, an equal group size cannot be obtained for this analysis. The power for unequal group sizes is expected to be lower. Table 3 shows the power as a function of effect size for $\alpha = 0.01$, $n = 13, 14, 15, 16$, and $k = 2, 3$. When there are two different haplotypes within a locus, 80% power can be achieved using 16 strains when effect size is greater than 0.49 or using 13 strains when the effect size is greater than 0.56.

With this background, we can now analyze the performance of this haplotype-based computational mapping method. It correctly predicted the genetic

Table 3
The Power of the One-Way ANOVA as a Function of the Genetic Effect
Size for Different Total Sample Size (*n*) and Number of Groups (*k*)

η^2	$n = 13$		$n = 14$		$n = 15$		$n = 16$	
	$k = 2$	$k = 3$	$k = 2$	$k = 3$	$k = 2$	$k = 3$	$k = 2$	$k = 3$
0.2	0.15	0.09	0.17	0.10	0.19	0.11	0.21	0.13
0.25	0.21	0.13	0.24	0.15	0.27	0.17	0.30	0.19
0.3	0.29	0.17	0.32	0.20	0.36	0.23	0.40	0.26
0.35	0.37	0.23	0.42	0.27	0.46	0.31	0.51	0.35
0.4	0.47	0.30	0.52	0.35	0.57	0.40	0.62	0.45
0.45	0.58	0.39	0.63	0.45	0.68	0.50	0.73	0.56
0.5	0.68	0.49	0.74	0.56	0.79	0.62	0.83	0.67
0.55	0.79	0.60	0.84	0.67	0.87	0.73	0.90	0.78
0.6	0.88	0.72	0.91	0.78	0.94	0.83	0.96	0.88
0.65	0.94	0.83	0.96	0.88	0.98	0.92	0.99	0.94
0.7	0.98	0.91	0.99	0.95	0.99	0.97	1.00	0.98
0.75	1.00	0.97	1.00	0.99	1.00	0.99	1.00	1.00

basis for strain-specific differences in several biologically important traits
(4). In one published example, haplotypic blocks associated with categorical
MHC phenotypes for the class Ia *K*, class III *S*, and the class Ib *Qa2* loci
were correctly identified. The identified blocks were contained within
regions of 27, 51, and 100 kb, respectively, which contained the actual MHC
genes corresponding to the trait. The MHC phenotypes represent a diverse
class of categorical phenotypes. The 16 strains were grouped into five phenotypic categories for the class Ia *K* and class III *S* traits. There are two categories for the class Ib *Qa2* phenotypes. Most importantly, there were no false
positives among top predictions for these traits. In another example, a binary
response phenotype—measuring the induction of cytochrome P450 enzymes
after treatment with aromatic hydrocarbons (AH) response—using data
obtained from 13 inbred mouse strains was computationally analyzed. The
phenotypic data was analyzed, and two adjacent haplotypic blocks within a
27-kb region, each containing three haplotypes, were computationally identified. The identified region contained the *Ahr* locus, a gene that contributes
to the AH response phenotype. The functional genetic element that contributes to the phenotype was easily identified by analysis of the polymorphisms within the region. In one other example, the pattern of expression of
a differentially expressed gene within the lungs of 10 inbred mouse strains
was computationally analyzed to identify a novel *cis*-acting allele-specific

enhancer element *(4)*. For this analysis, the level of expression of the *H2-Eα* gene in the lungs of 10 inbred strains was measured. A log transformation of this gene expression data was computationally analyzed to identify a 1-kb region within the first intron of the *H2-Eα* gene. This computational prediction led to the discovery of a novel functional element regulating the *H2-Eα* expression. Of note, only 10 strains were used in this computational mapping. When gene expression data from only eight or nine strains were used for the computational analysis, the same region was predicted, and no false-positive predictions were obtained. These examples demonstrate that the computational mapping can be achieved using phenotypic data from a relatively limited number of inbred strains.

To illustrate how haplotype-based computational mapping is performed, we provide a detailed description of how *H2-Eα* gene expression data was analyzed. For this analysis, the level of *H2-Eα* gene expression in female lung was measured three times for each of the 10 inbred strains analyzed (Table 4). An important assumption of haplotype-based analysis is that the residuals are normally distributed and the standard deviation is the same for groups of strains sharing haplotypes. However, the level of expression of this gene was quite different among the strains analyzed, and the standard deviation within each mouse strain was proportional to its level of expression. Therefore, the log transform was used, and the error distribution was closer to normal. The plot of the residual against the strain average (Fig. 2) shows that the assumptions used for the linear model are approximately true for the log-transformed data.

When replicate measurements are available, the data can be evaluated prospectively to determine whether the computational analysis is likely to correctly identify a genetic locus. The genetic influence of a single locus should be larger than the threshold determined by the power analysis. Even though it impossible to estimate the contribution of the primary locus based on the raw data, it is possible to estimate the total genetic effect. This is

Table 4
$H2-Eα$ Gene Expression in Female Lung: Three Independent Measurements Were Obtained for Each Mouse Strain

129/ SvJ	A/J	A/HeJ	AKR/J	B10.D2	Balb/ cJ	C3H/ He	C57BL/ 6J	DBA/ 2J	MRL/ MpJ
8	46	29	56	1078	999	37	10	1017	30
3	34	14	37	1158	1013	30	6	1370	40
6	46	27	40	929	1177	43	8	1642	46

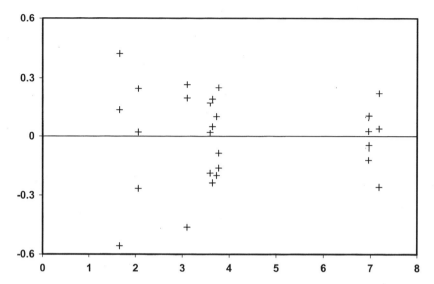

Fig. 2. Plot of residual of ln(expression) from the average level within the strain against the strain average.

accomplished by comparing the within-strain differences with the between-strain difference and check that the total effect exceeds the threshold. In this case, assuming the 10 strains are grouped into $k = 3$ haplotypes, the critical F statistics value with degree of freedom $(k - 1, n - k)$ and significance level $\alpha = 0.01$ is $F_{\text{crit}} = 9.55$. The power of the analysis, which is derived from equation (2), is greater than 80% for effect size $\eta^2 > 75\%$. One-way ANOVA of the log-transformed values asserts that means are different for different strains (Table 5). Because the between-strain differences can be completely attributed to genetic differences, the total genetics effect can be estimated as:

$$\omega^2 = \frac{\text{SSB} - (k-1) \times \text{MSE}}{\text{SST} + \text{MSE}} = \frac{112.40 - 9 \times 0.07}{113.84 + 0.07} = 98\% > 75\%.$$

The fact that gene expression data was available for only 10 strains was compensated by the large genetic effect. Therefore, if most of the total genetic effect comes from a single locus, the computational analysis is likely to detect it.

Using the strain average of the log-transformed gene expression level as the input phenotypic data, the computational analysis generated the results shown in Table 6. One predicted region, located between 32 and 33 Mb on

Table 5
One-Way ANOVA for Comparing the Strain Means of the Log-Transformed Expression Data[a]

Source	DF	Sum of squares	Mean square	F value	$Pr > F$
Model	9	112.3975994	12.4886222	173.57	<.0001
Error	20	1.43899	0.0719495		
Corrected total	29	113.8365894			

[a]DF, degrees of freedom. *See* also Table 3.

Table 6
Computational Genetic Analysis of *H2-Eα* Gene Expression Data[a]

129/ SvJ 1.66	C57BL/ 6J 2.06	A/ HeJ 3.10	C3H/ He 3.59	MRL/ MpJ 3.64	A/J 3.73	AKR/J 3.78	B10.D2 6.96	Balb/ cJ 6.97	DBA/ 2J 7.18

p-value	Genetic effect	Haplotype	Chr	Position (MB)	#SNPs
1.3e-7	0.98		17	32.57~33.26	244
8.4e-7	0.99		17	33.88	4
1.0e-6	0.98		17	32.91	15
1.3e-6	0.98		17	32.81	4
6.4e-5	0.85		17	32.91	4
7.9e-5	0.90		17	32.94	25
2.0e-4	0.98		13	20.72~20.73	10
5.8e-4	0.84		17	32.54~32.78	9

[a]The mean of the log of *H2-Eα* expression in lung was calculated. In the table, each row is a haplotypic block that may be a single single nucleotide polymorphism (SNP) or a composite of multiple SNPs. Each square represents the haplotype of a different mouse strain, and the strains are arranged in the same order as in the data table across the top. Each unique haplotype within a block is represented by a different color square; and strains sharing a haplotype are represented by a square of the same color. A blank square indicates that haplotype data is missing for that strain.

chromosome 17, was most closely associated with the gene expression phenotype. The three haplotypes within this region corresponded to the three different levels of log-transformed gene expression. Some predicted regions appear to overlap with this region. This overlap occurred because this region may consist of multiple blocks each having regions with the same strain distribution pattern that were separated by regions with a different pattern.

4. FUTURE DIRECTIONS

A number of phenotypic traits of biomedical importance can be rapidly characterized using commonly available inbred mouse strains. The genetic basis for these trait differences can then be rapidly analyzed using this haplotype-based computational analysis method. For example, a large amount of gene expression data can be obtained using oligonucleotide microarrays. This enables allele-specific functional genomic elements regulating strain-specific differences in expression for many different genes to be identified. As the number of genes analyzed and the number of strains for which allelic data are available increases, many of the current limitations caused by a lack of strain-specific genetic data will decrease. However, a remaining concern is the relatively limited genetic complexity that can be analyzed by this computational method. As shown in the analysis in Section 3, haplotype-based mapping is most effective when the genetic contribution from a single locus accounts for 50% or more of the total observed trait variance among the inbred strains. For many quantitative traits of biomedical interest, multiple genetic loci, each with a small effect, contribute to the overall trait value. Three factors will significantly increase the ability of this computational method to analyze genetic traits and its ability to correctly identify genetic loci of small effect size. First, increasing the number of inbred strains that have been genetically characterized in our SNP database will improve its ability to identify genetic loci with a small effect. The statistical power of the computational analysis increased as the number of strains analyzed was increased (Table 3). Second, more sophisticated experimental dissection of a phenotypic trait of interest will make complex biological differences more amenable to this type of computational genetic analysis. Although we may not be able to analyze a very complex trait directly, clever experimental design can reduce the complexity of a selected phenotype. As one example, we have been characterizing pharmacokinetic parameters for various drugs after administration to different inbred mouse strains. This computational genetic analysis was used to identify factors affecting the metabolisms of commonly used prescription drugs. The rate of disappearance of the administered drug was measured as a function of time after dosing. Unfortunately, the metabolic profiles were rather complicated for a number of the drugs tested, and we could not identify the factors regulating the metabolism of these drugs. However, we administered a radiolabeled form of one compound and measured the rate of formation of 10 different intermediate metabolites across 13 different inbred mouse strains. Computational analysis of the rate of formation of selected intermediate metabolites enabled identification of a genetic factor regulating the metabolism of this test drug. Therefore, creatively designed experimental protocols can reduce the complexity of a number of traits, and this will widen the application of this computational genetic analysis method. Lastly, our method for haplotype block construction will also be improved. Currently, our method does not allow for any mismatches within the blocks it identifies. Two strains share a haplotype only if they have the same allele at every marker position within the region. This method has worked reasonably well for constructing the current version of our high-resolution haplotypic map for the inbred mouse strains. However, allowing for the inclusion of an occasional allelic mismatch within a larger block structure may improve the quality of the haplotypic map used for computational mapping. This is especially true for model organisms in which point mutations are likely to occur between strains that share a common ancestral chromosomal region.

REFERENCES

1. Doerge RW, Zeng Z-B, Wier BS. Statistical issues in the search for genes affecting quantitative traits in experimental populations. Stat Sci 1997;12:195–219.
2. Darvasi A. Experimental strategies for the genetic dissection of complex traits in animal models. Nat Genet 1998;18:19–24.
3. Darvasi A, Soller MA simple method to calculate resolving power and confidence interval of qtl map location. Behav Genet 1997;27:125–132.
4. Liao G, Wang J, Guo J, et al. In silico genetics: identification of a novel functional element regulating H2-Ea gene expression. Science 2004;306: 690–695.
5. Grupe A, Germer S, Usuka J, et al. In silico mapping of complex disease-related traits in mice [see comments]. Science 2001;292:1915–1918.
6. Wade CM, Kulbokas EJ, Kirby AW, et al. The mosaic structure of variation in the laboratory mouse genome. Nature 2002;420:574–578.
7. Patil N, Berno AJ, Hinds DA, et al. Blocks of limited haplotype diversity revealed by high-resolution scanning of human chromosome 21 [see comments]. Science 2001;294:1719–1723.
8. Johnson GC, Esposito L, Barratt BJ, et al. Haplotype tagging for the identification of common disease genes. Nat Genet 2001;29:233–237.
9. Daly MJ, Rioux JD, Schaffner SF, et al. High-resolution haplotype structure in the human genome. Nat Genet 2001;29:229–232.
10. Zhang K, Deng M, Chen T, et al. A dynamic programming algorithm for haplotype block partitioning. Proc Natl Acad Sci USA 2002;99:7335–7339.
11. Mcqueen JB. Some methods for classification and analysis of multivariate observations. In: Le Cam LM, Neyman J, eds. Proceedings of the fifth Berkeley symposium on mathematical statistics and probability. Berkeley, CA: University Of California Press, 1967:pp. 281–297.

12. Milligan GW, Cooper MC. An examination of procedures for determining the number of clusters in a data set. Psychometrika 1985;50:159–179.
13. Churchill GA, Doerge RW. Empirical threshold values for quantitative trait mapping. Genetics 1994;138:963–971.
14. Fisher RA. The design of experiments. London: Oliver & Boyd Ltd., 1995.
15. Jackson Labs. Mhc haplotypes. Jackson Laboratory Notes. 1998;475.
16. Calinski T, Harabasz J. A dendrite method for cluster analysis. Commun Stat 1974;3:1–27.
17. Cohen J. Statistical power analysis for the behavioral sciences. Hillsdale, NJ: Lawrence Erlbaum Associates, Inc., 1988.

4

Haplotype Structure of the Mouse Genome

Jianmei Wang, Guochun Liao, Janet Cheng,
Anh Nguyen, Jingshu Guo, Christopher Chou,
Steven Hu, Sharon Jiang, John Allard, Steve Shafer,
Anne Puech, John D. McPherson, Dorothee Foernzler,
Gary Peltz, and Jonathan Usuka

1. INTRODUCTION

Commonly available inbred mouse strains can be used to genetically model traits that vary in the human population, including those associated with disease susceptibility. In order to understand how genetic differences regulate trait variation in humans, we must first develop a detailed understanding of how genetic variation in the mouse produces the phenotypic differences among inbred mouse strains. The information obtained from analysis of experimental murine genetic models can direct biological experimentation, clinical research, and human genetic analysis. This "mouse to man" approach will increase our knowledge of the genes and pathways regulating important biological processes and disease susceptibility.

The availability of the complete sequence of the mouse genome *(1)* enables the genetic differences among commonly studied inbred strains to be characterized. This will facilitate identification of the genetic basis for phenotypic trait differences among the inbred strains. To do this, we have analyzed the pattern of genetic variation among 18 inbred mouse strains and have produced a high-resolution haplotypic map of the inbred mouse genome. This haplotypic map covers 75 Mb of the mouse genome. An additional 99 Mb of the mouse genome, which was not polymorphic among the 16 *Mus musculus* strains, was also analyzed. Analysis of the genetic distance between inbred strains and of the haplotypic blocks generated using different strains demonstrated that inclusion of only the 16 *M. musculus* strains

From: *Computational Genetics and Genomics*
Edited by: G. Peltz © Humana Press Inc., Totowa, NJ

produced balanced haplotypic block structures that reflected extensive allele sharing among closely related inbred strains. Although haplotypic blocks in the inbred mouse genome had similarities with those described in humans, there are important differences that increase the likelihood that genetic variants underlying phenotypic trait differences can be successfully identified in the mouse.

2. CHARACTERIZATION OF GENETIC VARIATION AMONG INBRED STRAINS

Polymorphisms were identified by resequencing targeted genomic regions in 1672 genes across 18 inbred mouse strains *(2)*: 129/Sv, A/HeJ, A/J, AKR/J, B10.D2-H2/oSnJ, BALB/cByJ, BALB/cJ, C3H/HeJ, C57BL/6J, CAST/Ei, DBA/2J, LG/J, LP/J, MRL/MpJ, NZB/BinJ, NZW/LaC, and SM/J SPRET/Ei. Identification of single nucleotide polymorphisms (SNPs) was performed by targeted resequencing of genomic regions using methods that have been described previously *(2)*. For genes that were less than 5 kb in size, the entire gene was analyzed for polymorphisms. For genes greater than 5 kb in size, a 1-kb region surrounding each exon, a 2-kb region at 5' of the transcriptional start site, and a 500-bp segment downstream of the 3' end of the transcript were analyzed. Both strands of a selected genomic region were sequenced, and sequence waveforms were analyzed using Phred and Phrap *(3,4)*. Potential polymorphisms were identified, and sequence quality was assessed in an automated fashion. Only SNPs with very high-quality sequence were accepted: those with either single stranded sequence with Phred scores equal to or above 30 or (more commonly) double stranded DNA sequence with Phred scores equal to or above 20 for both strands. The mouse SNP database (*see* http:\\mouseSNP.roche.com) used in this study contained 105,064 unique SNPs, and a total of 1,440,349 alleles were characterized for these 18 strains. The number of SNPs on each chromosome ranged from a low value of 1083 SNPs on chromosome 18 to 16,615 SNPs on chromosome 7 (Table 1).

The genetic distance between the inbred mouse strains was assessed using this allelic information. To measure this, the percent allelic difference was calculated as the ratio of the number of SNPs identified using only a selected pair of strains to the total number of SNPs identified among all 18 inbred strains. The CAST/Ei and SPRET/Ei strains were derived from wild mice of Asian and European origin, respectively. The 16 other *M. musculus* strains were bred from a small group of mice at the beginning of the last century (reviewed in ref. 5). Consistent with their independent origin, the CAST/Ei and SPRET/Ei strains have more than 39 and 70%, respectively,

Table 1
The Number of Genes Analyzed and SNPs Identified on Each Chromosome

Chromosome	SNP number	Gene number
1	9171	125 (1504)
2	7495	105 (2058)
3	3666	90 (1237)
4	3671	72 (1499)
5	9078	82 (1478)
6	6160	66 (1282)
7	16,615	193 (2003)
8	5602	81 (1189)
9	5057	111 (1394)
10	3719	98 (1205)
11	5343	103 (1877)
12	2376	44 (852)
13	2084	62 (1012)
14	3363	60 (898)
15	3084	63 (953)
16	4250	50 (811)
17	5520	123 (1157)
18	1083	37 (628)
19	4066	49 (795)
X	3661	58 (1116)
Total	105,064	1672 (24,948)

The numbers within parenthesis indicate the total number of genes on each chromosome. SNP, single nucleotide polymorphism.

allelic differences when compared with any one of the 16 other *M. musculus* strains (Table 2). In contrast, the 16 other *M. musculus* strains were far more genetically similar. The allelic differences among *M. musculus* strain pairs ranged from 0.8% (A/HeJ:A/J) to 16.4% (NZW/LaC:Balb/cJ) (Table 2). The genetic distance revealed by SNP allelic information is consistent with published genealogies of mouse inbred strains *(5)*.

3. THE STRUCTURE OF HAPLOTYPIC BLOCKS IN THE MURINE GENOME

In order to analyze genetic variation among inbred murine strains, we developed a novel method (*see* Chapter 3) to define the high-resolution haplotypic block structure of the inbred mouse genome. Relative to the

Table 2
Allelic Differences Between Inbred Strain Pairs

	A/He	A/J	AKR	B10	C57	B/B	B/c	C3H	MRL	LGJ	SMJ	129	LPJ	DBA	NZB	NZW	CAS	SPR
A/He		0.8	8.9	11.7	13.2	7.5	8.3	8.6	9.7	8.7	10.9	13.1	12.4	12.4	14.7	14.9	40.2	72.2
A/J	0.8		8.7	11.7	13.5	7.5	8.2	8.6	10.1	8.8	11.6	12.6	12.4	12.4	15	14.5	44.2	72.3
AKR	8.9	8.7		12.1	13.5	9.5	9.9	9.1	7.1	8.5	10	12.6	12.7	12.3	15	15.1	42.8	71.3
B10.D2	11.7	11.7	12.1		2.7	9.6	9.7	12.5	10	8.7	14.1	13.2	13.6	13.9	13.1	15.3	42	72.2
C57B6	13.2	13.5	13.5	2.7		11.6	11.3	12.5	10.6	9.4	13.5	13.5	14	15.9	12.7	15.8	43.2	72.5
BALB/B	7.5	7.5	9.5	9.6	11.6		1.5	10.1	7.5	7.6	13.1	12.6	11.3	12.5	13.3	15.1	42.3	72.5
BALB/c	8.3	8.2	9.9	9.7	11.3	1.5		9.4	7.1	6.8	11.8	13.4	11.9	12.8	13.1	16.4	43.3	72.5
C3H	8.6	8.6	9.1	12.5	12.5	10.1	9.4		8.3	9	10.1	12.9	13.2	12	13.5	15.6	44.6	72.1
MRL	9.7	10.1	7.1	10	10.6	7.5	7.1	8.3		3.8	10.7	12.9	13.5	13.1	12.4	14.6	42.8	72.3
LGJ	8.7	8.8	8.5	8.7	9.4	7.6	6.8	9	3.8		10.1	12.8	13	12.5	10.7	14.4	41.8	71.9
SMJ	10.9	11.6	10	14.1	13.5	13.1	11.8	10.1	10.7	10.1		15.1	14.9	14.2	12.7	16.1	40.3	71.6
129/Sv	13.1	12.6	12.6	13.2	13.5	12.6	13.4	12.9	12.9	12.8	15.1		4.9	13.5	13	13.1	43.8	71.6
LPJ	12.4	12.4	12.7	13.6	14	11.3	11.9	13.2	13.5	13	14.9	4.9		14.7	12.9	13.7	39.1	72.2
DBA/2	12.4	12.4	12.3	13.9	15.9	12.5	12.8	12	13.1	12.5	14.2	13.5	14.7		16.1	13.9	42.5	71.8
NZB	14.7	15	15	13.1	12.7	13.3	13.1	13.5	12.4	10.7	12.7	13	12.9	16.1		11.2	40.6	72.2
NZW	14.9	14.5	15.1	15.3	15.8	15.1	16.4	15.6	14.6	14.4	16.1	13.1	13.7	13.9	11.2		39.4	72.5
CAST	40.2	44.2	42.8	42	43.2	42.3	43.3	44.6	42.8	41.8	40.3	43.8	39.1	42.5	40.6	39.4		70.1
SPRET	72.2	72.3	71.3	72.2	72.5	72.5	72.5	72.1	72.3	71.9	71.6	71.6	72.2	71.8	72.2	72.5	70.1	

The 18 strains used in this analysis are listed across the rows and columns. Within each cell is the percentage of single neucleotide polymorphisms (SNPs) for which each corresponding strain-pair has different alleles. The percentage of different alleles was calculated using all 105,064 SNPs for which allelic data was available for both strains being compared. *See* beginning of Section 2 for full names of the mouse strains.

algorithms used for generating human haplotypic blocks *(6,7)*, our algorithm generated haplotypic blocks with stronger lethal dose. We present the haplotypic block structure constructed using 16 inbred strains, the most extensive high-resolution haplotype analysis to date. The detailed view of the haplotypic block structure can be found at http://mousesnp.roche.com. Note that the haplotypic block map is not yet constructed for the whole genome. Currently, it covers 75 Mb of the genomic region, containing selected genes of interest. The coverage is increasing steadily as more genes are sequenced.

The type of strains used to generate the haplotypic blocks had a very significant effect on their structure. Analysis of the genetic variation present in only four strains (129/SvJ, A/J, C57BL/6J, and CAST/Ei), identical to those used by Wade et al. *(9)*, generated a skewed haplotypic block structure (Fig. 1A). In this case, the minor allele haplotype consisted of only the single CAST/Ei strain, the most distant lineage from the other three strains, in 33% of the haplotypic blocks. Our genetic distance estimates (Table 2) indicated that the CAST/Ei and SPRET/Ei strains were significantly different from the other 16 *M. musculus* strains. When genetic variation unique to the CAST/Ei and SPRET/Ei strains was included in the haplotypic map, the natural block structure was disrupted by the SNPs introduced by inclusion of CAST/Ei and SPRET/Ei, the haplotypic blocks were shortened, and the extent of allele sharing among the *M. musculus* strains could not be delineated. As one example, comparison of the haplotypic map for chromosome 7 generated using 16 *M. musculus* strains to that produced after replacing 2 of the 16 *M. musculus* strains (129/Sv and A/HeJ) with the CAST/Ei and SPRET/Ei strains revealed the important differences (Fig. 1C). Although inclusion of SPRET/Ei and CAST/Ei strains increased the number of SNPs analyzed from 21,255 to 62,939, CAST/Ei (SPRET/Ei) strain had a unique haplotype in 27% (45%) of the blocks generated. In contrast, each of the 16 *M. musculus* strains had unique haplotype in only 1.1–7.6% of the blocks.

Because of this, the haplotypic analysis was confined to the 16 *M. musculus* strains, and SNPs that were uniquely found in the CAST/Ei and SPRET/Ei strains were excluded. Even then, the number of strains included in the analysis significantly affected the results. As the number of strains analyzed increased from 4 to 16, the general structure of the haplotypic blocks stabilized (Table 3). Any effect caused by potential bias in the selection of inbred strains was diminished by inclusion of this large number of strains. The number of unique haplotypes within a block increased by only 0.03 for each additional strain (Fig. 2). This indicates that each additional strain had a pattern of polymorphism that fit within an existing haplotype for most of the blocks. When only a few strains were used in haplotypic map construction, less

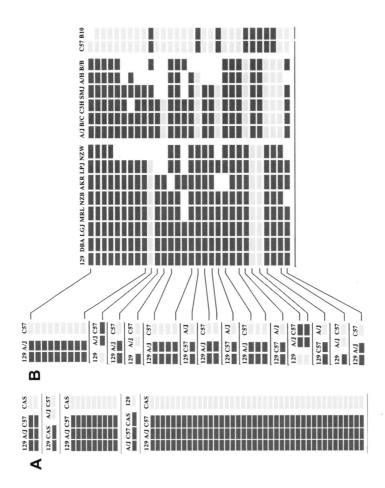

Fig. 1. The inbred strains analyzed affect haplotypic block structure. Each row represents a single nucleotide polymorphism (SNP); the alleles are colored blue or yellow, or left blank when data is missing. Within each block, the strains are ordered such that strains sharing the same haplotype are next to each other. Strains with ambiguous haplotypes because of missing data are colored gray. (**A**) A representative haplotypic block on chromosome 7 (22.7 Mb) constructed using *A/J*, *129*, *C57BL/6* and *CAST/Ei* strains. (**B**) Comparison of haplotypic blocks constructed on chromosome 12 (29.6 Mb) using 3 (*A/J*, *129* and *C57BL/6*) or 16 *Mus musculus* strains. SNPs present at the boundary of blocks are joined by lines. Identical regions are indicated by dots. The map on the left has fewer SNPs than the map on the right because fewer strains (3 vs 16) were used in its construction.

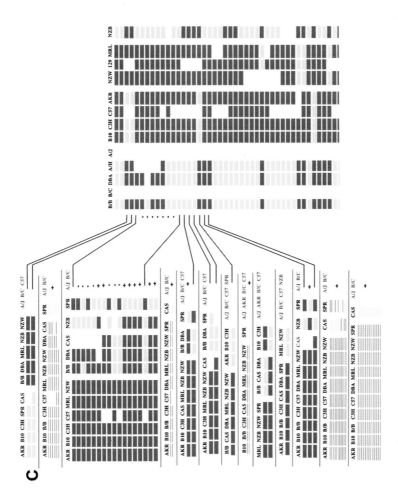

Fig. 1. (*Continued*) (C) Comparison of haplotypic blocks on chromosome 7 (22.1 Mb) generated using 13 *M. musculus* strains, or when two strains are replaced by *CAST/Ei* and *SPRET/Ei* strains "+" signs on the left panel indicate new SNPs introduced by inclusion of the strains *CAST/Ei* and *SPRET/Ei*.

Table 3
Analysis of the Properties of Haplotypic Blocks Constructed Using
Allelic Information for 16 *Mus musculus* Strains

# Strains	Minimum strain #	Total # of SNPs	# Blocks	Average # SNPs per block[a]	Haplotypes per block[a]	% SNPs in block[a]
16	9	21,255	2796	16.42	2.62	88
15	9	20,156	2489	17.71	2.59	88
14	9	18,251	2152	18.42	2.56	89
13	9	15,879	1746	20.21	2.50	90
12	8	16,262	1790	20.31	2.49	90
11	8	14,781	1594	20.86	2.49	90
10	7	16,245	2036	19.67	2.45	88
9	6	14,871	1860	20.16	2.42	88
8	6	12,644	1696	18.97	2.37	87
7	5	12,410	1662	20.11	2.33	87
6	4	13,090	1810	19.99	2.29	86
5	4	10,577	1804	17.77	2.16	82
4	3	9,440	1590	19.48	2	82

[a]Only blocks of 4 SNPs or more are included in the calculation. SNPs, single nucleotide polymorphisms.

genetic diversity was present, and the true structure of the haplotypic blocks could not be identified. An extreme case, in which the haplotypic block structure generated using only three strains was compared with that from 16 strains, is illustrated in Fig. 1B.

To construct haplotype blocks that reflect the extensive allele sharing found among closely related inbred strains, SNPs in which the minor allele was unique to the CAST/Ei or SPRET/Ei strains were excluded. The resulting haplotypic blocks were based on analysis of genetic variation among the 16 *M. musculus* strains. Furthermore, only biallelic SNPs for which allelic information was available for at least nine strains were used. Out of the 35,458 SNPs identified among the 16 strains evaluated, 7385 SNPs involving a nucleotide deletion were removed (because they could result from a sequence misalignment). Also, 6651 other SNPs were removed because allelic information for less than nine strains was available, and 167 other SNPs were removed because they were not biallelic. The remaining 21,255 SNPs formed 2796 haplotypic blocks. Of these, 1133 haplotypic blocks had four or more SNPs, and 88% of all SNPs analyzed were contained within blocks. Haplotypic blocks with at least four SNPs had an average of 16 SNPs per block and 2.6

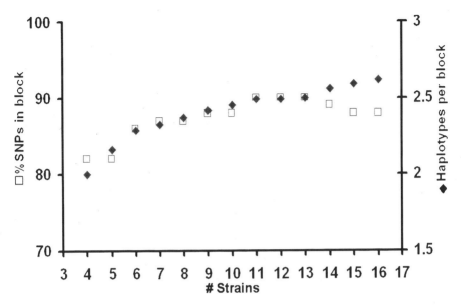

Fig. 2. The number of inbred strains analyzed effects the haplotypic block structure. The percentage of single nucleotide polymorphisms (SNPs) included within a block, and the number of haplotypes within a block is shown as a function of the number of strains analyzed. Only blocks with four SNPs or more are counted. As the number of strains analyzed is increased, the percent of SNPs included within a block stabilizes around 88~90%. The number of haplotypes within a block increased by 0.03 haplotypes per strain added.

haplotypes per block and covered 47 Mb of the mouse genome. Haplotypic blocks with two SNPs or more covered more than 75 Mb of genomic sequence (Table 4). There was a large variation in block size ranging from 2 bases to 2 Mb. The average block length was 39 kb with a standard deviation of 155 kb. Most blocks contained SNPs located within a single gene, but some blocks contained multiple genes. For example, a block located on chromosome 7 (33.18–33.21 Mb) contains the *Pold1*, *Nr1h2*, and *Kdap* genes. More often, an individual gene was separated into several different blocks. As an extreme example, the 50-kb *Capn2* gene contains 33 distinct blocks. The haplotypic maps for each of the 20 chromosomes constructed using these 16 *M. musculus* strains are available at http:\\mouseSNP.roche.com.

To evaluate the extent of linkage disequilibrium within the haplotypic blocks, we applied our algorithm to a randomly reordered SNP map on chromosome 1. The 2272 SNPs on chromosome 1 were used for construction of the randomized haplotypic block structure. A random order for the 2272 SNPs was generated by randomly drawing integers from the set (1, 2, …, 2272) one

Table 4
Strain Analysis Effects on Haplotypic Block Properties

SNPs per block	# Blocks	kb per block	Haplotypes per block	% SNPs	Total block size (Mb)
>10	498	48	2.72	69	23.9
4–10	635	36	2.53	18	23.0
2–3	790	36	2.55	8	28.6
1	873	N/A	2	4	N/A
Total	2796	39.3	2.40	100	75.5

The number of strains analyzed affects haplotypic block properties. As the number of strains analyzed is increased, the number of single nucleotide polymorphisms included within a block and the number of haplotypic blocks increases; the number of haplotypes within a block does not significantly increase. On average, the number of different haplotypes within a block increased by only 0.03 per strain added.

at a time until all numbers were drawn. The structure of the randomized blocks was generated by rearranging the SNP allele information in random order, whereas retaining the original chromosome location. Neighboring SNPs in a block were within 1 Mb apart. This randomization process was repeated 10 times. The properties of the resulting blocks were evaluated after each iteration. Among the 10 haplotypic maps generated with the SNPs in random order, the percent of SNPs in blocks containing a minimum of four SNPs (23% ± 3%) and the average number of SNPs per block (5.7 ± 0.4) were markedly decreased relative to that in haplotypic blocks generated using properly ordered SNPs. In addition, the average number of haplotypes per block (3.8 ± 0.2) was also significantly increased. The strong contrast between the properties of haplotypic blocks generated using sequential and randomly ordered SNPs shows the extent of the linkage disequilibrium for SNPs within the same linkage group. This high level of linkage disequilibrium is a result of relatively simple genealogy of the commonly used laboratory mouse strains.

4. DISCUSSION

There are several methods for defining a haplotypic block, and the ideal method depends on the anticipated application. For analyses of human genetic variation, haplotype blocks have been generated with the goal of minimizing the total number of SNPs required to characterize a significant percentage of the haplotypic diversity present within each block *(7)*. This haplotypic block structure produced by these methods is useful for human genetic studies, in which association studies require genotyping of a large number of individuals. However, this approach does not produce an optimal block structure for experimental murine genetics, which always involves characterization of a much smaller number of inbred strains. Haplotype-based association studies in mice can generate much more precise results when blocks that are smaller in size, and which have a less diverse haplotypic composition, are examined.

Haplotype blocks in the genome of inbred mouse strains were also constructed by three other groups *(8–10)*. In one analysis, three pair-wise comparisons of genomic sequence data from four inbred strains (129, C3H, Balb/c, and C57/BL6) identified long segments with extremely high or extremely low polymorphism rates *(9)*. In another analysis, 3900 SNPs were obtained from analysis of small genomic regions (<500 bp) within 2630 evenly spaced loci in six inbred strains *(8)*. Genome-wide haplotype block patterns were then constructed by pair-wise comparison of marker alleles among the six inbred strains. Yalcin et al. analyzed the frequency of polymorphisms within a 4.8-Mb region among eight inbred strains *(10)*. They reported that sparse sampling of genomic sequence within a region may falsely identify regions with a low frequency of polymorphism (SNP deserts). They also found that the haplotype block structures produced by their method were not robust. However, the lack of robustness in the blocks they produced resulted from two factors. Their algorithm allowed for only two haplotypes within each block, and all regions analyzed were organized into haplotype blocks. Compared to these previous studies, our current analysis is based on a much larger set of SNPs and alleles that were obtained from a larger set of strains, and a different method for haplotype construction was used. In contrast to the pair-wise comparisons used in some of the previous studies, our haplotypic block structure was produced by simultaneous comparison of allelic data obtained from all strains. For the genes that we analyzed, 10 kb per gene on average was resequenced across each of the 16 strains. To allow for the possibility of multiallelic local sequence variation, our haplotypic block construction algorithm allowed for more than two haplotypes within a block. This produced a haplotype block map with much higher resolution and a more stable structure that could be used for association studies.

The inbred *M. musculus* strains are much more closely genetically related than are individuals in a human population. The mouse strains were bred from a small group of "fancy" mice at the beginning of the last century (reviewed in refs. *5* and *11*). Consistent with their origin, the haplotype block structure of the inbred mouse strains is far more ordered relative to that of humans. The structure of the murine haplotypic blocks can be compared with those described on human chromosome 21 *(6)*. On one level, they appear to have similar properties. The percentage of murine and human SNPs contained within identified blocks and the average numbers of SNPs per haplotypic block were very similar. However, there are very significant differences between the haplotypic blocks of human and inbred mouse. Human haplotypic blocks have significantly more haplotypes per block (3.5) than the inbred mouse strains (2.6). In addition, the murine and human haplotypic blocks were constructed under very different conditions. Human haplotypic blocks were produced by counting only those haplotypes that were relatively common in the population and by including only SNPs whose minor allele frequency was above 0.1. In contrast, all SNPs and all haplotypes were used for construction of inbred mouse haplotypic blocks. If the conditions used for inbred mouse were applied to human, at least one, and possibly several, additional haplotype(s) would be added to each human block, and the average size of a human block would decrease. If the same minimum cutoff of four SNPs per block that was used in mouse haplotypic block generation was applied to human haplotypic block generation, the average number of haplotypes within a human haplotypic block would be further increased. The inbred mouse haplotypic block structure was generated by analyzing 16 individual strains, whereas 20 different human chromosomes were evaluated to generate the human haplotypic blocks. Therefore, this comparison of haplotypic block structure of mouse and human is still valid, especially because there was a very small increase in the number of haplotypes per block as the number of different murine strains evaluated increased (Table 3, Fig. 2).

Relative to human genetic analysis, there are two significant advantages that make it likely that many of the basic principles underlying the genetic basis for phenotypic trait variation will be understood by genetic analysis of inbred mouse strains. There is far less ambiguity in the haplotypic map of the mouse genome, and higher quality phenotypic data can be easily obtained using inbred strains of mice. First, inbred mice are homozygous at all loci, making it relatively easy to generate haplotypic information that has almost 100% accuracy. In humans, pedigree analysis or statistical methods, such as maximum likelihood or Bayesian analyses, must be used to infer the haplotypes. Second, the higher level of linkage disequilibrium among inbred mice results in clean and stable haplotypic block structure. The lack of ambiguity in the haplotypic map increases its potential utility. Phenotypic data can be more easily obtained under controlled experimental conditions from mice than could possibly be obtained from humans. The homozygosity of the inbred mouse strains eliminates the confounding effect of allelic interactions at the same locus, and the lower genetic diversity of the inbred strains reduces the number of genetic factors underlying the phenotypic differences. As shown here, haplotype-based association studies can be performed using phenotypic data obtained from inbred mouse strains. This high-resolution map of the haplotypic block structure of the mouse genome will facilitate identification of genetic loci underlying genetic traits. The power of this map will be further enhanced as additional inbred strains are included and as it covers a larger fraction of the mouse genome. Also, this map will enable the development of a new haplotype-based computational method for genetic analysis of phenotypic traits varying among inbred mouse strains.

ACKNOWLEDGMENTS

Janet Cheng, Anh Nguyen, and Jianmei Wang were partially supported by an National Human Genome Research Institute grant (1 R01 HG02322-01) awarded to Gary Peltz. We also want to thank Michael Ott of the Roche Center for Medical Genomics for his help.

REFERENCES

1. Waterston RH, Lindblad-Toh K, Birney E, et al. Initial sequencing and comparative analysis of the mouse genome [Review]. Nature 2002;420:520–562.
2. Grupe A, Germer S, Usuka J, et al. In silico mapping of complex disease-related traits in mice [see comments]. Science 2001;292:1915–1918.
3. Ewing B, Green P. Base-calling of automated sequencer traces using phred. II. Error probabilities. Genome Res 1998;8:186–194.
4. Ewing B, Hillier L, Wendl MC, et al. Base-calling of automated sequencer traces using phred. I. Accuracy assessment. Genome Res 1998;8:175–185.
5. Beck JA, Lloyd S, Hafezparast M, et al. Genealogies of mouse inbred strains. Nat Genet 2000;24:23–25.
6. Patil N, Berno AJ, Hinds DA, et al. Blocks of limited haplotype diversity revealed by high-resolution scanning of human chromosome 21 [see comments]. Science 2001;294:1719–1723.
7. Zhang K, Deng M, Chen T, et al. A dynamic programming algorithm for haplotype block partitioning. Proc Natl Acad Sci USA 2002;99:7335–7339.
8. Wiltshire T, Pletcher MT, Batalov S, et al. Genome-wide single-nucleotide polymorphism analysis defines haplotype patterns in mouse. Proc Natl Acad Sci USA 2003;100:3380–3385.
9. Wade CM, Kulbokas EJ, Kirby AW, et al. The mosaic structure of variation in the laboratory mouse genome. Nature 2002;420:574–578.
10. Yalcin B, Fullerton J, Miller S, et al. Unexpected complexity in the haplotypes of commonly used inbred strains of laboratory mice. Proc Natl Acad Sci USA 2004;101:9734–9739.
11. Silver LM. Mouse genetics. New York: Oxford University Press, 1995;3–14.

5

SNP Discovery and Genotyping

Methods and Applications

Jun Wang, Dee Aud, Soren Germer, and Russell Higuchi

1. INTRODUCTION

The identification of genes affecting complex traits (i.e., biological traits affected by several genetic and environmental factors) is a very difficult and challenging task *(1–3)*. For many complex traits, the observable variation between individuals is quantitative; hence, loci affecting such traits are generally termed quantitative trait loci *(*QTLs*)*. In contrast with monogenic traits, it is impossible to identify all the genomic regions responsible for complex trait variation without additional information on how these regions segregate *(1,4)*. A key development in complex trait analysis was the establishment of large collections of molecular/genetic markers. With the discovery of a large amount of single nucleotide polymorphisms (SNPs) in human and model organisms, correlating SNP markers with phenotype in a segregating population has become a useful tool in QTL studies *(5)*. In both linkage and association mapping, the development of high-throughput methods to discover and genotype polymorphism markers has enabled whole-genome scanning to detect individual loci possible *(2)*.

2. SNP DISCOVERY

SNPs are single base differences observed when sequences from different genomes are compared. Among human genomes these changes occur at the frequency of about 1 in every 1000 bases *(6)*. This high density of SNP markers facilitated the fine mapping of genes and prompted large-scale efforts to identify and map new SNPs (for review *see* refs. *7* and *8*).

From: *Computational Genetics and Genomics*
Edited by: G. Peltz © Humana Press Inc., Totowa, NJ

The discovery of new polymorphisms has been most rapid in the human and mouse genomes. Although it is often still useful to perform *de novo* SNP discovery, the constantly growing number of validated human SNPs deposited in public databases makes a search of these databases an important first step in any study of human SNPs.

Most human SNPs are deposited in a database ("dbSNP") that is maintained and curated by the National Center for Biotechnology Information (NCBI). In its most recent build (build 110, January 2003), dbSNP contained more than three million human SNPs. This database can be queried in a variety of ways using the excellent NCBI search interfaces. Although most of the dbSNP polymorphisms derive from computational analysis of aligned sequence traces, more than half a million of the SNPs have additionally been validated experimentally. Many of the SNPs in dbSNP were identified by the SNP Consortium, which itself maintains an excellent website with a search interface.

For alternative search tools (and to some extent informational content), the Human Genome Variation Database can be used as it contains most of the SNPs available through dbSNP. A number of more specific public databases contain information and SNPs related to specific projects, and though most of them also deposit their data in dbSNP, their own search interfaces can sometimes be useful tools. These include the Human Gene Mutation Database, which lists phenotypically related polymorphisms; the Japanese SNP database, which contains SNPs mapped in Japanese populations; the Cancer Genome Anatomy Project database; the National Institute of Environmental Health Sciences (GenesSNPs); and several others. In addition, some companies (e.g., Sequenom, San Diego, CA; ABI, Foster City, CA) maintain proprietary databases with comprehensive SNP information related to the SNP genotyping technologies they sell. A database of mouse SNPs, the Mouse SNP Database at http://mouseSNP.roche.com/, is described in Heading 4.

Because of the variable quality of high-throughput sequence reads, unvalidated SNPs from purely *in silico* searches are frequently false. Although an increasing number of SNPs are being validated, the density of validated SNPs within a particular gene of interest is likely to be too low to enable thorough association studies to be performed. Also, SNPs in the particular disease group or ethnic group (or in our case, model organism) under investigation are likely to be underrepresented or missing. For these and other reasons, SNP discovery for particular research needs will remain an active area.

Our own SNP discovery efforts, predominantly in inbred mouse strains, have been polymerase chain reaction (PCR)-based (as opposed to the recombinant deoxyribonucleic acid [DNA] methods used to generate most whole-genome sequences). A nearly complete mouse genome sequence allowed the facile design of PCR primers resulting in SNP discovery that was evenly distributed along chromosomes. PCR amplicons can be assessed for SNPs in a number of different ways, including denaturing high-performance liquid chromatography (*see* ref. *9*), single-stranded conformational polymorphism analysis (*see* ref. *10*), and denaturation gradient gel electrophoresis (*see* ref. *11*). All these methods detect heteroduplexes generated during the PCR reaction by the presence of an SNP in the heterozygous state. These methods maximize sequencing efficiency by targeting DNA sequences containing one or more polymorphism. However, DNA sequencing itself, because of the development of reusable and high-speed capillary gels and the automation of sample loading, has become rapid enough that it is now usually possible to proceed directly to DNA sequencing.

Although it may seem obvious, it is worthwhile to note that when PCR primers are designed to amplify a known gene, the resulting polymorphisms identified will have all the information available for that gene, such as chromosomal position, gene name, gene function, and any annotation that is available for that gene. Also, the position of the polymorphism within the gene itself will be available as well as information, such as coding vs non-coding sequence, or promoter sequence vs 3′ untranslated region (UTR). In some cases, a readily identified functional mutation may be discovered, such as the introduction of a premature stop codon into the resulting messenger ribonucleic acid (mRNA).

Historically, the sequencing of complementary DNA (cDNA) libraries had the advantage of focusing on expressed sequences. The discovered SNPs were located in the coding sequence or in the 3′ UTR. This area often contains important regulatory elements for each gene *(12,13)*. As whole-genome sequences became available, PCR-directed sequencing became more useful than cDNA libraries, requiring less work and allowing for detection of polymorphisms in genes that are expressed at levels too low for representation in the libraries.

Recently, we used the PCR-based approach to assemble a murine SNP database that includes annotation and mapping information for all the polymorphisms contained in the database *(14)*. Currently, the database contains more than 70,000 SNPs among 21 commonly used inbred mouse strains. The sequencing is performed using an ABI-3700 capillary sequencer with an autoloading attachment. Currently, two operators can sequence about 5000 PCR amplicons, each with 500 bp, in a week, and about half the sequenced amplicons contain SNPs. PCR primers are designed automatically by computer from batch-loaded, genome sequence files; the sequences are automatically entered into an electronic file for ordering oligonucleotides which are delivered as pairs in 96-well plates. Each PCR amplicon is sequenced with the same primers used for PCR amplification. A Qiagen Robot 3000 is used for primer dilution, PCR reaction setup, amplicon clean-up (using Qiaqick PCR Purification kits), and sequence template preparation. The amplicons are analyzed by gel electrophoresis to assess primer specificity. The major costs for this project have been the capital investment in the sequencer and robot and the ongoing expense of primers, thermostable polymerase, and plastic disposables. Although perhaps more expensive than most small labs could afford on their own, this approach is well within the means of most "core" sequencing facilities that are now present at many academic and industrial institutions. For human SNPs discovery, sequencing of 5000 amplicons per week from 50 individuals would identify about 50 new SNPs per week.

3. GENOTYPING

In an influential article, Risch and Merikangas *(15)* argued that association studies based on linkage disequilibrium, such as case-control studies, had greater statistical power to detect genetic variants associated with common, complex disorders than did linkage or positional cloning approaches *(1,5,15,16)*. However, even using the most optimistic estimates of average linkage disequilibrium, genotyping of 100,000 or more SNPs would be needed to cover the whole genome in order to detect the relatively weak associations between genetic variants and disease; at least 1000 samples would need to be genotyped *(5,17,18)*. Thus, a whole-genome scan would require on the order of 100 million genotypes. There are a few very large-scale genotyping facilities with the potential throughput to complete such a study within a reasonable time. Yet, for most groups such genome-wide scans remain unaffordable. Recently, an international research consortium was established to identify the most common haplotypes across the whole genome with the intent to reduce the number of SNPs needed to capture the genetic diversity in many genomic regions *(17,19–22)*.

Until now, mostly candidate genes and candidate chromosomal regions identified in whole-genome linkage scans have been tested in association studies. Most often, investigators have chosen SNPs in candidate genes *(23–26)* that are known or thought to have functional consequences *(27)* (i.e., affect transcription, splicing, or coding of a gene). To more efficiently identify new candidate genes involved in disease, we and others have used model organisms, such as mouse, in which facile breeding experiments and functional tests can be done, including transgenic and gene-knockout experiments and high-throughput expression analysis.

Rather than typing a large number of SNPs one sample at a time, our strategy has been to first construct pools for cases and controls of equal amounts of DNA from each individual. The allele frequencies for each SNP are then measured for each pool using an allele-specific, quantitative PCR method (described under Heading 4). The initial screening of a very large number of SNPs can then be followed up by genotyping for each individual a much smaller subset of SNPs that show the largest estimated allele frequency differences. The pooling approach was first suggested many years ago *(28)* and has been successfully employed with restriction fragment length polymorphisms (RFLPs) and microsatellites *(29–31)*. Pooling for SNP mapping has gained popularity and sparked a large number of publications in the last few years *(32–44)*. The first studies reporting significant associations using pooling for SNP allele frequency determination have appeared *(14,45–47)*.

Most of the common methods used for genotyping have recently been reviewed *(8,48,49)*. An ideal genotyping system would (a) be able to perform with high-throughput capacity; (b) generate genotypes at a low cost; and (c) provide robust and reliable data. In actual practice, trade-offs must be made, depending mainly on the number of samples and the number of SNPs that need to be genotyped. Some older methods (e.g., RFLP) are suitable for genotyping relatively few samples, are simple to use, and do not require extensive instrument or reagent investments. However, for larger studies or applications involving hundreds to thousands of samples and SNPs, these methods are too slow and labor intensive. Some of the newer methods (e.g., hybridization to microarrays) are particularly well suited for typing large numbers of different SNPs. However, the high cost of such microarrays can make analyzing a large number of samples prohibitively expensive. Other methods (e.g., TaqMan) are more cost-effective for genotyping a large number of samples but are less useful for genotyping large numbers of SNPs, because of the expense of generating new assays.

Although costs as low as $0.01 per genotype have been reported, this does not always take into account all the costs associated with a genotyping project. For example, the up-front instrument investments, the cost of all consumables, the informatic costs associated with processing large amounts of genotyping data, the labor costs or robotic system requirements, or the costs associated with developing new genotyping assays are often not factored into these low estimates. Note also that expensive reagents (e.g., probes and primers) may not be completely consumed in real life situations and then cannot be amortized over an ideal number of genotypes.

Though methods of genotyping vary, most of them have enzymatic amplification of DNA as a step in the process, and for this almost all use PCR. In our research, we determine the genotypes and allele frequencies in the PCR amplification itself (a "homogenous" PCR), thus eliminating the need for post-PCR manipulation and processing *(33,50)*. The minimal processing also reduces the potential for sample cross-contamination. Our homogeneous detection system uses an SYBR green dye in the PCR reactions: the dye binds double-stranded DNA, and the fluorescence increases as the PCR product increases; the increase in fluorescence can be monitored with a number of commercially available, fluorescence-reading thermocyclers. Including a fluorescent DNA binding dye in the reaction eliminates the need for expensive labeled primer or probe systems.

The PCR reaction becomes allele-specific when primers are designed that bind at the 3′ end to the SNP. For SNP with two alleles, three primers are required for genotyping, one for each allele and a common primer. The common primer plus the primer specific for each allele will amplify in the presence of that allele. Theoretically, only the correct primer–allele combination will produce a PCR product, but in actual practice, there is always some nonspecific amplification *(51)*. To increase specificity we used a "hot-start," "Gold" version of the Stoffel fragment of *Taq* DNA polymerase *(52–54)* and recently derived a new variant, CEA2, which also increased efficiency (Elfstrom C and Higuchi R, unpublished data). We have developed hundreds of genotyping assays for both murine and human SNPs using a single set of amplification conditions, without the need to optimize each reaction *(14)*. Using only standard primers at low synthesis scale without purification allows us to develop high-throughput, low-cost genotyping assays.

The genotyping method we developed accelerates the genotyping process because it works on pooled samples. To generate the pools, equal aliquots of DNA from each sample in the group are added to the pool. The pool is split into two genotyping reactions, one for each allele-specific primer combination. The allele that is in the majority will amplify earlier (lower Ct value) than the allele that is in the minority for that pool of samples (higher Ct value for a later amplification). The difference between the Ct values between the two reactions for that pool is proportional to the difference in frequency between the two alleles in the pool (*see* refs. *33, 55,* and *57* for further details).

The SNP-based pooled DNA sample method of genotyping SNPs has been used with great success for both human and murine samples in genome-wide scans (mouse) and in candidate gene studies (mouse and human) *(14,46)*. It is an especially useful method when the number of samples is large enough that pooling saves a significant amount of labor and material (mostly the PCR enzyme). However, for large pool sizes (about

500 samples per pool), small allele frequency differences (0.05–0.1) may become statistically significant, and the errors generated by constructing pools and measuring the allele frequencies may make distinguishing these small differences difficult. Pooling samples allows a huge reduction in the number of genotyping reactions required for a large study, so the advantages to pooling are still very significant. For example, a study using 2000 SNPs for genotyping 500 cases and 500 controls would require 2 million individual genotyping reactions but only 32,000 reactions when pooling the samples and using four replicates for each allele frequency determination.

To genotype an individual DNA sample for a single SNP, the same procedure used for allele frequency measurement can be performed—the delay in amplification caused by primer mismatch is used simply to note the absence of that allele. In addition, we have also developed a single-tube approach to genotyping individual samples, which uses a GC-tail added to one of the allele-specific primers; the genotype of the sample is detected by analyzing a continuous dissociation curve ("melting curve") subsequent to the PCR reaction. Amplifications with the GC-tail will show a different dissociation pattern than amplifications with the other allele-specific primer *(50)*.

As technology advances, cheaper and easier genotyping methods may emerge, but for now, SNP-based amplification of pooled samples provides a low-cost method of large-scale genotyping. There are now several different pooling methods that are reportedly quite accurate *(34,57,58)*. For human case-control studies, using a pooling approach also has the unappreciated advantage in that it consumes only a small percentage of the amount of often precious DNA; the DNA available is often so limited that individual genotyping over a large number of markers may be impossible.

4. GENOTYPING STUDIES IN THE MOUSE

Among all the model organisms, the mouse is unsurpassed as a tool for analyzing mammalian biology and human disease *(59,60)*. The unique advantages of the mouse include a century of genetic studies, hundreds of spontaneous mutations, scores of inbred strains, practical techniques for random mutagenesis, and the generation of transgenic and knockout/knockin mice *(61–63)*. Most importantly, high-quality genomic sequence information for the mouse is currently available in the public domain *(64)*. There is extensive organizational and functional similarity between the mouse and human genomes in addition to large regions of sequence similarity. More than 90% of the mouse genome is partitioned into sections of homology or synteny with the human genome, more than 40% of the human genome aligns to that of the mouse at the nucleotide level, and 80% of the mouse genes have strict orthologs in the human genome *(64)*. Because the genes, biochemical pathways, and physiological and organ functions in mice are closely related to those of humans, the mouse is a very important and useful experimental system to study the genetics and biology of human disease *(59)*.

A map of closely spaced genetic polymorphisms is a valuable tool to allow mouse geneticists to fully exploit inherited trait models. Toward this end, we have made a mouse SNP database (http://mouseSNP.roche.com) available to the public. The mouse SNP database has grown from the originally published 2848 SNPs *(65)* to more than 70,000 unique SNPs and a total of nearly 800,000 alleles. For each SNP, allelic information is available for up to 21 commonly used inbred mouse strains. More than 95% of the SNPs in the database have been mapped to a specific chromosome and to a specific base pair on the ENSMBL mouse version 3 scaffold (http://www.ensembl.org/). The mouse SNP database is web accessible and allows real-time queries of SNP, mouse strain, and allele information. The query results are provided through a graphical user interface. In addition, 740 SNP genotyping assays based on allele-specific kinetic PCR have been developed. The oligonucleotide primer sequences and conditions for performing the genotyping assays are also provided. This SNP database allowed us to perform genome scans in mouse genetic models of osteoporosis, emphysema, viral bronchitis, and breast cancer. Some of our work on the osteoporosis model is outlined here as an example.

We undertook a large genotyping study involving eight phenotypic traits in collaboration with Robert Klein et al. of Oregon Health Sciences University *(14)*. His group generated a C57BL/6 × DBA/2 cross, in which 994 F2 progeny were phenotyped at 16 wk of age for eight skeletal traits. These skeletal traits included bone mineral density, moment of inertia, cortical thickness, cortical area, marrow area, weight, and femur length. In addition, the femoral cross-sectional area was analyzed separately in males and females. The most extreme F2 progeny with the top and bottom 15% phenotypic values were selected for each trait. Equal amounts of DNA from each phenotypically extreme sample were collected to construct two pools (high and low) for each trait. For a total of 18 pools, differences in allele frequency were determined between related pairs of pools for 140 SNPs across the whole genome using the allele-specific kinetic PCR genotyping method. The results from this genome scan identified a large number of QTLs related to bone quality (*see* Fig.1 for results of scan using bone mineral density). We identified candidate genes in many of these loci, some of which we validated with in vivo and in vitro experiments *(66)*. Using these methods, one person was able to obtain the equivalent of 280,000 genotypes in 3 mo. This method accelerated SNP analysis, improved traditional QTL detection, and made

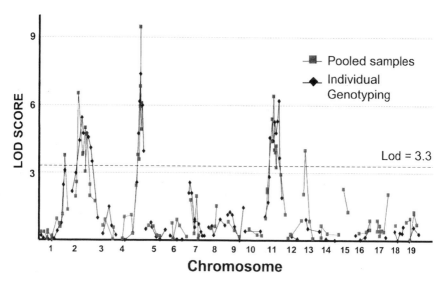

Fig. 1. Comparison of SNP-based genotyping of pooled DNA samples with microsatellite genotyping of individual DNA samples. Phenotypically extreme F2 progeny from a B6D2 intercross with the highest and lowest bone mineral density (BMD) were subjected to whole-genome scanning for association with BMD by genotyping either individual DNA samples (from 299 mice) with 112 microsatellite markers or two pooled DNA samples (150 mice per pool) with 109 SNP markers. The significance of each allele frequency difference was calculated using the *z*-test and plotted as a logarithm of the odds (lod) score for all chromosomes. Dashed line indicates a lod score of 3.3, the threshold for genome-wide significance. (Reprinted with permission from ref. *14*)

large-scale studies feasible. This method is easily performed using reagents and equipment that are available and affordable to small-scale and academic laboratories.

Conventional genotyping can be replaced altogether by an alternative QTL mapping method. This is a computational method for predicting chromosomal regions regulating phenotypic traits *(14)* based on the mouse SNP database and phenotypic differences between the commonly used inbred mouse strains. The computational method calculates genotypic distances between a pair of mouse strains based on allelic differences. The genotypic distances are then compared with phenotypic differences between the two mouse strains. This process is repeated for all strain pairs with phenotypic information available, and a correlation value is derived using linear regression on the phenotypic and genotypic distances for each genome locus. This method has been demonstrated to successfully predict several phenotypic traits (*see* details in ref. *14*).

To improve the precision of the computational method, a haplotype map has been generated for 13 commonly used *Mus musculus* strains and is being expanded to include 21 strains *(67)*. The computational method has been modified to correlate phenotypic data obtained from inbred mouse strains with haplotypic blocks. This method evaluates how well the occurrence of haplotype alleles within a block correlates with the phenotypic data. A matching score is assigned to the haplotypic block, which is then adjusted on the size and structure of the block. This process is repeated for all the haplotypic blocks until the best matching blocks are generated. With this new algorithm, our ability to effectively analyze complex traits in mouse genetic models will be greatly improved.

5. FUNCTIONAL STUDIES: TYPING mRNA IN F1 CROSSES TO STUDY GENE REGULATION

Polymorphisms that are transcribed into the coding region or 3' UTR of a gene can have profound effects on the production of a functional protein or on regulation of the RNA or protein encoded by a gene *(12)*. One such transcribed polymorphism affected susceptibility to asthma in a mouse genetic model, a deletion in the coding region of the gene resulted in C5-deficiency that correlated with susceptibility *(68)*. In humans, a polymorphism in the *TCF7* gene, C883A, was associated with type 1 diabetes *(69)*.

In addition to direct functional effects, a transcribed polymorphism can be used to analyze transcriptional regulation of a gene. If two mouse strains differ in the allele present in a transcribed gene, the F1 generation derived from a cross of these strains can be used to study *cis*- vs *trans*-regulation *(70)* (Fig. 2).

In F1 mice, the transcription factors, polymerases, and other *trans*-acting factors that will affect transcription of the RNA in question are derived equally from each parental strain. If the mRNA level is regulated by *trans*-acting factors, then the F1 mice should have equal levels of the two alleles represented in the mRNA transcribed by this gene, (allele 1/allele 2) = 1. If however, the mRNA expression is controlled in a *cis* manner, in other words, if this gene controls its own expression, then the proportion of allele 1 to allele 2 will not equal 1 *(70)*.

The following example is from an animal model for T-helper cell differentiation. The expression of TCF7 mRNA is about threefold higher in the B10.D2 mouse strain than Balb/c. An SNP was identified in the second exon of the *TCF7* gene. After converting the mRNA to cDNA, the ratio of cDNA of one genotype to the other was determined by quantitative, allele-specific PCR (Fig. 3).

In this case, the ratio of allele 1 to allele 2 was not equal to one, indicating that the transcriptional control is caused by *cis*-acting factors.

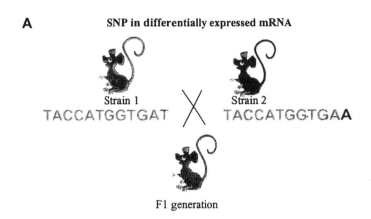

B   CTACCCACCGGCCT[C/G]GGAGCAGGGCAGC

G=B10.D2 allele
C=Balb/c allele

B10.D2	Balb/c	F1	
100	0	66	% G allele
0	100	34	% C allele

Fig. 2. The messenger RNA (mRNA) level for *TCF7* is controlled in a *cis*-acting manner. (**A**) A depiction of breeding two inbred parents to generate a first filial (F1) generation. The F1 mouse receives equal contribution from each parent. (**B**) The level of two alleles (C/G) of the *TCF7* single nucleotide polymorphisms in F1 mouse. The F1 mouse would have equal C or G allele from both parents that is transcribed into mRNA. If the RNA level is controlled in a *cis*-dependent manner, the levels would be different from 50/50 as seen in this figure.

Cowles et al. *(70)* analyzed allele-specific transcription in F1 mice and in different tissues for these mice. This allowed them to study *cis*-regulated expression in conjunction with tissue-specific expression. Gene regulation plays an important role in mammalian biology, so the interest in gene regulation will continue to increase, and SNP-based assays allow easy analysis of transcriptional regulation.

6. CONCLUSIONS

The number of human SNPs available in the public databases continues to grow at a very rapid rate. More importantly, the quality of the information available for each SNP is improving even faster. Between June and November of 2003, the number of uniquely mapped human SNPs grew from approx 4.1 to 5.8 million, whereas the number of experimentally validated SNPs grew from approx half a million to an impressive 2.4 million. The number of SNPs with a known allele frequency increased at a much slower rate, but as data from the international haplotype map project becomes available in 2004, this should change dramatically. For the individual researcher, additional human SNP discovery will only be conducted on limited regions for which a higher SNP density may be required. For these purposes, existing SNP discovery technologies would be sufficient. For most model organisms, however, the SNP coverage is still too low. Except for the commonly used inbred mouse strains, only a handful to a few thousand SNPs have been deposited in NCBI dbSNP for other organisms. For example, dbSNP build 118 only contains two reference SNPs for the chimpanzee *Pan troglodytes*. As additional genomes from other organisms are sequenced, and *in silico* computational biology takes off, generation of extensive polymorphism data will become a priority.

Impressive progress has been made in the area of SNP genotyping in recent years, yet, in terms of throughput and pricing, whole-genome scans of sufficiently large numbers of cases and controls for association studies continue to be beyond the reach of all but a few institutions. Although the price per single genotype has decreased to close to $0.01 for some technologies, the comprehensive or actual price of genotyping in real life situations including labor costs, consumables, and up-front instrumentation investments are more realistically in the range of $0.1–$1. In addition, such prices are most often only achievable in sustained ultra-high-throughput operations processing 10–100 thousands of genotypes per day. At a comprehensive price of $0.05 per genotype, generating 100 thousand genotypes per day would entail yearly expense of roughly 1 million dollars. Similarly, a 100,000 SNP whole-genome scan of 500 cases and 500 controls would cost $5 million. As with sequencing, progress in SNP genotyping prices and throughput has been incremental rather than exponential in recent years. Promising developments in the field of genome sequencing bear close monitoring; if it does indeed become possible, as some have projected, to sequence a whole mammalian genome for a few thousand dollars, these developments may make targeted genotyping of select polymorphisms unnecessary.

Finally, progress is being made in terms of understanding the functional relevance of SNPs and other polymorphisms. New and improved experimental and *in silico* methods for determining and predicting the biological function of polymorphisms transcribed into RNA (as discussed here), as well as intronic regulatory SNPs, are urgently needed.

REFERENCES

1. Risch NJ. Searching for genetic determinants in the new millennium. Nature 2000;405:847–856.
2. Mackay TF. The genetic architecture of quantitative traits. Annu Rev Genet 2001;35:303–339.
3. Darvasi A, Pisante-Shalom A. Complexities in the genetic dissection of quantitative trait loci. Trends Genet 2002;18:489–491.
4. Doerge RW. Mapping and analysis of quantitative trait loci in experimental populations. Nat Rev Genet 2002;3:43–52.
5. Collins FS, Guyer MS, Charkravarti A. Variations on a theme: cataloging human DNA sequence variation. Science 1997;278:1580–1581.
6. Taillon-Miller P, Piernot EE, Kwok PY. Efficient approach to unique single-nucleotide polymorphism discovery. Genome Res 1999;9:499–505.
7. Nowotny P, Kwon JM, Goate AM. SNP analysis to dissect human traits. Curr Opin Neurobiol 2001;11:637–641.
8. Carlson CS, Newman TL, Nickerson DA. SNPing in the human genome. Curr Opin Chem Biol 2001;5:78–85.
9. Underhill PA, Jin L, Lin AA, et al. Detection of numerous Y chromosome biallelic polymorphisms by denaturing high-performance liquid chromatography. Genome Res 1997;7:996–1005.
10. Orita M, Suzuki Y, Sekiya T, Hayashi K. Rapid and sensitive detection of point mutations and DNA polymorphisms using the polymerase chain reaction. Genomics 1989;5:874–879.
11. Petersen DC, Laten A, Zeier MD, Grimwood A, Rensburg EJ, Hayes VM. Novel mutations and SNPs identified in CCR2 using a new comprehensive denaturing gradient gel electrophoresis assay. Hum Mutat 2002;20:253–259.
12. Irizarry K, Kustanovich V, Li C, et al. Genome-wide analysis of single-nucleotide polymorphisms in human expressed sequences. Nat Genet 2000;26:233–236.
13. Picoult-Newberg L, Ideker TE, et al. Mining SNPs from EST databases. Genome Res 1999;9:167–174.
14. Grupe A, Germer S, Usuka J, et al. In silico mapping of complex disease-related traits in mice. Science 2001;292:1915–1918.
15. Risch N, Merikangas K. The future of genetic studies of complex human diseases. Science 1996;273:1516–1517.
16. Lander ES. The new genomics: global views of biology. Science 1996;274:536–539.
17. Gabriel SB, Schaffner SF, Nguyen H, et al. The structure of haplotype blocks in the human genome. Science 2002;296:2225–2229.
18. Kruglyak L. Prospects for whole-genome linkage disequilibrium mapping of common disease genes. Nat Genet 1999;22:139–144.

19. Daly MJ, Rioux JD, Schaffner SF, Hudson TJ, Lander ES. High-resolution haplotype structure in the human genome. Nat Genet 2001;29:229–232.
20. Reich DE, Cargill M, Bolk S, et al. Linkage disequilibrium in the human genome. Nature 2001;411:199–204.
21. Patil N, Berno AJ, Hinds DA, et al. Blocks of limited haplotype diversity revealed by high-resolution scanning of human chromosome 21. Science 2001; 294:1719–1723.
22. Dawson E, Abecasis GR, Bumpstead S, et al. A first-generation linkage disequilibrium map of human chromosome 22. Nature 2002;418:544–548.
23. Tabor HK, Risch NJ, Myers RM. Opinion: candidate-gene approaches for studying complex genetic traits: practical considerations. Nat Rev Genet 2002; 3:391–397.
24. Cheng S, Grow MA, Pallaud C, et al. A multilocus genotyping assay for candidate markers of cardiovascular disease risk. Genome Res 1999;9:936–949.
25. Ioannidis JP, Ntzani EE, Trikalinos TA. Contopoulos-ioannidis DG. Replication validity of genetic association studies. Nat Genet 2001;29:306–309.
26. Lohmueller KE, Pearce CL, Pike M, Lander ES, Hirschhorn JN. Meta-analysis of genetic association studies supports a contribution of common variants to susceptibility to common disease. Nat Genet 2003;33:177–182.
27. Sunyaev S, Ramensky V, Koch I, Lathe W, III, Kondrashov AS, Bork P. Prediction of deleterious human alleles. Hum Mol Genet 2001;10:591–597.
28. Arnheim N, Strange C, Erlich H. Use of pooled DNA samples to detect linkage disequilibrium of polymorphic restriction fragments and human disease: studies of the HLA class II loci. Proc Natl Acad Sci USA 1985;82:6970–6974.
29. Pacek P, Sajantila A, Syvanen AC. Determination of allele frequencies at loci with length polymorphism by quantitative analysis of DNA amplified from pooled samples. PCR Methods Appl 1993;2:313–317.
30. Shaw SH, Carrasquillo MM, Kashuk C, Puffenberger EG, Chakravarti A. Allele frequency distributions in pooled DNA samples: applications to mapping complex disease genes. Genome Res 1998;8:111–123.
31. Barcellos LF, Klitz W, Field LL, et al. Association mapping of disease loci, by use of a pooled DNA genomic screen. Am J Hum Genet 1997;61: 734–747.
32. Germer S, Holland MJ, Higuchi R. High-throughput SNP allele-frequency determination in pooled DNA samples by kinetic PCR. Genome Res 2000;10:258–266.
33. Chen J, Germer S, Higuchi R, Berkowitz G, Godbold J, Wetmur JG. Kinetic polymerase chain reaction on pooled DNA: a high-throughput, high-efficiency alternative in genetic epidemiological studies. Cancer Epidemiol Biomarkers Prev 2002;11:131–136.
34. Kwok PY. Approaches to allele frequency determination. Pharmacogenomics 2000;1:231–235.
35. Sham P, Bader JS, Craig I, O'Donovan M, Owen M. DNA pooling: a tool for large-scale association studies. Nat Rev Genet 2002;3:862–871.
36. Breen G, Harold D, Ralston S, Shaw D, St Clair D. Determining SNP allele frequencies in DNA pools. Biotechniques 2000;28:464–466, 468, 470.

37. Hoogendoorn B, Norton N, Kirov G, et al. Cheap, accurate and rapid allele frequency estimation of single nucleotide polymorphisms by primer extension and DHPLC in DNA pools. Hum Genet 2000;107:488–493.
38. Mohlke KL, Erdos MR, Scott LJ, et al. High-throughput screening for evidence of association by using mass spectrometry genotyping on DNA pools. Proc Natl Acad Sci USA 2002;99:16,928–16,933.
39. Neve B, Froguel P, Corset L, Vaillant E, Vatin V, Boutin P. Rapid SNP allele frequency determination in genomic DNA pools by pyrosequencing. Biotechniques 2002;32:1138–1142.
40. Norton N, Williams NM, Williams HJ, et al. Universal, robust, highly quantitative SNP allele frequency measurement in DNA pools. Hum Genet 2002; 110:471–478.
41. Sasaki T, Tahira T, Suzuki A, et al. Precise estimation of allele frequencies of single-nucleotide polymorphisms by a quantitative SSCP analysis of pooled DNA. Am J Hum Genet 2001;68:214–218.
42. Wasson J, Skolnick G, Love-Gregory L, Permutt MA. Assessing allele frequencies of single nucleotide polymorphisms in DNA pools by pyrosequencing technology. Biotechniques 2002;32:1144–1146, 1148, 1150 passim.
43. Werner M, Sych M, Herbon N, Illig T, Konig IR, Wjst M. Large-scale determination of SNP allele frequencies in DNA pools using MALDI-TOF mass spectrometry. Hum Mutat 2002;20:57–64.
44. Xiao M, Latif SM, Kwok PY. Kinetic FP-TDI assay for SNP allele frequency determination. Biotechniques 2003;34:190–197.
45. Bansal A, van den Boom D, Kammerer S, et al. Association testing by DNA pooling: an effective initial screen. Proc Natl Acad Sci USA 2002;99: 16,871–16,874.
46. Rollinson S, Allan JM, Law GR, et al. High-throughput association testing on DNA pools to identify genetic variants that confer susceptibility to acute myeloid leukemia. Cancer Epidemiol Biomarkers Prev 2004;13:795–800.
47. Shifman S, Bronstein M, Sternfeld M, et al. A highly significant association between a COMT haplotype and schizophrenia. Am J Hum Genet 2002;71: 1296–1302.
48. Kwok PY. Methods for genotyping single nucleotide polymorphisms. Annu Rev Genomics Hum Genet 2001;2:235–258.
49. Gut IG. Automation in genotyping of single nucleotide polymorphisms. Hum Mutat 2001;17:475–492.
50. Germer S, Higuchi R. Single-tube genotyping without oligonucleotide probes. Genome Res 1999;9:72–78.
51. Chou Q, Russell M, Birch DE, Raymond J, Bloch W. Prevention of pre-PCR mis-priming and primer dimerization improves low-copy-number amplifications. Nucleic Acids Res 1992;20:1717–1723.
52. Lawyer FC, Stoffel S, Saiki RK, et al. High-level expression, purification, and enzymatic characterization of full-length *Thermus aquaticus* DNA polymerase and a truncated form deficient in 5′ to 3′ exonuclease activity. PCR Methods Appl 1993;2:275–287.

53. Tada M, Omata M, Kawai S, et al. Detection of *ras* gene mutations in pancreatic juice and peripheral blood of patients with pancreatic adenocarcinoma. Cancer Res 1993;53:2472–2474.

54. Birch DE. Simplified hot start PCR. Nature 1996;381:445, 446.

55. Germer S, Higuchi R. Homogeneous allele-specific PCR in SNP genotyping. In: Kwok PY, ed. Single nucleotide polymorphisms: methods and protocols. Totowa, NJ: Humana, 2002.

56. Barcellos L, Germer, S, Klitz W. DNA pooling methods for association mapping of complex disease loci. In: Carrington M, Hoelzel AR, eds. Molecular epidemiology: a practical approach. Oxford: Oxford University Press, 2001.

57. Shifman S, Pisante-Shalom A, Yakir B, Darvasi A. Quantitative technologies for allele frequency estimation of SNPs in DNA pools. Mol Cell Probes 2002;16:429–434.

58. Le Hellard S, Ballereau SJ, Visscher PM, et al. SNP genotyping on pooled DNAs: comparison of genotyping technologies and a semi automated method for data storage and analysis. Nucleic Acids Res 2002;30:e74.

59. Rossant J, McKerlie C. Mouse-based phenogenomics for modelling human disease. Trends Mol Med 2001;7:502–507.

60. Paigen K. A miracle enough: the power of mice. Nat Med 1995;1:215–220.

61. Joyner AL. Gene targeting: a practical approach. New York: Oxford University Press, 1999.

62. Yu Y, Bradley A. Engineering chromosomal rearrangements in mice. Nat Rev Genet 2001;2:780–790.

63. Copeland NG, Jenkins NA, Court DL. Recombineering: a powerful new tool for mouse functional genomics. Nat Rev Genet 2001;2:769–779.

64. Waterston RH, Lindblad-Toh K, Birney E, et al. Initial sequencing and comparative analysis of the mouse genome. Nature 2002;420:520–562.

65. Lindblad-Toh K, Winchester E, Daly MJ, et al. Large-scale discovery and genotyping of single-nucleotide polymorphisms in the mouse. Nat Genet 2000;24:381–386.

66. Klein RF, Allard J, Avnur Z, et al. Regulation of bone mass in mice by the lipoxygenase gene Alox15. Science 2004;303:229–232.

67. Liao G, Wang J, Guo J, et al. In silico genetics: identification of a functional element regulating H2-Ealpha gene expression. Science 2004;306:690–695.

68. Karp CL, Grupe A, Schadt E, et al. Identification of complement factor 5 as a susceptibility locus for experimental allergic asthma. Nat Immunol 2000;1: 221–226.

69. Noble JA, White AM, Lazzeroni LC, et al. A polymorphism in the TCF7 gene, C883A, is associated with type 1 diabetes. Diabetes 2003;52:1579–1582.

70. Cowles CR, Hirschhorn JN, Altshuler D, et al. Detection of regulatory variation in mouse genes. Nat Genet 2002;32:432–437.

II

Selected Examples: Murine Models of Human Disease

6

Genetic and Genomic Approaches to Complex Lung Diseases Using Mouse Models

Michael J. Holtzman, Edy Y. Kim, and Jeffrey D. Morton

1. INTRODUCTION

Common lung diseases are likely to be multifactorial and multigenic. In addition, the lung exhibits a limited set of biological and physiological responses, so different lung diseases exhibit significant overlap in phenotype. This complexity in the development and manifestation of lung disease poses significant challenges for developing complete and accurate models of disease. Nonetheless, a layered strategy that includes in vitro and in vivo systems can offset these limitations. In vitro systems have evolved from simple organ culture to intricate procedures for cell culture that exhibit high fidelity to behavior in vivo. Similarly, in vivo systems have evolved from traditional physiology-based models in large animals and rodents to genetic modification of mice using targeted and conditional systems. Complex traits may be studied in inbred, recombinant, or congenic strains of mice, and single gene effects may be segregated naturally or experimentally. Ultimately, results from these in vitro and in vivo models identify candidate genes for further study in humans.

This chapter reviews the development and application of genetic and genomic approaches to complex lung diseases, focusing on the use of mouse model systems. Although the particular strength of the murine system has been its applicability to studies conducted in vivo, suitable cell culture systems have now been established for comparative work in vitro as well. Whenever possible, the extension and correlation of findings to human studies will also be noted. The chapter is organized by disease entity, using the examples of cystic fibrosis (CF), emphysema, tuberculosis, and asthma as illustrative of well-studied targets for multidisciplinary genetic and genomic

From: *Computational Genetics and Genomics*
Edited by: G. Peltz © Humana Press Inc., Totowa, NJ

approaches. In addition, the distinct characteristics of these diseases have shaped different approaches to defining underlying genetic mechanisms and so illustrate the range of available methods that can be used in mouse models of lung disease.

2. CYSTIC FIBROSIS

CF is the most common autosomal-recessive disorder in Caucasian populations, with an incidence of 1 in 2500 live births *(1)*. Thus, the identification of the CF transmembrane conductance regulator (CFTR) as the site of the underlying genetic abnormality for this disease was a seminal example of the positional cloning approach to identify and characterize a candidate gene in humans *(2–4)*. The CFTR gene has 27 exons that span 230 kb of the long arm of human chromosome 7 (7q31.2) and encodes a transmembrane glycoprotein of 1480 amino acid residues *(5)*. The gene product is a member of the adenosine triphosphate-binding cassette family of transporters that have conserved transmembrane and nucleotide-binding domains linked by a regulatory domain with phosphorylation sites for protein kinases A and C *(2,6)*.

Before the identification of the CFTR gene, physiological studies showed that CF epithelia have defective cyclic adenosine monophosphate (cAMP)-mediated chloride ion transport *(7–9)*. Subsequent studies indicated that CFTR was the major cAMP-regulated chloride channel in the apical membrane of epithelial cells *(10,11)* and so had a central role in transepithelial salt transport, fluid flow, and ion concentrations in the intestine, pancreas, sweat gland, and airway epithelia *(12)*. CF results from defective CFTR activity that disrupts transepithelial ion transport. In general, nonsense or stop mutations in CFTR result in severe disease, whereas missense mutations result in milder disease. More than 900 mutations have been identified within human CFTR. The most frequent CF mutation includes 66% of mutant CFTR alleles. This mutation deletes in-frame the phenylalanine at position 508 (ΔF508) *(13)*. The *ΔF508 CFTR* allele produces a misfolded protein that is trapped in the endoplasmic reticulum *(14–16)*. In contrast, another common mutation (G551D) results in a protein with normal processing but decreased chloride channel activity *(17)*.

2.1. Murine Models of CF

A number of mouse models of CF were developed based on targeted mutations of the *Cftr* gene (Table 1). Initial strategies were based on knockout technology that introduces a genomic construct into mouse embryonic stem cells. Clones that have undergone genetic recombination are implanted into pseudopregnant female mice. The resulting chimeric mice are crossed to

Table 1
Mouse Models of Cystic Fibrosis Generated by Gene Targeting[a]

Genetic change	Mouse name	Molecular approach	Reference
Cftr knockouts	cftr[tm1Unc]	In-frame stop (exon 10)	*19*
	cftr[tm1Hgu]	Insertion (exon 10)	*20*
	cftr[tm1Cam]	Insertion (exon 10)	*25*
	cftr[tm1Bay]	Duplication (exon 3)	*223*
	cftr[tm3Bay]	In-frame stop (exon 2)	*224*
	cftr[tm1Hsc]	Insertion (exon 1)	*26*
Cftr mutations	cftr[tm1Kth]	Homologous recombination (ΔF508)	*24*
	cftr[tm1Eur]	Homologous recombination (ΔF508)	*23*
	cftr[tm2Cam]	Homologous recombination (ΔF508)	*22*
	cftr[TgHm1G551D]	Homologous recombination (G551D)	*17*

[a]Modified with permission from ref. *47*. CFTR, cystic fibrosis transmembrane conductance regulator.

produce mice that are homozygous for the targeted gene deficiency. The first mouse model disrupted the *CFTR* gene by introducing a stop codon in exon 10 (strain CFTR[m1UNC]) *(12,18,19)*. These CFTR-deficient mice are viable but lack the lung inflammation found in human CF. Instead, these mice develop severe bowel disease that was fatal by 40 d of age. A second gene knockout model (CFTR[m1HGV]) used insertional mutagenesis rather than the strategy of gene replacement used for the CFTR[m1UNC] strain. The CFTR[m1HGV] mouse strain produces 10% of normal CFTR levels and has 90% long-term survival with abnormalities of the colon and vas deferens *(20)*. The CFTR[m1UNC] strain has been complemented by human CFTR driven by the rat intestinal fatty acid-binding protein promoter *(21)*. However, like the CFTR[m1UNC] strain, CFTR[m1HGV] mice exhibit normal lung histology.

Additional murine models duplicate human CF mutations. Two strains (CFTR[ΔF508ROT] and CFTR[ΔF508CAM]) contain the ΔF508 CFTR mutation, and a third line contains the G551D mutation *(17,22–24)*. These strains also show moderate (G551D) to severe (ΔF508) intestinal pathology, such as goblet cell hyperplasia (GCH) and concretions in the crypts of Liberkuhn. However, lung histology is again normal *(18–20,23,25)*. Thus, these models may be appropriate for the 10% of human newborns with CF and older patients who suffer similar intestinal obstruction and mucus accumulation, but they miss the major pulmonary pathology of the disease.

In each of these models, the severity of the intestinal pathology depends on the strain's genetic background. For example, one CFTR-null strain (CFTR^{m1HSC}) exhibits severe intestinal obstruction and only 30% survival, but this phenotype is altered when the original line is crossed with other inbred strains. This heterogeneity is a result of a separate locus on chromosome 7 that influences the intestinal phenotype. At least one genetic locus unlinked to *Cftr* can also modify the severity of CFTR-dependent lung disease in mice *(26)*. When the original CFTR^{m1UNC} strain was extensively backcrossed (18 generations) into the C57BL/6 strain, this congenic strain develops spontaneous and progressive lung disease at an early age *(27)*. The lung pathology is characterized by ineffective mucociliary transport, overinflation of alveoli, inflammation, and interstitial fibrosis, which resembles human CF. Future studies will need to identify genes besides *Cftr* that modulate the severity of CF. For example, other epithelial ion channels (e.g., calcium-dependent chloride channels) may minimize lung pathophysiology in *Cftr*-null mice. The strain-dependence of CFTR-induced pathology may be further defined in the mouse model using quantitative trait loci (QTL) to identify additional candidate genes.

CF mouse models also help to determine whether there is a heterozygote advantage that can explain the maintenance of CF alleles in the human population. For example, it has been proposed that the CF alleles mediate resistance to the secretory diarrhea caused by cholera. In support of this concept, the amount of chloride ion transport induced by cholera toxin correlates directly with functional levels of CFTR *(28)*. Similarly, *Salmonella typhi* uses CFTR to enter intestinal epithelial cells so that a CF heterozygote with decreased CFTR levels may have decreased susceptibility to typhoid fever *(29)*. These possibilities can now be tested in the mice with *Cftr* mutations.

2.2. Pseudomonas Infection

Although CFTR mutations are the principal genetic defect in CF patients, the major cause of morbidity and mortality among CF patients is chronic respiratory infection, especially with *Pseudomonas aeruginosa (30)*. An exaggerated, persistent, and predominantly neutrophilic inflammatory response to *P. aeruginosa* infection is a hallmark of lung disease in CF patients *(31)*.

Other opportunistic pathogens, including *Burkholderia cepacia*, nontuberculous mycobacteria, *Aspergillus fumigatus*, and *Strenotrophomonas maltophilia*, can also be cultured from the airways of CF patients *(32)*. Hypotheses to explain the link between defective CFTR and increased lung infection include the following:

1. The hyperabsorption of water by CF epithelia leads to mucociliary dysfunction and poor pathogen clearance from the airway *(33)*.
2. High salt concentration in the CF airway leads to inactivation of antimicrobial defensins *(34)*.
3. CFTR normally binds *P. aeruginosa*, so the loss of CFTR results in aberrant bacterial clearance *(35)*.

To date, however, none of these possibilities have yet provided an explanation for the chronic lung infection with *P. aeruginosa* (and its relation to CFTR expression or function). Mouse models exist for infection with *P. aeruginosa*, and as expected, *Cftr*-mutant mice are more susceptible than wild-type mice to infection *(36–38)*. A model of chronic infection with *P. aeruginosa* can be achieved by intratracheal instillation of agarose beads and bacteria. This model has been used to identify susceptible (DBA/2; C57BL/6) and resistant (Balb/c) mouse strains *(39–42)*. T-helper type 1 (Th1) CD4+ T-cells are protective, so this finding stands in contrast to the view that the resistant Balb/c strain tends to skew toward a T-helper type 2 (Th2) response *(43–45)*. Recent data show that CD1d-restricted T-cells are required to clear *P. aeruginosa* from infected lungs *(46)*, but the acquired immune response to *P. aeruginosa* still needs to be more fully defined. It is also possible that alterations in airway mucins (e.g., increased sialylation) may occur in CF and so increase the susceptibility of the host to infection *(47)*. Each of these possibilities can be addressed directly in the mouse model.

2.3. Gene Therapy

Mouse models of CF also provide a suitable system for the development of gene therapy. Intratracheal *(48)* and intranasal *(49)* administrations of liposomes have been used to deliver plasmids encoding the *Cftr* gene in vivo. This strategy has allowed for at least partial correction of defects in cAMP-mediated chloride secretion in treated mice. The use of adenoviral vectors for gene expression has proven difficult because of low level and transient expression and concomitant inflammation *(50)*. Subsequent human trials of adenoviral gene transfer have also been unsatisfactory because of similar problems *(51,52)*. Strategies under study include attempts to increase efficiency of expression (e.g., by increasing the accessibility of the adenoviral receptor) and to decrease airway inflammation (e.g., by eliminating further elements of the adenoviral backbone or using other viral vectors).

3. EMPHYSEMA

Chronic obstructive pulmonary disease affects 2 million individuals and contributes to more than 80,000 deaths per year in the United States *(53)*. This disease is defined as chronic airflow obstruction caused by chronic bronchitis or emphysema. Most cases of emphysema develop after cigarette smoking, but 2–5% of cases are familial and result from a deficiency in α-1-antitrypsin (AAT) *(53,54)*. In 1964, Eriksson et al. observed that even nonsmoking AAT-deficient patients are more susceptible to emphysema than the general population *(55)*. Because AAT inhibits proteases, such as neutrophil elastase *(56)*, it appeared likely that AAT-deficient patients were susceptible to uncontrolled degradation of elastin and consequent emphysema. This possibility has evolved into the more general concept that an imbalance between protease and antiprotease activity may lead to all forms of emphysema. Candidates include other neutrophil proteases, such as proteinase 3, cathepsin G, and other matrix metalloproteases (MMPs), as well as macrophage elastase (now known as MMP-12), and cysteine proteases. Recent data suggest that degradation of other extracellular matrix components, particularly collagen, may also contribute to emphysema *(57)*. Taken together, it appears likely that inflammatory stimuli, especially cigarette smoking, initiate a cascade that alters the balance of protease activities in the lung. Proteases released by activated macrophages and neutrophils mediate the degradation of collagen and elastin in the extracellular matrix. Inflammatory cytokines serve to recruit and activate additional immune cells and so further amplify the damage. The destruction of extracellular matrix leads to cell death and abnormal repair, and this whole process develops into permanent airspace enlargement and bronchiolar collapse in susceptible individuals.

Animal models support such a scheme for excessive protease activity. In one of the first animal models of emphysema, intratracheal delivery of a plant protease caused airspace enlargement in rats that resembled the pathology of emphysema in humans *(58)*. Intratracheal administration of neutrophil elastase, proteinase 3, pancreatic elastase, and vascular endothelial growth factor inhibitor causes similar emphysema in animal models *(59–64)*. After intratracheal treatment with an elastase or protease, neutrophils and macrophages infiltrate the lung and initiate a process that leaves the lung with a disorganized elastin matrix and permanent airway enlargement. However, a bolus of exogenous protease is of limited relevance to human disease. Intratracheal treatment with lipopolysaccharide also enlarges airspaces under experimental conditions *(63)*, but bacterial pneumonia does not cause emphysema in humans *(65)*. Thus, models with greater relevance and evidence of genetic susceptibility needed to be developed (as outlined in Subheadings 3.1.–3.5.).

3.1. Genetics of AAT Deficiency

Severe AAT deficiency occurs in 1 in 3500 people, and adults with mild deficiency (AAT levels less than 35% of normal) have a 20–50% higher risk of emphysema. Severe deficiency (AAT levels less than 10% of normal) confers at least 80% risk of developing emphysema *(66)*. Polymorphisms in the *AAT* gene are classified into three categories: M (with normal AAT levels), S (mild AAT deficiency, e.g., $Glu^{264} \rightarrow Val$), and Z (more severe AAT deficiency, e.g., $Glu^{342} \rightarrow Lys$). The significant mutations disrupt salt bridges and cause AAT polymerization with consequently low levels of secretion and impaired function *(67)*. In rodents, injection of D-galactosamine inhibits AAT *(68,69)*. Treated animals do not spontaneously develop emphysema, but these animals are more susceptible to lung damage from elastase treatment. Mice with null mutations in the *Aat* gene or knockin mutations for human M, S, and Z type alleles are currently under development and should provide significant insight into AAT deficiencies *(70)*. Experimental models are made more difficult because humans have only one AAT gene and a pseudogene on chromosome 14 *(71,72)*, whereas mice have a cluster of four to five *Aat* genes on chromosome 12 *(73)*. In addition, alveolar macrophages in mice (unlike humans) are normally AAT-deficient *(74)*. Nonetheless, AAT deficiency is an ideal target for gene therapy because it involves a single gene, a blood-borne product, and a phenotype that is restored with only 35% of normal levels *(65)*. Thus, the development of a mouse model for use in AAT gene therapy remains a useful endpoint.

3.2. Genetic Models of Emphysema

In humans, serum AAT levels and lifestyle do not completely predict emphysema *(75)*. Genetic polymorphism may contribute to this heterogeneous response. Novel emphysema genes may be found in spontaneously mutated mice, such as the beige, blotchy, tight-skin, and pallid strains *(76)*. Beige mice have airspace enlargement at all ages because of an autosomal-recessive defect on chromosome 13 *(77,78)*. Beige mice illustrate a typical strategy for finding genes. Perou et al. selected the smallest yeast artificial chromosome (YAC) contigs that can complement beige fibroblasts in vitro. Positional cloning isolated the *beige* gene and its human homolog *(79)*. Blotchy mice have panlobular emphysema because of defective copper metabolism that reduces lysyloxidase activity and causes abnormal collagen crosslinks *(80–82)*. Blotchy mice demonstrate fruitful feedback between human and murine genetics. Human complementary deoxyribonucleic acid (cDNA) probes identified the *blotchy* gene on chromosome 10 *(83)*. This mouse strain resembles a human disease that predisposes to emphysema *(cutis laxa*–loose, inelastic skin). With a defect in *Fibrillin-1*, tight-skin mice have abnormal airspace development and progressive emphysema *(84,85)*. Pallid mice develop mild airspace enlargement late in life *(86)*. Pallid mice have a nonsense mutation in a protein interacting with syntaxin-13 that regulates vesicle trafficking *(87)*. Inbred mouse strains also vary in their response to cigarette smoke *(65,73)*. For example, C57BL/6J and DBA/2 strains of mice develop airspace enlargement, but the ICR strain of mice does not exhibit any change after cigarette smoking *(88)*. The susceptibility may result from antielastase deficiency (C57BL/6J) or antioxidant deficiency (DBA/2). These strains are candidates for QTL analysis and determination of candidate genes. A particular challenge for each of these conditions will be to find the relevance to human disease.

3.3. Transgenic Mouse Models

Mouse models can provide proof-of-principle for new hypotheses. For example, previous research had focused on elastin degradation as the key step in emphysema. However, overexpression of human collagenase-1 (MMP-1) in mice using a lung-specific promoter haptoglobin was found to be sufficient to cause airspace enlargement *(89,90)*. Whether the role of collagenase is important only during lung development or can mediate disease is now under study. Support of a pathogenic role for collagenase has come with the finding of increased levels of collagenase messenger ribonucleic acid (mRNA) in the lungs of emphysema subjects *(91–93)*. These findings stand in contrast to those using lung-specific overexpression of platelet-derived growth factor-B (PDGF-B). These transgenic mice exhibit enlarged airspaces with fibrosis *(94)*, but there is no evidence for a similar role of PDGF-B in human emphysema.

One of the problems with transgenic mouse models is that the level of transgene expression depends on the site of transgene integration into the genome. By testing several founder mice, investigators can therefore determine the dose-dependence of a target gene and the physiological consequences of this effect. For example, in mice expressing the *Mmp 1* transgene, the founder lines with the earliest and highest gene expression show changes in lung morphology by 5 d of age *(90)*. However, other founder lines with lower expression exhibit normal lung development and do not develop airspace enlargement until later, a time course that fits better with a model of human emphysema. Similarly, mice with high levels of expression for a transgene encoding TGF-α exhibit lung fibrosis with alveolar enlargement. Mice with lower expression do not exhibit significant fibrosis and thereby provide a phenotype that is closer to human emphysema *(95)*. Thus, one can take advantage of the dose-dependence of transgene expression to develop a more suitable phenotype for modeling human disease.

3.4. Inducible and Conditional Expression Systems

Despite the utility of site-dependent expression in some transgenic models, it had remained difficult in other models to segregate transgene effects on lung development from ones that occur in the adult animal. To solve this problem, lung biologists have taken advantage of inducible promoter systems that can be activated at any time during or after development *(96)*. For example, the Clara cell 10-kDa protein (CC10) promoter can be used to drive lung-specific expression of a reverse tetracycline transactivator (rtTA) *(97)*. In the absence of a tetracycline-type drug (e.g., doxycycline), rtTA cannot bind to a tet-operator driving the target gene. However, when the animal is treated with doxycycline, then rtTA activates transcription of the target gene. If doxycycline treatment is provided *in utero* to adulthood, the phenotype may mimic the one manifested using a nonconditional promoter system. For example, continuous interleukin (IL)-11 expression causes alveolar enlargement and airway fibrosis *(96,98)*. However, if doxycycline treatment is stopped at birth, alveolar enlargement occurs without fibrosis, and if treatment begins in adulthood, the lungs show fibrosis but no airspace enlargement. Thus, the inducible promoter system indicates that IL-11 production may not be an appropriate mediator of emphysema in the adult. By contrast, transgenic expression of IL-13 in the adult causes protease generation (e.g., MMP-9 and MMP-12) in concert with enlarged airspaces, mucous cell metaplasia, and airway inflammation *(99)*. Induction of interferon (IFN)-γ in adulthood causes a similar phenotype *(100)*. By permitting normal lung development, an inducible promoter system can be used to generate a model of diseases that are acquired in the adult. These models demonstrate that cytokine production is sufficient to develop the disease phenotype, but the physiological relevance of high and continuous levels of these mediators from an unusual cellular source (e.g., Clara cells) remains uncertain.

3.5. Knockout Mice

Mice with targeted null mutations have been used to determine whether the expression of a specific target gene is necessary for the development of experimental emphysema. Several of these mice exert their effects on development rather than the adult lung. For example, a lack of alveolar development leads to airspace enlargement in mice with null mutations of *Pdgf-a, fibulin-1*, and fibroblast growth factor receptors 3 and 4 *(101–103)*. Although these models may represent the abnormal repair process that occurs in emphysema, a more convincing model exhibits normal lungs that only exhibit emphysema after chronic exposure to cigarette smoke. In this type of model, it appears that MMP-12-null mice are protected from the usual development of airspace enlargement *(104)*. However, the relevance of this finding for humans remains uncertain, especially because MMP-12 expression may not change in the lungs of human subjects with emphysema *(91–93)*. More recently, investigators aiming to create a hypertension model by overexpression of a sodium channel recognized that one line of these mice exhibited progressive airway enlargement *(105)*. The development of the emphysema phenotype in this line was because of fortuitous disruption and inactivation of the *klotho* gene, thereby implicating this gene as a previously unsuspected candidate for emphysema. Crossing null-mutation mice with transgenic mice can provide additional insights into emphysema pathogenesis. For example, IL-13 transgenic mice show less airspace enlargement after they are crossed with MMP-9- or MMP-12-null mice *(106)*. These types of genetic models can better define the interaction between susceptibility genes in vivo.

3.6. Genome-Wide Searches

Although genetically modified mice serve to test focused hypotheses, the use of genome-wide scans can uncover new candidate genes for mediating the emphysema phenotype. For example, a microarray-based screen provided initial evidence of increased levels of expression for the secreted frizzled-related protein 1 (SFRP-1) in emphysema vs healthy control subjects *(107,108)*. Subsequently, it was found that SFRP-1 mRNA levels are increased in mouse models of emphysema because of cigarette smoke or transgene expression, and overexpression of SFRP-1 causes apoptosis in cultured lung epithelial cells. Thus, studies of human subjects can lead to the development of better murine models with a biologically relevant mechanism.

4. TUBERCULOSIS

Tuberculosis is caused by infection with pathogenic *Mycobacterium* and affects one-third of the world population causing more than 2 million deaths per year *(109)*. Efforts at control are hampered by increasing multidrug resistance in certain populations *(110)*. Worldwide, active tuberculosis is fatal in 50% of patients *(111)*. The predominant organism, *Mycobacterium tuberculosis* is a Gram-positive bacterium with a peptidoglycan wall containing complex lipidoglycans that help the microbe to resist desiccation *(112)*. The lung is the main entry point and the usual focus of disease. Alveolar macrophages phagocytose inhaled bacteria and trigger a characteristic inflammatory response. Mononuclear cells accumulate to form a granuloma, or tubercle, that has a central zone of infected macrophages surrounded by giant cells, uninfected macrophages, and lymphocytes. Infection with *M. tuberculosis* is latent and contained in the tubercle, so the vast majority of infected individuals are asymptomatic and noninfectious over the course of their lifetime. However, a weakened immune system (e.g., because of human immunodeficiency virus infection, glucocorticoid treatment, or aging) renders the host more vulnerable to reactivation of tuberculosis from the latent state.

4.1. Bacillus Calmette-Guerin Vaccination

The bacillus Calmette-Guerin (BCG) is an attenuated strain of *Mycobacterium bovis* that has been used as a tuberculosis vaccine for the past century. It is the world's most commonly used vaccine and may reduce disease morbidity and mortality, but it has had less than ideal efficacy in recent trials *(113,114)*. The United States does not administer BCG because it converts the tuberculin skin test to positive and so voids its use for detecting recent infection. The basis for poor efficacy of BCG includes the following:

1. Immune responses to environmental mycobacteria prior to immunization.
2. Genetic variability in the human population.
3. Differences in strains, doses, and vaccination schedules.
4. Administration to previously infected individuals *(114)*.

Reemergence of tuberculosis as a health problem has mandated a more thorough understanding of both the host and microbial genetics that underlie the disease.

4.2. Microbial Genetics

Research on tuberculosis has been advanced by the availability of the genome sequence for *M. tuberculosis*. This microbial genome contains 4000 genes encoding proteins and 50 genes coding for stable RNA *(115)*, and at least in principle, this data contains the sequence of all possible targets for antimycobacterial agents. Regions of particular interest include sequences for novel proteins, such as the PE (glycine–alanine-rich) and PPE (glycine–asparagine-rich) families *(116)*. Genome sequence also allows for comparative analysis that can identify virulence factors common to virulent strains or absent in nonvirulent strains *(117,118)*. This information may also aid in choosing the proper microbe strain for use in animal models. Similarly, the recent definition of the mouse genome and the availability for genetic modification in this species should allow for the development of appropriate mouse models of tuberculosis. As developed in Subheadings 4.3. and 4.4., clearance of infection is a dynamic and complex multigenic process.

4.3. Host Genetics

Immunity to mycobacterial infection has been studied in several animal models, including mouse *(119,120)*. The advantage of the mouse model relies on differential susceptibilities to infection across homogenous inbred strains. Most studies aim to test several parameters of susceptibility with various *M. tuberculosis* isolates, doses, and routes of infection. Initial studies linked *Bcg*, a locus on murine chromosome 1, to resistance to infection with BCG *(121)*. Resistance to other intracellular parasites were also linked to loci on chromosome 1. For example, the locus *Lsh* is linked to resistance to *Leishmania donovani*, and *Ity* is linked to resistance to lethal *Salmonella typhimurium*. Macrophages from susceptible mouse strains showed an impaired ability to restrict the growth of intracellular mycobacteria in vivo *(122)*. In the *Bcg* locus, *Nramp1* (natural resistance-associated macrophage protein) was identified as the BCG-resistance gene. *Nramp1* is also termed *Slc11a1* (solute carrier family 11a member 1). The *Nramp1* gene consists of 15 exons that span 11.5 kb of genomic DNA and encode a 90-100 kDa integral membrane protein *(123,124)*. Targeted disruption of *Nramp1* eliminated resistance to BCG, *L. donovani*, and *S. typhimurium*. This result established that *Bcg*, *Lsh*, and *Ity* loci are linked to the same gene *(125)*. Biochemical studies showed that *Nramp1* is localized to the late endosomal compartment of resting macrophages and is recruited to phagosomes and lysosomes *(126)*. To combat bacterial infection, Nramp1 may either provide iron that becomes multivalent in the presence of reactive oxygen and nitrogen radicals or it may block the availability of iron or manganese required for bacterial enzymes. The gene for *Nramp1* maps to human chromosome 2q35, and polymorphisms found in human populations may explain variable susceptibility to tuberculosis *(127,128)*. For example, NRAMP1 polymorphisms in intron 4 and the 3′-untranslated region is strongly linked to increased susceptibility in a West African human cohort *(129)*. Thus, the Nramp1 paradigm illustrates how studies can move from phenotype to genotype in mice and then be extended to human subjects.

Despite this information, subsequent studies of Nramp1 have provided evidence that additional genes may also confer susceptibility to tuberculosis. In particular, development and comparison of a strain of mice that was resistant to BCG infection (i.e., Bcg^r in a DBA/2 background) to one that was susceptible (i.e., Bcg^s in a Balb/c background) provided the unexpected finding that the BCG-resistant strain was more susceptible to infection with *M. tuberculosis (130)*. In addition to new questions over the role of Nramp1, these results also raise significant concern over the use of BCG infection as a model for virulent mycobacterial infection in humans.

Subsequent studies have used QTL analysis to identify additional genes that might mediate susceptibility to tuberculosis in mice. For example, this type of analysis was applied to the F2 intercross of mouse strains that were susceptible (DBA/2) and resistant (C57BL/6) to infection with *M. tuberculosis*. In this case, three loci (*Trl 1*, *Trl 2*, and *Trl 3*) account for half of the phenotypic variation in the F2 hybrid strain. Several candidate genes of immunological relevance are localized to *Trl 1* and *Trl 2*, and these now need to be analyzed for function *(131)*. In another study of QTL analysis, F1 hybrid and F2 intercross progeny from susceptible (C3HeB/Fe) and resistant C57BL/6 strains were used to identify the sst1 (susceptibility to tuberculosis 1) locus. This linkage site is distinct from *Nramp1*, which is located at a distance of 10–19 cM, but candidate genes have not yet been identified *(132)*.

4.4. Immune Response

Both the innate and adaptive immune responses mediate resistance to *M. tuberculosis*. For instance, the innate immune system is responsible for generating nitric oxide that is needed to kill the microbial organism, and mice deficient for inducible nitric oxide synthase are more susceptible to tuberculosis than their wild-type counterparts *(133)*. An influence of adaptive immunity in host defense against tuberculosis comes from the finding that mice with the H-2^k major histocompatibility complex (MHC) haplotype are protected against infection compared to ones with H-2^b *(134,135)*. Similar to mice, human susceptibility to tuberculosis is also linked to MHC haplotypes (HLA-DR2 and HLA-DQB1) *(136,137)*.

The cascade of events required for a successful immune response likely begins with the MHC-dependent presentation of antigen and generation of CD4$^+$ T-cells specific for *M. tuberculosis* antigen. The consequent activation of Th1 cells leads to the production of IFN-γ, which in turn activates infected macrophages and causes nitric oxide production and death of the pathogen. In strains of mice (e.g., Balb/c) that tend toward a Th2 response, the administration of IL-12 can act to increase the Th1 response and improve clearance of infection (*138*). The class of CD8$^+$ T-cells may also contribute to host defense in this setting, because β_2-microglobulin-deficient mice that lack functional MHC class I and CD8$^+$ T-cells are also more susceptible to infection with *M. tuberculosis (139)*. The murine system therefore offers an opportunity to check the influence of each of these steps using selective deficiencies and complementation of the immune response.

Despite their utility, mouse models of tuberculosis do offer some limitations for application to human immune responses. For example, mice uniformly lack group 1 CD1 molecules that can present *M. tuberculosis* antigen to T-cells (*140*). Thus, mouse models of tuberculosis require attention to idiosyncrasies of this species compared to the human model. Nonetheless, insight into pathogenesis and treatment of tuberculosis will likely be greatly advanced with studies of mouse, human, and microbial genomes, as well as modifications of these genomes and specific deficiencies of the host immune system.

5. ASTHMA

Asthma is characterized by reversible obstruction, hyperreactivity, and inflammation of the pulmonary airways. The corresponding histopathology includes overproduction of mucus and hyperplasia of mucous cells, hyperplasia and hypertrophy of airway smooth muscle, and subepithelial fibrosis (*53*). In addition, airways of asthmatic subjects exhibit chronic and acute-on-chronic inflammation that involves immune cells (e.g., eosinophils, mast cells, and lymphocytes) and parenchymal cells (e.g., bronchial epithelial cells) (*141*). Individual asthmatic subjects vary considerably in the type, severity, and frequency of symptoms, although correlations between phenotype and histopathology are still under study. The cause of this pathology remains uncertain. Traditional proposals are based on excessive Th2 production of cytokines (especially IL-4, IL-5, IL-9, and IL-13) that serve to drive the asthma phenotype, but this simplistic proposal has been challenged by several lines of evidence in experimental models and humans (*142*). In addition, although there is no question of a genetic influence on the development of asthma, there is still no agreement on even a single candidate gene for mediating susceptibility to the disease. Thus, experimental models of asthma must address each of these uncertainties over pathogenesis of asthma, as well as its increasing incidence, in the populations of Western countries (*143*). To date, a variety of experimental animal models have been used for asthma pathogenesis and treatment (*144–146*). The use of mouse models is tempered by the fact that mouse airways have increased Clara cells (*147*), decreased mast cells, distinct eosinophil behavior, as well as decreased airway branching and neurogenic control compared to the human models *(148,149)*. Nonetheless, as noted under Headings 2–4, the well-developed database for murine immunology and the capacity for genetic modification of the mouse genome offer significant advantages over other species.

5.1. Mouse Models of Asthma

The endogenous Th2 response is often driven by allergen, so models of asthma most commonly use allergen challenge as a stimulus to induce the asthma phenotype. In the usual mouse model of allergic asthma, intraperitoneal delivery of allergen is used for sensitization and intranasal delivery or aerosolization is used for subsequent allergen challenge. Commonly used antigens include ovalbumin, *Schistosoma mansoni* egg, and *A. fumigatus* *(150)*. After allergen challenge, mice develop airway inflammation, airway hyperreactivity (AHR), and mucous cell (i.e., GCH) hyperplasia. The inflammatory response includes increased numbers of neutrophils, macrophages, lymphocytes, and eosinophils *(151)*, but the response is highly influenced by the choice of mouse strain and protocols for sensitization and challenge. Because short-term antigen challenge may not accurately reflect the chronic antigen exposure in humans, new models of chronic antigen challenge have also been developed. These models subject mice to allergen challenge with ovalbumin three times per week for 2 mo *(152)*. In contrast to models with short-term challenge, chronic delivery may also cause epithelial thickening and subepithelial fibrosis similar to the case in asthmatic subjects *(152)*. Chronic allergen challenge can also eventually suppress some features of the acute allergic response (e.g., increased serum levels of IgE and airway eosinophilia). The effect of chronic challenge on airway reactivity is still uncertain and may be influenced by the dose of allergen *(153)*. In addition, chronic allergen challenge may elicit AHR and GCH in some strains (e.g., BALB/c) but not others (e.g., C57BL/6 mice) *(154)*.

An additional development in acute allergen challenge models involves the role of the Th1 response. Traditional Th2-based proposals for asthma pathogenesis implied that Th1 responses were decreased in this setting and in asthma. This view was supported by evidence that Th1 cytokines, such as IFN-γ and IL-12, may downregulate the allergic response *(155)*. Similarly, infection with murine cytomegalovirus (which typically increases Th1 over Th2 responses) also decreases allergen-induced AHR and tissue eosinophilia *(156)*. However, additional work in the mouse system indicates that this view of the Th1 response may also be too simplistic. For example, adoptive transfer of Th1 cells in ovalbumin-sensitized mice causes an increase rather than the expected decrease in airway inflammation *(157)*. These findings have led to a revision of the Th2 hypothesis to better account for a contribution of Th1 cells *(142,158,159)*. It appears that Th1 cells are more capable of traffic to the airways and so are required to assist Th2 cell recruitment in response to allergen challenge *(160,161)*. A similar mechanism may underlie the capacity of viral infection, which normally triggers a Th1 response, to nonspecifically set the allergic response into motion *(162)*.

In addition to allergen, an infection with certain types of respiratory viruses can also trigger acute exacerbations of asthma, and respiratory infections in childhood can predispose individuals to developing the disease. In particular, paramyxoviruses, such as respiratory syncytial virus (RSV), are the predominant cause of serious respiratory illness in infants; infants hospitalized for RSV bronchiolitis later develop asthma at 10 times the rate of control infants *(163)*. In view of these findings, mouse models of asthma are being developed that rely on respiratory infection as a stimulus. For example, some studies indicate that BALB/c mice infected with RSV may acutely develop airway eosinophilia and hyperreactivity, and infection with RSV may increase the effect of allergen on these asthma traits *(164)*. However, this type of viral model causes only transient changes in airway behavior. The subsequent development of a model that relies on Sendai virus infection of C57BL/6 mice resembles human asthma because the mice exhibit a permanent switch to a complex asthma phenotype that includes AHR and GCH *(165)*. Moreover, these chronic asthma traits are closely associated in a single susceptible genotype, so the model provides a basis for next segregating these traits using mouse strains that are susceptible rather than resistant to these chronic virus-inducible events (Fig. 1).

5.2. Measurement of Asthma Traits: Airway Reactivity

Assessment of airway reactivity requires monitoring airway caliber before and after delivery of nonspecific stimuli (e.g., acetylcholine or methacholine) that cause airway smooth muscle constriction. Measurements of airway function in mice are limited by the small size of the animal, and in some cases, the need for large numbers of assessments that must be determined in a chronic setting. Earlier work sometimes relied on measurement of pulmonary resistance done ex vivo using excised lungs or determinations of airway smooth muscle behavior performed in vitro using tracheal rings *(166,167)*. To preserve the critical controls over airway behavior that are established in vivo, additional techniques were developed and later modified to measure pulmonary resistance in anesthetized and ventilated mice *(168)*. In an alternative method, the tracheal airway is occluded at the end of inspiration, and the immediate decrease in pressure is a measure of

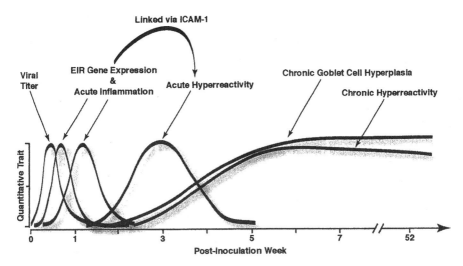

Fig. 1. Time course of quantitative events that occur during the development of the asthma phenotype induced by experimental viral infection in a susceptible strain of mice. Events begin with viral replication (that peaks at 3–5 d after inoculation) that is later cleared from the lung (by 2 wk after inoculation). This initial infection is followed by induction of epithelial immune-response gene expression (that peaks at 5 d after inoculation) and is followed by immune cell infiltration (that peaks at various times depending on cell type, e.g., at 8–12 d for lymphocytes). Each of these events is linked to the subsequent development of acute airway hyperreactivity that depends on *ICAM-1* gene expression and peaks on approx 21 d after inoculation. After this time, there is progressive and chronic goblet cell hyperplasia and hyperreactivity that persist for at least 1 yr after infection. Within a single susceptible genotype, these two chronic asthma phenotypes can be difficult to segregate based solely on time course, so other approaches (e.g., definition of mouse strains with distinct genetic susceptibilities) are needed. ICAM-1, intercellular adhesion molecule-1. (Modified with permission from ref. *142.*)

airway resistance. In another variation, peak inspiratory pressures are determined over time, and the area under the pressure-time curve is expressed as an airway pressure time index (APTI) that can correlate with airway resistance *(169)*. Each of these methods requires the use of general anesthesia that can alter airway behavior and surgery that does not permit a chronic preparation to obtain repeated experiments in the same animal. However, this problem has been overcome by the use of other noninvasive means of assessing airway caliber. In particular, barometric plethysmography allows for measurements in unanesthetized animals that provide indirect assessments of airway caliber. A commonly used method is based on a breath-by-breath calculation of enhanced pause (Penh) that appears to correlate with measurements of pulmonary resistance after methacholine challenge *(170)*. However, Penh can be influenced by factors other than airway resistance, such as breathing pattern and nasal resistance *(168)*.

5.3. Genetic Determinants of Airway Reactivity

Inbred mouse strains have been used to define genetic differences in base-line airway reactivity to acetylcholine or serotonin, as well as increases in reactivity (AHR), after exposure to ozone or diesel exhaust particles *(171–175)*. In an initial study to identify genetic determinants of airway reactivity in mice, hyperreactive A/J mice were crossed with hyporeactive C3H/HeJ mice to generate F1 offspring, and these were then used to create an F2 intercross (F1 × F1) generation *(169)*. A 1:3 ratio of normal to hyper-reactive mice in the F2 generation suggested that reactivity may depend on a single recessive locus, but no quantitative analysis was done to better define this possibility. A similar strategy was applied to platelet-activating factor induced AHR *(176)*, as well as baseline breathing patterns *(177)*. In the allergen-challenge model, asthma traits (e.g., AHR, eosinophilia, and increased serum immunoglobulin-E [IgE]). are also strain-dependent and can be segregated using congenic mouse strains *(178,179)*. Congenic mice that differ in a single genomic region can simplify and extend comparisons of inbred mouse strains by linking one allergen-induced trait (e.g., AHR), but not others (e.g., tissue eosinophilia and increased serum IgE), to a limited region of the genome *(180,181)*. To date, linkage data for AHR has been variable among different studies of inbred strains, likely caused at least in part by differences in experimental methods for phenotype assessment *(169,171,172,175)*.

5.4. QTL Analysis of AHR

QTL analysis requires that phenotype be quantified and be variable in magnitude over a continuous distribution *(182)*. Thus, in a typical QTL analysis, high- and low-responder strains are crossed, and this F1 hybrid generation is either backcrossed to a parental strain or intercrossed to create a population with a wide distribution of the quantitative phenotype. A large number of progeny are needed to allow for frequent enough genetic recombination events to permit informative genotyping. Progeny are genotyped using simple sequence length polymorphisms or single nucleotide polymorphisms (SNPs) that span the mouse genome and then target regions of interest with more closely spaced genomic markers *(183,184)*. Genotype–phenotype linkages are determined by calculating the probability that the data occurs by linkage rather than chance and are expressed as the negative log of the odds ratio or logarithm of the odds (lod) score. QTL analysis procedures include interval mapping, regression mapping, and marker regression *(185,186)*. Additional methods find minor QTL linkages that are overshadowed by the major QTL. For example, permutation-based methods empirically estimate the threshold value for significance *(187,188)*. Computer programs for QTL analysis include QTL Café and QTL/MAPMAKER *(189,190)*. A lod score of 3 or greater indicates statistically significant linkage of the genotype with the phenotype, and a score of 2–3 is suggestive of linkage but not significant. A locus is also evaluated by its contribution to variance. For an F1 backcross to a parent strain, the effect of the locus on phenotypic variation equals half of the difference in phenotype between mice heterozygous for the locus (resembling F1 at that locus) and mice homozygous for that locus (resembling the parent at that locus). For loci with no effect on phenotype, the average heterozygous mouse has the same phenotype as a homozygous mouse. Assuming independent segregation, the effect of other loci will cancel out. For an F2 intercross, each locus has two effects on phenotypic variation—an additive effect and dominance deviation. The additive effect is half of the phenotypic difference between mice homozygous for one parental allele and mice homozygous for the other allele. The dominance deviation is the difference between the phenotype of heterozygous mice and the calculated average of the parental phenotypes. In essence, heterozygous mice will be skewed toward the phenotype of the parent with the dominant allele.

5.5. QTL Analysis of AHR in Naïve Mice

Perhaps the simplest approach to defining genetic determinants of airway reactivity is represented by QTL analysis of baseline reactivity in inbred mouse strains that have not been experimentally altered by allergen or toxin exposure. In studies by De Sanctis et al., airway reactivity was quantified by determining the dose of methacholine that was required to double the baseline level of pulmonary resistance in hyperreactive A/J and hyporeactive C57BL/6 strains of mice *(191–193)*. The F1 cross from these strains was hyperreactive, but the F2 intercross and C57BL/6 backcross generations had a normal distribution that was suitable for analysis of a multigenic trait. Phenotypic extremes in the backcross progeny were genotyped with markers spaced 9 cM apart, and three genomic regions of interest were examined in all backcross mice with markers at 1 cM apart (Table 2). Two loci, *Bhr1* and *Bhr2*, were identified by linkage to AHR, and a third locus *Bhr3* was suggestive of linkage and exhibited epistasis (genetic interaction) with the other two loci that might lower its independent lod score.

Table 2
Identification of QTLs Linked to Airway Reactivity in Mice

Mouse strain	Parameter	Locus	Chr	Functional associations	Reference
Baseline studies of naïve mice					
A/J × C57BL/6	TPP	*Bhr1*	2	IL-1β	*191*
		Bhr2	15	IL-2R, IL-3R, PDGF-R	
		Bhr3[a]	17	TNFα, mast cell proteases	
A/J × C3H/HeJ	APTI/EIO	QTL[a]	6	IL-5R	*194*
A/J × C3H/HeJ	TPP	QTL[a]	6		*195*
		QTL[b]	7	Kallikrein	
		QTL[a]	17		
DBA/2 × Balb/c	Penh	*Tapr*	11	Human 5q23–35	*198*
DBA/2J × C57BL/6	APTI	QTL[b]	13	Human 5q31–33	*207*
Allergen challenge studies of sensitized mice					
BP2 × Balb/c	Penh	QTL[b]	10	IFNγ, Human 12q21.1–12q24.22	*189*
		QTL[b]	11	Eotaxin, iNOS, Human 17q12–22	
		QTL[a]	9		
		QTL[a]	17		
A/J × C3H/HeJ	APTI	*Abhr1*	2	Human 10p11-13, 2q12–14, 9q22–34	*180*
		Abhr2	2	Human 9q33–34, 2q14–24	
		QTL[a]	7	Human 19q13	

APTI, airway pressure time index; EIO, end-inspiratory occlusion; Penh, enhanced pause; TPP, transpulmonary pressure; IL-2R, Interleukin-2 receptor; PDGF-R, platelet-derived growth factor receptor, iNOS, inducible nitric oxide synthase; QTL, quantitative trait loci.

[a]QTL with possible but not significant linkage (lod score < 3).

[b]QTL with significant linkage (lod score > 2.95, $p < 0.05$).

A similar strategy was also used to analyze AHR in hyperreactive A/J and hyporeactive C3H/HeJ strains of mice. In this case, AHR was assessed by acetylcholine responsiveness and measurements of APTI and total respiratory resistance (R_{rs}) *(194)*. For the F1, F2, and F1 backcross mice, the distribution of APTI differed from the one for R_{rs}, perhaps because APTI reflects the behavior of small airways, whereas R_{rs} reflects function in larger conducting airways. Which of these parameters correlates best with the site of airway obstruction in humans with asthma is also uncertain. The APTI data fit with a model that calls for a major locus that is modified by a multigenic component, whereas the R_{rs} data does not fit with any model of genetic inheritance. Analysis of the F1 backcross to A/J indicated that APTI and R_{rs} have a common QTL on chromosome 6, but there was no linkage between AHR and murine homologs of human genes previously linked to asthma (e.g., on human *5q31–q33*). A large region of chromosome 6 lacks crossover events, perhaps because of chromosomal inversions, and makes it difficult to perform higher resolution mapping of this region.

In a subsequent study of the same strains (i.e., A/J and C3H/HeJ), methacholine-induced AHR was quantified by changes in lung resistance (RL), and male A/J × female C3H/HeJ F1 generation was significantly different from male C3H/HeJ × female A/J F1 mice *(195)*. This gender-dependence of AHR occurred in several studies and underscores the complexity of asthma-like traits. The QTL analysis of the F1 backcross to the C3H/HeJ parental strain indicated linkage of AHR to loci on chromosomes 6, 7, and 17. The locus on chromosome 6 was the same as the one identified in earlier studies *(194)*.

5.6. QTL Analysis in the Allergen Model

QTL analysis was first applied to the allergen challenge model in A/J × C3H/HeJ F1 mice that were backcrossed to the A/J parental strain. Mice were phenotyped for AHR using APTI, and the allergic response was monitored by levels of Bronchoalveolar lavage fluid eosinophils and serum IgE *(180)*. For AHR, two significant QTLs (*Abhr1* and *Abhr2*) and one possible QTL were found that appear distinct from ones found in naïve mice from the same A/J0 × C3H/HeJ cross *(194,196)*. This result suggests that different mechanisms determine AHR in naïve mice and in mice with allergen challenge. To achieve greater genetic diversity, others have intercrossed five strains with a high antibody response to ovalbumin, and high-responders were further bred to increase the antibody response *(197)*. Subsequently, Zhang et al. studied one of these strains (BP2) with allergen-induced AHR and eosinophilia *(189)*. In the F2 mice derived from BP2 × Balb/c, AHR and eosinophilia segregated separately, and genotyping with 180 microsatellite markers indicated that AHR was linked to at least two significant loci. In this case (and other complex traits), not every allele from the high-responder strain will increase the strength of the phenotype. For example, when one locus was examined in isolation, the allele from the high responder BP2 strain decreased AHR. The locus on chromosome 17 had no additive effect, so mice homozygous for the *Bp2* allele showed the same phenotype as the Balb/c allele. However, the locus on chromosome 17 has a large dominance deviance. The heterozygotes have AHR values closer to the low responder strain (Balb/c). These data suggest that chromosome 17 may contain two closely spaced loci. For both parental strains, these two loci oppose each other's effect on AHR, so their net additive effect is zero. However, both these loci have a dominance deviation that results in decreased AHR. For example, the locus that reduces AHR is dominant for both parental strains.

Congenic strains are useful to limit the QTL analysis to a small genomic region and to isolate one locus from the epistatic effects of other loci. For example, McIntire et al. backcrossed hyporeactive DBA/2 mice to hyperreactive Balb/c for multiple generations so that, except for a small region of DBA/2, the progeny were genetically identical to Balb/c *(198)*. Following immunization, these congenic strains were screened for decreased IL-4 levels, and one strain (HBA) exhibited decreased AHR and lower levels of Th2 cytokines. A genome-wide scan indicated that HBA had a segment of chromosome 11 from DBA/2. This recessive locus was designated Tapr (T-cell and airway phenotype regulator) and was used to define linkage to *Tim* genes.

5.7. Identifying Candidate Genes

After linkage is established for a genetic locus, candidate genes for AHR must be identified. Positional cloning often requires linkage to a region of approx 1 cM (equivalent to 1000 kb or 300 meiotic events) *(199)*. Linked markers can be used to screen a library of large genomic inserts (e.g., those contained on YACs). The ends of the first positive clones are used as probes for the second round of screening, so that by walking down the chromosome, one creates a physical map of the genetic region of interest. A multigenic trait makes positional cloning difficult because any one gene may exert a small effect on the overall phenotype.

An alternative approach uses radiation hybrid (RH) maps to locate a QTL in the genome. In this case, a murine RH map uses a panel of cell lines that have random fragments of mouse (donor) genome fused to hamster (recipient) genome. The random fragments are generated by irradiation of genomic DNA instead of relying on crossover events. Cell lines are genotyped to establish physical relationships between DNA markers and genomic fragments *(200)*. The RH map and the physical map of the mouse genome were used to identify candidate genes in the *Tapr* QTL *(201)*. A cluster of expressed sequence tags exhibited polymorphisms in the parent strains, and in the F1 backcross, the (T-cell, immunoglobulin domain, mucin domain) *Tim1* and *Tim3* polymorphisms co-segregated with the QTL *Tapr*. Further work will be needed to determine the function of *Tim* genes and to follow-up on the relevance of *Tim* homology with human *hHAVcr1* (Hepatitis A virus receptor).

In addition to positional cloning approaches, some have selected a candidate gene based on physiological or biological rationales and then sought evidence of localization to established QTLs. For example, the QTL *Abhr1* contained the *C5* gene and so suggested that the *complement factor 5 receptor (C5r1)* gene may be a candidate. In fact, *C5r1* genomic sequence contains several polymorphisms between hyperreactive A/J and hyporeactive C3H/HeJ strains *(202)*. The F1 × A/J backcross mice were genotyped, and *C5r1* was localized to a QTL that was previously linked to AHR on chromosome 7 *(180)*.

A useful strategy to limit the number of candidate genes in a QTL is based on the corresponding levels of gene expression. Levels of gene expression can be quantified by mRNA levels from oligonucleotide microarray or multiplex kinetic polymerase chain reaction (PCR) assays *(203)*. For example, A/J × C3H/HeJ mice were used to identify a QTL linked to allergen-induced AHR, and following this microarrays were applied to the F1 backcross to A/J mice to identify genes with the QTL that exhibited altered expression between high and low responders *(204)*. The *C5* gene was the only candidate that was both localized to a QTL and differentially expressed in microarrays comparing high to low responders to allergen. Subsequent PCR analysis indicated that expression levels of C5 were correlated with genotype and were inversely correlated with phenotype (AHR). In hyperreactive A/J mice, a deletion in C5 caused a deficiency in C5 protein, and 2/3 of the high-responder mice were homozygous for the *A/J* allele. This significant but incomplete correlation reflects the multigenic nature of AHR. Nonetheless, the results suggested that C5 deficiency causes an imbalance of Th2 over Th1 responses in this system, although the functional pathway for this possibility still needs to be defined. In using expression levels to screen for candidates, it is critical to recognize that altered expression may be directly responsible for genetic susceptibility or may simply reflect a genetic abnormality that is upstream of gene expression. Nonetheless, expression screening compensates for two drawbacks of QTL analysis—the inability to identify specific genes and changes in gene function. Thus, combining expression screening with the QTL analysis provides for a more informative genetic approach.

Studies of AHR-linked candidate genes should be considered incomplete without studies of function, and this deficiency has been illustrated in several instances. For example, IL-9 affects mast cells and IgE release and has been linked to asthma in humans *(205,206)*. In addition, Nicolaides et al. identified *IL-9* as a candidate gene using a model of atracurium-induced AHR *(207)*. Lung levels of IL-9 were increased in hyperreactive DBA/2J compared to hyporeactive C57BL/6J mice and were found at an intermediate level in F1 mice with intermediate levels of AHR. However, IL-9-null mice exhibit no change in allergen-induced increases in airway reactivity *(208)*. Taken together, the results suggest that IL-9 expression may be associated with AHR but may not be necessary in the pathway that leads to AHR.

5.8. High-Throughput QTL Analysis

New approaches to increase the efficiency of linkage analysis have been developed and can be applied to asthma traits. For example, genotyping with SNPs may be faster than using simple-sequence length polymorphisms or microsatellite markers, and SNPs are just as informative in crosses aimed to differentiate two alleles. To achieve finer mapping, new SNPs are being developed at a high rate based on massive sequencing efforts, and DNA microarrays with possible polymorphisms allow for large-scale screening of candidate SNPs *(209)*. For genotyping in QTL analysis, traditional methods include gel-based restriction fragment length polymorphism and allele-specific oligonucleotide hybridization *(210)*. More recently, microarrays and kinetic PCR, with primers specific for each SNP allele, have been used to increase efficiency by multiplexing many reactions in parallel *(204,209)*. Single-base extension (SBE) forms the basis for other high-throughput methods. In SBE, a primer at the SNP incorporates a single fluorescently labeled dideoxynucleotide that is complementary to the polymorphic nucleotide. Several methods use microarrays or labeled microspheres to perform multiple SBE reactions in parallel *(211–214)*.

Additional methodologies have been developed to help decrease the investment in animals and time that is needed to generate intercrosses for QTL analysis. A computer database with genotypes for 15 inbred mouse strains at more than 500 SNPs has been developed and may be useful for mapping some traits to specific genomic regions *(215)*. In this approach, phenotypes of inbred strains are quantified, and following this, they are used in pairwise comparisons of phenotype and genotype. Linear regression tests the correlation of a phenotype with genotype across all the strains. This method was used to correctly identify the loci linked to AHR in two previous studies that used QTL analysis *(180,189)*. At its current average resolution of 38 cM, *in silico* mapping cannot replace intercrosses and QTL analysis, but the panel of inbred strains can significantly accelerate the investigation.

In addition, it appears that SNPs tend to cosegregate based on a limited number of haplotypes in humans *(216)*. If a similar pattern is found in mice, it may be possible to generate highly informative maps with a smaller but well-positioned number of SNPs in interstrain comparisons.

5.9. Interspecies Methods

Comparisons between species may use conserved genomic elements to identify regulatory elements. In a study of human, dog, and murine genomes, two-thirds of regulatory elements were conserved across species *(217)*. Human chromosome 5q31 contains genes for several Th2 cytokines (IL-4, IL-5, and IL-13) and has been linked to asthma, so Loots et al. searched for sequences that were conserved between human 5q31 and the murine ortholog on chromosome 11 *(218)*. A conserved noncoding sequence (CNS-1) located between the *IL-4* and *IL-13* genes was identified as a candidate regulatory element. This possibility was developed in transgenic mice that were made to express a large (450 kb) segment of human 5q31 using a YAC clone. The Th2 cells from these transgenic mice produced human IL-4 and IL-13, and this capacity was lost in transgenic mice with a CNS-1 deletion, suggesting that CNS-1 is a necessary regulatory element for Th2 cytokine production. A panel of YAC transgenic mice containing human 5q31 was screened for elevated serum IgE after allergen challenge *(219,220)*, suggesting that YAC transgenic mice can be a general tool to screen human genomic loci for mediating asthma-like traits. In a simpler interspecies comparison, a specific human gene sequence can be used to search for a mouse homolog, and this approach was used to identify the murine *Muc5b* gene that encodes for a mucus glycoprotein that is inducible by allergen challenge *(221)*.

5.10. Functional Assessments Using Transgenic Mice

The final step in assessments of genetic elements is one of the most difficult, i.e., assessment of function in vivo. Frequently, validation is approached by genetic modification of the mouse genome and subsequent assessment of phenotype. In the asthma model, this approach has offered significant insight but has also been marked by inherent contradictions. For example, IL-9 transgenic mouse exhibited increases in baseline airway reactivity, suggesting that *IL-9* is a candidate gene for mediating AHR. However, IL-9-deficient mice exhibit the usual increase in reactivity after allergen challenge *(208,222)*. As noted in Subheading 3.4., it is difficult to ascertain the physiological significance of transgenic expression using gene promoter elements that may not reflect the nature of endogenous gene expression. Nonetheless, a variety of transgenic and targeted mice have been generated, focusing mostly on the candidates that

Table 3
Phenotypes of Genetic Modification in Mouse Models of Asthma

Target	AHR	GCH	EOS	IgE	References
IFN-γ	NN	I	I	I	*165,225–227*
IL-4	C	C	C	C	*228–231*
IL-5	NN	C	C	C	*230,232–234*
IL-6	I	ND	I	ND	*235,236*
IL-8	C	ND	NN	I	*237*
IL-9	NC	NC	NC	NC	*208,222*
IL-10	C	NN	C	I	*238*
IL-11	C	ND	ND	ND	*98*
IL-12	I	ND	I	ND	*239*
IL-13	NC	NC	ND	NN	*240,241*
IL-18	I	I	I	ND	*242*
GATA-3	C	C	C	C	*243,244*
Tbet	I	ND	ND	ND	*245*
STAT-6	C	C	C	C	*246,247*
IgE	NN	ND	NN	N	*248*
ICAM-1	C	NN	C	I	*249*
C3a	C	ND	NN	ND	*250*
CD40/CD40L	NN	ND	NN	C	*230*
B-cell	C	NN	NN	N	*170,251,252*
Mast cell	NN	ND	NN	NN	*253*

AHR, airway hyperreactivity; EOS, eosinophils; GCH, goblet cell hyperplasia; IgE, serum immunoglobulin E; C, contributes; I, inhibits; NC, not certain; ND, not determined; NN, not necessary; IL, interleukin; IFN, interferon; ICAM, intercellular adhesion molecule.

control the Th2 pathway, and these provide significant insight into gene function in the allergic asthma model (as summarized in Table 3). A particular challenge of future studies will be to segregate complex asthma traits (e.g., AHR, GCH, and subepithelial fibrosis) in order to define individual genetic controls.

6. SUMMARY

The genetic basis for common lung diseases has been difficult to determine in studies of human subjects, at least in part because of the complexity of disease phenotypes and the phenotypic overlap among common diseases. In that context, investigators have turned to mouse models of lung disease to more precisely define a disease trait and to take advantage of homogenous inbred strains that might allow for segregating complex traits and for defining the genetic basis of individual traits. The field is continuing to develop high-fidelity mouse models of disease and beginning to subject these model systems to linkage (QTL) analysis and genetic modification. These approaches are evolving to take better advantage of the sequence for the human and mouse genomes, as well as the capacity for whole-genome scanning, using informative markers (especially SNPs), improved techniques for analyzing gene expression (especially oligonucleotide microarray), and new methods for conditional and more specific gene expression and targeting. By integrating results from these different methodologies, it is now possible to devise a rationale scheme for progressing from the identification of a human disease trait through analysis in a mouse genetic model of this trait and then return to verification of the findings in a human subject (Fig. 2). This

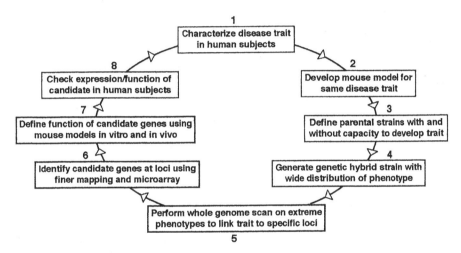

Fig. 2. Schematic approach to defining the genetic basis of complex lung diseases. This scheme begins with (1) characterizing disease traits in human subjects (uppermost box) and proceeds clockwise through; (2) developing a mouse model that exhibits the same disease trait; (3) defining parental strains that do or do not exhibit the trait but are otherwise well-matched for other traits; (4) generating genetic hybrid strains that exhibit a broad distribution of the same phenotypic trait, e.g., an F2 intercross; (5) performing a whole-genome scan, e.g., using allele-specific single nucleotide polymorphism markers, on phenotypic extremes to identify loci that are linked to the trait; (6) identifying specific candidate genes at the locus either by finer mapping and sequencing or screening for altered gene expression by oligonucleotide microarray; (7) defining the function of the new candidate gene using a mouse model that exhibits expression of the corresponding trait in vivo and if possible in vitro to better establish molecular mechanism; and (8) returning to human subjects to check for altered expression and/or function of the candidate gene to the extent that is possible in research on humans, especially in relationship to the trait under study (1).

integration is critical to bridge the gap between genetic mapping and biological function. Further progress will depend on the development of additional mouse models that accurately reflect human disease phenotypes and the coordinated assessment of mouse and human genetic and biological data. Significant progress has already been made in defining the genetic basis for lung diseases, such as CF, but new genetic and genomic methods are likely to next be successful in defining more complex lung diseases, such as asthma and emphysema. These studies should aim to define diseases in molecular, as well as clinical terms, and so provide more specific targets for diagnosis and treatment of lung diseases.

REFERENCES

1. Davis PB, Drumm M, Konstan MW. Cystic fibrosis. Am J Respir Crit Care Med 1996;154:1229–1256.
2. Riordan JR, Rommens JM, Kerem B, et al. Identification of the cystic fibrosis gene: cloning and characterization of complementary DNA. Science 1989;245:1066–1073.
3. Rommens JM, Iannuzzi MC, Kerem B, et al. Identification of the cystic fibrosis gene: chromosome walking and jumping. Science 1989;245:1059–1065.
4. Kerem B, Rommens JM, Buchanan JA, et al. Identification of the cystic fibrosis gene: genetic analysis. Science 1989;245:1073–1080.
5. Davidson DJ, Porteous DJ. Genetics and pulmonary medicine. 1. The genetics of cystic fibrosis lung disease. Thorax 1998;53:389–397.
6. Jentsch TJ, Stein V, Weinreich F, Zdebik AA. Molecular structure and physiological function of chloride channels. Physiol Rev 2002;82:503–568.
7. Knowles M, Gatzy J, Boucher R. Increased bioelectric potential difference across respiratory epithelia in cystic fibrosis. N Engl J Med 1981;305:1489–1495.
8. Knowles MR, Stutts MJ, Spock A, Fischer N, Gatzy JT, Boucher RC. Abnormal ion permeation through cystic fibrosis respiratory epithelium. Science 1983;221:1067–1070.
9. Knowles M, Gatzy J, Boucher R. Relative ion permeability of normal and cystic fibrosis nasal epithelium. J Clin Invest 1983;71:1410–1417.
10. Anderson MP, Gregory RJ, Thompson S, et al. Demonstration that CFTR is a chloride channel by alteration of its anion selectivity. Science 1991;253:202–205.
11. Anderson MP, Rich DP, Gregory RJ, Smith AE, Welsh MJ. Generation of cAMP-activated chloride currents by expression of CFTR. Science 1991;251:679–682.
12. Sheppard DN, Welsh MJ. Structure and function of the CFTR chloride channel. Physiol Rev 1999;79:S23–S45.
13. McIntosh I, Lorenzo ML, Brock DJ. Frequency of delta F508 mutation on cystic fibrosis chromosomes in UK. Lancet 1989;2:1404–1405.
14. Gilbert A, Jadot M, Leontieva E, Wattiaux-De Coninck S, Wattiaux R. Delta F508 CFTR localizes in the endoplasmic reticulum-Golgi intermediate compartment in cystic fibrosis cells. Exp Cell Res 1998;242:144–152.

15. Pind S, Riordan JR, Williams DB. Participation of the endoplasmic reticulum chaperone calnexin (p88, IP90) in the biogenesis of the cystic fibrosis transmembrane conductance regulator. J Biol Chem 1994;269:12,784–12,788.
16. Fuller W, Cuthbert AW. Posttranslational disruption of the delta F508 cystic fibrosis transmembrane conductance regulator (CFTR)-molecular chaperone complex with geldanamycin stabilizes delta F508 CFTR in the rabbit reticulocyte lysate. J Biol Chem 2000;275:37,462–37,468.
17. Delaney SJ, Alton EW, Smith SN, et al. Cystic fibrosis mice carrying the missense mutation G551D replicate human genotype-phenotype correlations. Embo J 1996;15:955–963.
18. Clarke LL, Grubb BR, Gabriel SE, Smithies O, Koller BH, Boucher RC. Defective epithelial chloride transport in a gene-targeted mouse model of cystic fibrosis. Science 1992;257:1125–1128.
19. Snouwaert JN, Brigman KK, Latour AM, et al. An animal model for cystic fibrosis made by gene targeting. Science 1992;257:1083–1088.
20. Dorin JR, Dickinson P, Alton EW, et al. Cystic fibrosis in the mouse by targeted insertional mutagenesis. Nature 1992;359:211–215.
21. Zhou L, Dey CR, Wert SE, DuVall MD, Frizzell RA, Whitsett JA. Correction of lethal intestinal defect in a mouse model of cystic fibrosis by human CFTR. Science 1994;266:1705–1708.
22. Colledge WH, Abella BS, Southern KW, et al. Generation and characterization of a delta F508 cystic fibrosis mouse model. Nat Genet 1995;10:445–452.
23. van Doorninck JH, French PJ, Verbeek E, et al. A mouse model for the cystic fibrosis delta F508 mutation. EMBO J 1995;14:4403–4411.
24. Zeiher BG, Eichwald E, Zabner J, et al. A mouse model for the delta F508 allele of cystic fibrosis. J Clin Invest 1995;96:2051–2064.
25. Ratcliff R, Evans MJ, Cuthbert AW, et al. Production of a severe cystic fibrosis mutation in mice by gene targeting. Nat Genet 1993;4:35–41.
26. Rozmahel R, Wilschanski M, Matin A, et al. Modulation of disease severity in cystic fibrosis transmembrane conductance regulator deficient mice by a secondary genetic factor. Nat Genet 1996;12:280–287.
27. Kent G, Iles R, Bear CE, et al. Lung disease in mice with cystic fibrosis. J Clin Invest 1997;100:3060–3069.
28. Gabriel SE, Brigman KN, Koller BH, Boucher RC, Stutts MJ. Cystic fibrosis heterozygote resistance to cholera toxin in the cystic fibrosis mouse model. Science 1994;266:107–109.
29. Pier GB, Grout M, Zaidi T, et al. *Salmonella typhi* uses CFTR to enter intestinal epithelial cells. Nature 1998;393:79–82.
30. Koch C, Hoiby N. Pathogenesis of cystic fibrosis. Lancet 1993;341: 1065–1069.
31. Konstan MW, Berger M. Current understanding of the inflammatory process in cystic fibrosis: onset and etiology. Pediatr Pulmonol 1997;24:137–142; discussion 159–161.
32. Goldberg JB, Pier GB. The role of the CFTR in susceptibility to *Pseudomonas aeruginosa* infections in cystic fibrosis. Trends Microbiol 2000;8:514–520.

33. Matsui H, Grubb BR, Tarran R, et al. Evidence for periciliary liquid layer depletion, not abnormal ion composition, in the pathogenesis of cystic fibrosis airways disease. Cell 1998;95:1005–1015.
34. Zabner J, Smith JJ, Karp PH, Widdicombe JH, Welsh MJ. Loss of CFTR chloride channels alters salt absorption by cystic fibrosis airway epithelia in vitro. Mol Cell 1998;2:397–403.
35. Pier GB, Grout M, Zaidi TS, et al. Role of mutant CFTR in hypersusceptibility of cystic fibrosis patients to lung infections. Science 1996;271:64–67.
36. Pier GB, Meluleni G, Neuger E. A murine model of chronic mucosal colonization by *Pseudomonas aeruginosa*. Infect Immun 1992;60:4768–4776.
37. Davidson DJ, Dorin JR, McLachlan G, et al. Lung disease in the cystic fibrosis mouse exposed to bacterial pathogens. Nat Genet 1995;9:351–357.
38. Heeckeren A, Walenga R, Konstan MW, Bonfield T, Davis PB, Ferkol T. Excessive inflammatory response of cystic fibrosis mice to bronchopulmonary infection with *Pseudomonas aeruginosa*. J Clin Invest 1997; 100:2810–2815.
39. Starke JR, Edwards MS, Langston C, Baker CJ. A mouse model of chronic pulmonary infection with *Pseudomonas aeruginosa* and *Pseudomonas cepacia*. Pediatr Res 1987;22:698–702.
40. Morissette C, Skamene E, Gervais F. Endobronchial inflammation following *Pseudomonas aeruginosa* infection in resistant and susceptible strains of mice. Infect Immun 1995;63:1718–1724.
41. Sapru K, Stotland PK, Stevenson MM. Quantitative and qualitative differences in bronchoalveolar inflammatory cells in *Pseudomonas aeruginosa*-resistant and -susceptible mice. Clin Exp Immunol 1999;115:103–109.
42. Tam M, Snipes GJ, Stevenson MM. Characterization of chronic bronchopulmonary *Pseudomonas aeruginosa* infection in resistant and susceptible inbred mouse strains. Am J Respir Cell Mol Biol 1999;20:710–719.
43. Moser C, Jensen PO, Kobayashi O, et al. Improved outcome of chronic *Pseudomonas aeruginosa* lung infection is associated with induction of a Th1-dominated cytokine response. Clin Exp Immunol 2002;127:206–213.
44. Hsieh CS, Macatonia SE, O'Garra A, Murphy KM. T cell genetic background determines default T helper phenotype development in vitro. J Exp Med 1995;181:713–721.
45. Moser C, Johansen HK, Song Z, Hougen HP, Rygaard J, Hoiby N. Chronic *Pseudomonas aeruginosa* lung infection is more severe in Th2 responding BALB/c mice compared to Th1 responding C3H/HeN mice. APMIS 1997; 105:838–842.
46. Nieuwenhuis EE, Matsumoto T, Exley M, et al. CD1d-dependent macrophage-mediated clearance of *Pseudomonas aeruginosa* from lung. Nat Med 2002;8: 588–593.
47. Grubb BR, Boucher RC. Pathophysiology of gene-targeted mouse models for cystic fibrosis. Physiol Rev 1999;79:S193–S214.
48. Hyde SC, Gill DR, Higgins CF, et al. Correction of the ion transport defect in cystic fibrosis transgenic mice by gene therapy. Nature 1993;362:250–255.

49. Alton EW, Middleton PG, Caplen NJ, et al. Non-invasive liposome-mediated gene delivery can correct the ion transport defect in cystic fibrosis mutant mice. Nat Genet 1993;5:135–142.

50. Grubb BR, Pickles RJ, Ye H, et al. Inefficient gene transfer by adenovirus vector to cystic fibrosis airway epithelia of mice and humans. Nature 1994;371:802–806.

51. Zabner J, Ramsey BW, Meeker DP, et al. Repeat administration of an adenovirus vector encoding cystic fibrosis transmembrane conductance regulator to the nasal epithelium of patients with cystic fibrosis. J Clin Invest 1996;97:1504–1511.

52. Knowles MR, Hohneker KW, Zhou Z, et al. A controlled study of adenoviral-vector-mediated gene transfer in the nasal epithelium of patients with cystic fibrosis. N Engl J Med 1995;333:823–831.

53. Beers MH, Berkow R. The Merck manual of diagnosis and therapy. Whitehouse Station, NJ: Merck Research Laboratories, 1999.

54. Piitulainen E, Eriksson S. Decline in FEV1 related to smoking status in individuals with severe alpha1-antitrypsin deficiency (PiZZ). Eur Respir J 1999; 13:247–251.

55. Eriksson S. Pulmonary emphysema and alpha1-antitrypsin deficiency. Acta Med Scand 1964;175:197–205.

56. Parmar JS, Mahadeva R, Reed BJ, et al. Polymers of alpha(1)-antitrypsin are chemotactic for human neutrophils: a new paradigm for the pathogenesis of emphysema. Am J Respir Cell Mol Biol 2002;26:723–730.

57. Foronjy R, D'Armiento J. The role of collagenase in emphysema. Respir Res 2001;2:348–352.

58. Gross P, Pfitzer EA, Tolker E, Babyak MA, Kaschak M. Experimental emphysema: its production with papain in normal and silicotic rats. Arch Environ Health 1965;11:50–58.

59. Janoff A, Sloan B, Weinbaum G, et al. Experimental emphysema induced with purified human neutrophil elastase: tissue localization of the instilled protease. Am Rev Respir Dis 1977;115:461–478.

60. Senior RM, Tegner H, Kuhn C, Ohlsson K, Starcher BC, Pierce JA. The induction of pulmonary emphysema with human leukocyte elastase. Am Rev Respir Dis 1977;116:469–475.

61. Kao RC, Wehner NG, Skubitz KM, Gray BH, Hoidal JR. Proteinase 3. A distinct human polymorphonuclear leukocyte proteinase that produces emphysema in hamsters. J Clin Invest 1988;82:1963–1973.

62. Kuhn C, Yu SY, Chraplyvy M, Linder HE, Senior RM. The induction of emphysema with elastase. II. Changes in connective tissue. Lab Invest 1976; 34:372–380.

63. Snider GL, Lucey EC, Stone PJ. Animal models of emphysema. Am Rev Respir Dis 1986;133:149–169.

64. Kasahara Y, Tuder RM, Taraseviciene-Stewart L, et al. Inhibition of VEGF receptors causes lung cell apoptosis and emphysema. J Clin Invest 2000;106: 1311–1319.

65. Shapiro SD. Animal models for COPD. Chest 2000;117:223S-227S.
66. Brantly M, Nukiwa T, Crystal RG. Molecular basis of alpha-1-antitrypsin deficiency. Am J Med 1988;84:13–31.
67. Mahadeva R, Lomas DA. Genetics and respiratory disease. 2. Alpha 1-antitrypsin deficiency, cirrhosis and emphysema. Thorax 1998;53:501–505.
68. Blackwood RA, Cerreta JM, Mandl I, Turino GM. Alpha 1-antitrypsin deficiency and increased susceptibility to elastase-induced experimental emphysema in a rat model. Am Rev Respir Dis 1979;120:1375–1379.
69. Blackwood RA, Moret J, Mandl I, Turino GM. Emphysema induced by intravenously administered endotoxin in an alpha 1-antitrypsin-deficient rat model. Am Rev Respir Dis 1984;130:231–236.
70. Campbell EJ. Animal models of emphysema: the next generations. J Clin Invest 2000; 106:1445, 1446.
71. Long GL, Chandra T, Woo SL, Davie EW, Kurachi K. Complete sequence of the cDNA for human alpha 1-antitrypsin and the gene for the S variant. Biochemistry 1984;23:4828–4837.
72. Bao JJ, Reed-Fourquet L, Sifers RN, Kidd VJ, Woo SL. Molecular structure and sequence homology of a gene related to alpha 1-antitrypsin in the human genome. Genomics 1988;2:165–173.
73. Dawkins PA, Stockley RA. Animal models of chronic obstructive pulmonary disease. Thorax 2001;56:972–977.
74. Tardiff J, Krauter KS. Divergent expression of alpha1-protease inhibitor genes in mouse and human. Nucleic Acids Res 1998;26:3794–3799.
75. Janus ED, Phillips NT, Carrell RW. Smoking, lung function, and alpha1-antitrypsin deficiency. Lancet 1985;1:152–154.
76. Keil M, Lungarella G, Cavarra E, van Even P, Martorana PA. A scanning electron microscopic investigation of genetic emphysema in tight-skin, pallid, and beige mice, three different C57 BL/6J mutants. Lab Invest 1996;74:353–362.
77. Perou CM, Justice MJ, Pryor RJ, Kaplan J. Complementation of the beige mutation in cultured cells by episomally replicating murine yeast artificial chromosomes. Proc Natl Acad Sci USA 1996;93:5905–5909.
78. Nagle DL, Karim MA, Woolf EA, et al. Identification and mutation analysis of the complete gene for Chediak-Higashi syndrome. Nat Genet 1996;14:307–311.
79. Perou CM, Moore KJ, Nagle DL, et al. Identification of the murine beige gene by YAC complementation and positional cloning. Nat Genet 1996;13:303–308.
80. Fisk DE, Kuhn C. Emphysema-like changes in the lungs of the blotchy mouse. Am Rev Respir Dis 1976;113:787–797.
81. Mechanic GL, Farb RM, Henmi M, Ranga V, Bromberg PA, Yamauchi M. Structural crosslinking of lung connective tissue collagen in the blotchy mouse. Exp Lung Res 1987;12:109–117.
82. McCartney AC, Fox B, Partridge TA, et al. Emphysema in the blotchy mouse: a morphometric study. J Pathol 1988;156:77–81.
83. Mercer JF, Grimes A, Ambrosini L, et al. Mutations in the murine homologue of the Menkes gene in dappled and blotchy mice. Nat Genet 1994;6:374–378.

84. Martorana PA, van Even P, Gardi C, Lungarella G. A 16-month study of the development of genetic emphysema in tight-skin mice. Am Rev Respir Dis 1989;139:226–232.

85. Kielty CM, Raghunath M, Siracusa LD, et al. The tight skin mouse: demonstration of mutant fibrillin-1 production and assembly into abnormal microfibrils. J Cell Biol 1998;140:1159–1166.

86. Martorana PA, Brand T, Gardi C, et al. The pallid mouse. A model of genetic alpha 1-antitrypsin deficiency. Lab Invest 1993;68:233–241.

87. Huang L, Kuo YM, Gitschier J. The pallid gene encodes a novel, syntaxin 13-interacting protein involved in platelet storage pool deficiency. Nat Genet 1999;23:329–332.

88. Cavarra E, Bartalesi B, Lucattelli M, et al. Effects of cigarette smoke in mice with different levels of alpha(1)-proteinase inhibitor and sensitivity to oxidants. Am J Respir Crit Care Med 2001;164:886–890.

89. D'Armiento J, Dalal SS, Okada Y, Berg RA, Chada K. Collagenase expression in the lungs of transgenic mice causes pulmonary emphysema. Cell 1992;71: 955–961.

90. Dalal S, Imai K, Mercer B, Okada Y, Chada K, D'Armiento JM. A role for collagenase (Matrix metalloproteinase-1) in pulmonary emphysema. Chest 2000; 117:227S–228S.

91. Finlay GA, Russell KJ, McMahon KJ, et al. Elevated levels of matrix metalloproteinases in bronchoalveolar lavage fluid of emphysematous patients. Thorax 1997;52:502–506.

92. Finlay GA, O'Driscoll LR, Russell KJ, et al. Matrix metalloproteinase expression and production by alveolar macrophages in emphysema. Am J Respir Crit Care Med 1997;156:240–247.

93. Imai K, Dalal SS, Chen ES, et al. Human collagenase (matrix metalloproteinase-1) expression in the lungs of patients with emphysema. Am J Respir Crit Care Med 2001;163:786–791.

94. Hoyle GW, Li J, Finkelstein JB, et al. Emphysematous lesions, inflammation, and fibrosis in the lungs of transgenic mice overexpressing platelet-derived growth factor. Am J Pathol 1999;154:1763–1775.

95. Hardie WD, Piljan-Gentle A, Dunlavy MR, Ikegami M, Korfhagen TR. Dose-dependent lung remodeling in transgenic mice expressing transforming growth factor-alpha. Am J Physiol Lung Cell Mol Physiol 2001;281:L1088–L1094.

96. Ray P, Tang W, Wang P, et al. Regulated overexpression of interleukin 11 in the lung. Use to dissociate development-dependent and -independent phenotypes. J Clin Invest 1997;100:2501–2511.

97. Stripp BR, Sawaya PL, Luse DS, et al. *cis*-acting elements that confer lung epithelial cell expression of the *CC10* gene. J Biol Chem 1992;267:14,703–14,712.

98. Tang W, Geba GP, Zheng T, et al. Targeted expression of IL-11 in the murine airway causes lymphocytic inflammation, bronchial remodeling, and airways obstruction. J Clin Invest 1996;98:2845–2853.

99. Zheng T, Zhu Z, Wang Z, et al. Inducible targeting of IL-13 to the adult lung causes matrix metalloproteinase- and cathepsin-dependent emphysema. J Clin Invest 2000;106:1081–1093.

100. Wang Z, Zheng T, Zhu Z, et al. Interferon gamma induction of pulmonary emphysema in the adult murine lung. J Exp Med 2000;192:1587–1600.

101. Bostrom H, Willetts K, Pekny M, et al. PDGF-A signaling is a critical event in lung alveolar myofibroblast development and alveogenesis. Cell 1996;85: 863– 873.

102. Nakamura T, Lozano PR, Ikeda Y, et al. Fibulin-5/DANCE is essential for elastogenesis in vivo. Nature 2002;415:171–175.

103. Weinstein M, Xu X, Ohyama K, Deng CX. FGFR-3 and FGFR-4 function cooperatively to direct alveogenesis in the murine lung. Development 1998;125:3615–3623.

104. Hautamaki RD, Kobayashi DK, Senior RM, Shapiro SD. Requirement for macrophage elastase for cigarette smoke-induced emphysema in mice. Science 1997;277:2002–2004.

105. Suga T, Kurabayashi M, Sando Y, et al. Disruption of the *klotho* gene causes pulmonary emphysema in mice. Defect in maintenance of pulmonary integrity during postnatal life. Am J Respir Cell Mol Biol 2000;22:26–33.

106. Lanone S, Zheng T, Zhu Z, et al. Overlapping and enzyme-specific contributions of matrix metalloproteinases-9 and -12 in IL-13-induced inflammation and remodeling. J Clin Invest 2002;110:463–474.

107. Imai K, D'Armiento J. Activation of an embryonic gene product in pulmonary emphysema: identification of the secreted frizzled-related protein. Chest 2000; 117S:229S.

108. Imai K, D'Armiento J. Differential gene expression of sFRP-1 and apoptosis in pulmonary emphysema. Chest 2002;121:7S.

109. Dolin PJ, Raviglione MC, Kochi A. Global tuberculosis incidence and mortality during 1990–2000. Bull World Health Organ 1994;72:213–220.

110. Young DB, Duncan K. Prospects for new interventions in the treatment and prevention of mycobacterial disease. Annu Rev Microbiol 1995;49:641– 673.

111. Kaufmann SH. How can immunology contribute to the control of tuberculosis? Nat Rev Immunol 2001;1:20–30.

112. Russell DG. *Mycobacterium tuberculosis*: here today, and here tomorrow. Nat Rev Mol Cell Biol 2001;2:569–577.

113. Bloom BR, Murray CJ. Tuberculosis: commentary on a reemergent killer. Science 1992;257:1055–1064.

114. Andersen P. TB vaccines: progress and problems. Trends Immunol 2001;22: 160–168.

115. Cole ST, Brosch R, Parkhill J, et al. Deciphering the biology of *Mycobacterium tuberculosis* from the complete genome sequence. Nature 1998;393:537–544.

116. Domenech P, Barry CE, 3rd, Cole ST. *Mycobacterium tuberculosis* in the postgenomic age. Curr Opin Microbiol 2001;4:28–34.

117. Gordon SV, Brosch R, Billault A, Garnier T, Eiglmeier K, Cole ST. Identification of variable regions in the genomes of tubercle bacilli using bacterial artificial chromosome arrays. Mol Microbiol 1999;32:643–655.
118. Behr MA, Wilson MA, Gill WP, et al. Comparative genomics of BCG vaccines by whole-genome DNA microarray. Science 1999;284:1520–1523.
119. McMurray DN. Disease model: pulmonary tuberculosis. Trends Mol Med 2001;7:135–137.
120. Casanova JL, Abel L. Genetic dissection of immunity to mycobacteria: the human model. Annu Rev Immunol 2002;20:581–620.
121. Gros P, Skamene E, Forget A. Genetic control of natural resistance to *Mycobacterium bovis* (BCG) in mice. J Immunol 1981;127:2417–2421.
122. Stach JL, Gros P, Forget A, Skamene E. Phenotypic expression of genetically-controlled natural resistance to *Mycobacterium bovis* (BCG). J Immunol 1984;132:888–892.
123. Govoni G, Vidal S, Cellier M, Lepage P, Malo D, Gros P. Genomic structure, promoter sequence, and induction of expression of the mouse Nramp1 gene in macrophages. Genomics 1995;27:9–19.
124. Vidal SM, Malo D, Vogan K, Skamene E, Gros P. Natural resistance to infection with intracellular parasites: isolation of a candidate for Bcg. Cell 1993;73: 469–485.
125. Vidal S, Tremblay ML, Govoni G, et al. The Ity/Lsh/Bcg locus: natural resistance to infection with intracellular parasites is abrogated by disruption of the Nramp1 gene. J Exp Med 1995;182:655–666.
126. Gruenheid S, Pinner E, Desjardins M, Gros P. Natural resistance to infection with intracellular pathogens: the Nramp1 protein is recruited to the membrane of the phagosome. J Exp Med 1997;185:717–730.
127. Cellier M, Govoni G, Vidal S, et al. Human natural resistance-associated macrophage protein: cDNA cloning, chromosomal mapping, genomic organization, and tissue-specific expression. J Exp Med 1994;180:1741–1752.
128. Liu J, Fujiwara TM, Buu NT, et al. Identification of polymorphisms and sequence variants in the human homologue of the mouse natural resistance-associated macrophage protein gene. Am J Hum Genet 1995;56:845–853.
129. Bellamy R, Ruwende C, Corrah T, McAdam KP, Whittle HC, Hill AV. Variations in the NRAMP1 gene and susceptibility to tuberculosis in West Africans. N Engl J Med 1998;338:640–644.
130. Medina E, North RJ. The Bcg gene (Nramp1) does not determine resistance of mice to virulent *Mycobacterium tuberculosis*. Ann NY Acad Sci 1996;797:257–259.
131. Mitsos LM, Cardon LR, Fortin A, et al. Genetic control of susceptibility to infection with *Mycobacterium tuberculosis* in mice. Genes Immun 2000;1:467–477.
132. Kramnik I, Dietrich WF, Demant P, Bloom BR. Genetic control of resistance to experimental infection with virulent *Mycobacterium tuberculosis*. Proc Natl Acad Sci USA 2000;97:8560–8565.
133. MacMicking JD, North RJ, LaCourse R, Mudgett JS, Shah SK, Nathan CF. Identification of nitric oxide synthase as a protective locus against tuberculosis. Proc Natl Acad Sci USA 1997;94:5243–5248.

134. Brett S, Orrell JM, Swanson Beck J, Ivanyi J. Influence of H-2 genes on growth of *Mycobacterium tuberculosis* in the lungs of chronically infected mice. Immunology 1992;76:129–132.
135. Medina E, North RJ. Resistance ranking of some common inbred mouse strains to *Mycobacterium tuberculosis* and relationship to major histocompatibility complex haplotype and Nramp1 genotype. Immunology 1998;93: 270–274.
136. Bothamley GH, Beck JS, Schreuder GM, et al. Association of tuberculosis and *M. tuberculosis*-specific antibody levels with HLA. J Infect Dis 1989;159:549–555.
137. Goldfeld AE, Delgado JC, Thim S, et al. Association of an HLA-DQ allele with clinical tuberculosis. JAMA 1998;279:226–228.
138. Mehta PK, King CH, White EH, Murtagh JJ, Jr., Quinn FD. Comparison of in vitro models for the study of *Mycobacterium tuberculosis* invasion and intracellular replication. Infect Immun 1996;64:2673–2679.
139. Flynn JL, Goldstein MM, Triebold KJ, Koller B, Bloom BR. Major histocompatibility complex class I-restricted T cells are required for resistance to *Mycobacterium tuberculosis* infection. Proc Natl Acad Sci USA 1992;89: 12,013–12,017.
140. Balk S. MHC evolution. Nature 1995;374:505–506.
141. Lordan JL, Bucchieri F, Richter A, et al. Cooperative effects of Th2 cytokines and allergen on normal and asthmatic bronchial epithelial cells. J Immunol 2002;169:407–414.
142. Holtzman MJ, Morton JD, Shornick LP, et al. Immunity, inflammation, and remodeling in the airway epithelial barrier: epithelial-viral-allergic paradigm. Physiol Rev 2002;82:19–46.
143. National Institutes of Health, National Heart, Lung, and Blood Institute. Data Fact Sheet: Asthma Statistics, Vol 2002, 2002.
144. Morse B, Sypek JP, Donaldson DD, Haley KJ, Lilly CM. Effects of IL-13 on airway responses in the guinea pig. Am J Physiol Lung Cell Mol Physiol 2002;282:L44–L49.
145. Elwood W, Lotvall JO, Barnes PJ, Chung KF. Characterization of allergen-induced bronchial hyperresponsiveness and airway inflammation in actively sensitized brown-Norway rats. J Allergy Clin Immunol 1991;88:951–960.
146. de Weck AL, Mayer P, Stumper B, Schiessl B, Pickart L. Dog allergy, a model for allergy genetics. Int Arch Allergy Immunol 1997;113:55–57.
147. Persson CG. Con: mice are not a good model of human airway disease. Am J Respir Crit Care Med 2002;166:6, 7; discussion 8.
148. Malm-Erjefalt M, Persson CG, Erjefalt JS. Degranulation status of airway tissue eosinophils in mouse models of allergic airway inflammation. Am J Respir Cell Mol Biol 2001;24:352–359.
149. Gelfand EW. Pro: mice are a good model of human airway disease. Am J Respir Crit Care Med 2002;166:5, 6; discussion 7, 8.
150. Hogaboam CM, Blease K, Mehrad B, et al. Chronic airway hyperreactivity, goblet cell hyperplasia, and peribronchial fibrosis during allergic airway disease induced by *Aspergillus fumigatus*. Am J Pathol 2000;156:723–732.

151. Wills-Karp M, Ewart SL. The genetics of allergen-induced airway hyperresponsiveness in mice. Am J Respir Crit Care Med 1997;156:S89–S96.
152. Temelkovski J, Hogan SP, Shepherd DP, Foster PS, Kumar RK. An improved murine model of asthma: selective airway inflammation, epithelial lesions and increased methacholine responsiveness following chronic exposure to aerosolised allergen. Thorax 1998;53:849–856.
153. Sakai K, Yokoyama A, Kohno N, Hamada H, Hiwada K. Prolonged antigen exposure ameliorates airway inflammation but not remodeling in a mouse model of bronchial asthma. Int Arch Allergy Immunol 2001;126:126–134.
154. Kumar RK, Foster PS. Modeling allergic asthma in mice: pitfalls and opportunities. Am J Respir Cell Mol Biol 2002;27:267–272.
155. Louahed J, Toda M, Jen J, et al. Interleukin-9 upregulates mucus expression in the airways. Am J Respir Cell Mol Biol 2000;22:649–656.
156. Wu CA, Puddington L, Whiteley HE, et al. Murine cytomegalovirus infection alters Th1/Th2 cytokine expression, decreases airway eosinophilia, and enhances mucus production in allergic airway disease. J Immunol 2001;167: 2798–2807.
157. Hansen G, Berry G, DeKruyff RH, Umetsu DT. Allergen-specific Th1 cells fail to counterbalance Th2 cell-induced airway hyperreactivity but cause severe airway inflammation. J Clin Invest 1999;103:175–183.
158. Castro M, Walter MJ, Chaplin DD, Holtzman MJ. Could asthma worsen by stimulating the T helper type 1 (Th1) response? Am J Respir Cell Mol Biol 2000;22:143–146.
159. Holtzman MJ, Agapov E, Kim E, Kim J, Morton JD. Developing the epitheial-viral-allergic (Epi-vir-all) paradigm for asthma. Chest 2003;123(Suppl 3):377S–384S.
160. Randolph DA, Carruthers CJ, Szabo SJ, Murphy KM, Chaplin DD. Modulation of airway inflammation by passive transfer of allergen-specific Th1 and Th2 cells in a mouse model of asthma. J Immunol 1999;162:2375–2383.
161. Randolph DA, Stephens R, Carruthers CJ, Chaplin DD. Cooperation between Th1 and Th2 cells in a murine model of eosinophilic airway inflammation. J Clin Invest 1999;104:1021–1029.
162. Stephens R, Randolph DA, Huang G, Holtzman MJ, Chaplin DD. Antigen-nonspecific recruitment of Th2 cells to the lung as a mechanism for viral infection-induced allergic asthma. J Immunol 2002;169:5458–5467.
163. Sigurs N, Bjarnason R, Sigurbergsson F, Kjellman B. Respiratory syncytial virus bronchiolitis in infancy is an important risk factor for asthma and allergy at age 7. Am J Respir Crit Care Med 2000;161:1501–1507.
164. Schwarze J, Hamelmann E, Bradley KL, Takeda K, Gelfand EW. Respiratory syncytial virus infection results in airway hyperresponsiveness and enhanced airway sensitization to allergen. J Clin Invest 1997;100:226–233.
165. Walter MJ, Morton JD, Kajiwara N, Agapov E, Holtzman MJ. Viral induction of a chronic asthma phenotype and genetic segregation from the acute response. J Clin Invest 2002;110:165–175.
166. Fan T, Yang M, Halayko A, Mohapatra SS, Stephens NL. Airway responsiveness in two inbred strains of mouse disparate in IgE and IL-4 production. Am J Respir Cell Mol Biol 1997;17:156–163.

167. Duguet A, Biyah K, Minshall E, et al. Bronchial responsiveness among inbred mouse strains. Role of airway smooth-muscle shortening velocity. Am J Respir Crit Care Med 2000;161:839–848.

168. Drazen JM, Finn PW, De Sanctis GT. Mouse models of airway responsiveness: physiological basis of observed outcomes and analysis of selected examples using these outcome indicators. Annu Rev Physiol 1999;61:593–625.

169. Levitt RC, Mitzner W. Expression of airway hyperreactivity to acetylcholine as a simple autosomal recessive trait in mice. FASEB J 1988;2:2605–2608.

170. Hamelmann E, Schwarze J, Takeda K, et al. Noninvasive measurement of airway responsiveness in allergic mice using barometric plethysmography. Am J Respir Crit Care Med 1997;156:766–775.

171. Chiba Y, Yanagisawa R, Sagai M. Strain and route differences in airway responsiveness to acetylcholine in mice. Res Commun Mol Pathol Pharmacol 1995;90:169–172.

172. Levitt RC, Mitzner W. Autosomal recessive inheritance of airway hyperreactivity to 5-hydroxytryptamine. J Appl Physiol 1989;67:1125–1132.

173. Zhang LY, Levitt RC, Kleeberger SR. Differential susceptibility to ozone-induced airways hyperreactivity in inbred strains of mice. Exp Lung Res 1995;21:503–518.

174. Miyabara Y, Yanagisawa R, Shimojo N, et al. Murine strain differences in airway inflammation caused by diesel exhaust particles. Eur Respir J 1998;11: 291–298.

175. Konno S, Adachi M, Matsuura T, et al. Bronchial reactivity to methacholine and serotonin in six inbred mouse strains. Arerugi 1993;42:42–47.

176. Longphre M, Kleeberger SR. Susceptibility to platelet-activating factor-induced airway hyperreactivity and hyperpermeability: interstrain variation and genetic control. Am J Respir Cell Mol Biol 1995;13:586–594.

177. Tankersley CG, Fitzgerald RS, Levitt RC, Mitzner WA, Ewart SL, Kleeberger SR. Genetic control of differential baseline breathing pattern. J Appl Physiol 1997;82:874–881.

178. Gavett SH, Wills-Karp M. Elevated lung G protein levels and muscarinic receptor affinity in a mouse model of airway hyperreactivity. Am J Physiol 1993;265:L493–L500.

179. Brewer JP, Kisselgof AB, Martin TR. Genetic variability in pulmonary physiological, cellular, and antibody responses to antigen in mice. Am J Respir Crit Care Med 1999;160:1150–1156.

180. Ewart SL, Kuperman D, Schadt E, et al. Quantitative trait loci controlling allergen-induced airway hyperresponsiveness in inbred mice. Am J Respir Cell Mol Biol 2000;23:537–545.

181. Van Oosterhout AJ, Jeurink PV, Groot PC, Hofman GA, Nijkamp FP, Demant P. Genetic analysis of antigen-induced airway manifestations of asthma using recombinant congenic mouse strains. Chest 2002;121:13S.

182. Moore KJ, Nagle DL. Complex trait analysis in the mouse: The strengths, the limitations and the promise yet to come. Annu Rev Genet 2000;34:653–686.

183. Dietrich WF, Miller JC, Steen RG, et al. A genetic map of the mouse with 4,006 simple sequence length polymorphisms. Nat Genet 1994;7:220–245.

184. Wade CM, Kulbokas EJI, Kirby AW, et al. The mosaic structure of variation in the laboratory mouse genome. Nature 2002;420:574–578.
185. Stuber CW, Lincoln SE, Wolff DW, Helentjaris T, Lander ES. Identification of genetic factors contributing to heterosis in a hybrid from two elite maize inbred lines using molecular markers. Genetics 1992;132:823–839.
186. Knott SA, Haley CS, Thompson R. Methods of segregation analysis for animal breeding data: a comparison of power. Heredity 1992;68:299–311.
187. Churchill GA, Doerge RW. Empirical threshold values for quantitative trait mapping. Genetics 1994;138:963–971.
188. Doerge RW, Churchill GA. Permutation tests for multiple loci affecting a quantitative character. Genetics 1996;142:285–294.
189. Zhang Y, Lefort J, Kearsey V, Lapa e Silva JR, Cookson WO, Vargaftig BB. A genome-wide screen for asthma-associated quantitative trait loci in a mouse model of allergic asthma. Hum Mol Genet 1999;8:601–605.
190. Lander ES, Green P, Abrahamson J, et al. MAPMAKER: an interactive computer package for constructing primary genetic linkage maps of experimental and natural populations. Genomics 1987;1:174–181.
191. De Sanctis GT, Merchant M, Beier DR, et al. Quantitative locus analysis of airway hyperresponsiveness in A/J and C57BL/6J mice. Nat Genet 1995;11:150–154.
192. De Sanctis GT, Drazen JM. Genetics of native airway responsiveness in mice. Am J Respir Crit Care Med 1997;156:S82–S88.
193. Drazen JM, Takebayashi T, Long NC, De Sanctis GT, Shore SA. Animal models of asthma and chronic bronchitis. Clin Exp Allergy 1999;29(Suppl 2): 37–47.
194. Ewart SL, Mitzner W, DiSilvestre DA, Meyers DA, Levitt RC. Airway hyperresponsiveness to acetylcholine: segregation analysis and evidence for linkage to murine chromosome 6. Am J Respir Cell Mol Biol 1996;14:487–495.
195. De Sanctis GT, Singer JB, Jiao A, et al. Quantitative trait locus mapping of airway responsiveness to chromosomes 6 and 7 in inbred mice. Am J Physiol 1999;277:L1118–L1123.
196. De Sanctis GT, Singer JB, Jiao A, et al. Quantitative trait locus mapping of airway responsiveness to chromosomes 6 and 7 in inbred mice. Am J Physiol 1999;277:L1118–L1123.
197. Mouton D, Siqueira M, Sant'Anna OA, et al. Genetic regulation of multispecific antibody responsiveness: improvement of "high" and "low" characters. Eur J Immunol 1988;18:41–49.
198. McIntire JJ, Umetsu SE, Akbari O, et al. Identification of Tapr (an airway hyperreactivity regulatory locus) and the linked Tim gene family. Nat Immunol 2001;2:1109–1116.
199. Silver LM. Mouse genetics: concepts and applications. Oxford, UK: Oxford University Press, 1995.
200. Van Etten WJ, Steen RG, Nguyen H, et al. Radiation hybrid map of the mouse genome. Nat Genet 1999;22:384–387.
201. Gregory SG, Sekhon M, Schein J, et al. A physical map of the mouse genome. Nature 2002;418:743–750.

202. Shubitowski DM, Wills-Karp M, Ewart SL. The complement factor 5a receptor gene maps to murine chromosome 7. Cytogenet Genome Res 2002;97: 133–135.
203. Mills JC, Roth KA, Cagan RL, Gordon JI. DNA microarrays and beyond: completing the journey from tissue to cell. Nat Cell Biol 2001;3:E175–E178.
204. Karp CL, Grupe A, Schadt E, et al. Identification of complement factor 5 as a susceptibility locus for experimental allergic asthma. Nat Immunol 2000;1: 221–226.
205. Doull IJ, Lawrence S, Watson M, et al. Allelic association of gene markers on chromosomes 5q and 11q with atopy and bronchial hyperresponsiveness. Am J Respir Crit Care Med 1996;153:1280–1284.
206. Renauld JC, Kermouni A, Vink A, Louahed J, Van Snick J. Interleukin-9 and its receptor: involvement in mast cell differentiation and T cell oncogenesis. J Leukoc Biol 1995;57:353–360.
207. Nicolaides NC, Holroyd KJ, Ewart SL, et al. Interleukin 9: a candidate gene for asthma. Proc Natl Acad Sci USA 1997;94:13,175–13,180.
208. McMillan SJ, Bishop B, Townsend MJ, McKenzie AN, Lloyd CM. The absence of interleukin 9 does not affect the development of allergen-induced pulmonary inflammation nor airway hyperreactivity. J Exp Med 2002;195:51–57.
209. Wang DG, Fan JB, Siao CJ, et al. Large-scale identification, mapping, and genotyping of single-nucleotide polymorphisms in the human genome. Science 1998;280:1077–1082.
210. Saiki RK, Walsh PS, Levenson CH, Erlich HA. Genetic analysis of amplified DNA with immobilized sequence-specific oligonucleotide probes. Proc Natl Acad Sci USA 1989;86:6230–6234.
211. Lindblad-Toh K, Winchester E, Daly MJ, et al. Large-scale discovery and genotyping of single-nucleotide polymorphisms in the mouse. Nat Genet 2000; 24:381–386.
212. Chen J, Iannone MA, Li MS, et al. A microsphere-based assay for multiplexed single nucleotide polymorphism analysis using single base chain extension. Genome Res 2000;10:549–557.
213. Hirschhorn JN, Sklar P, Lindblad-Toh K, et al. SBE-TAGS: an array-based method for efficient single-nucleotide polymorphism genotyping. Proc Natl Acad Sci USA 2000;97:12,164–12,169.
214. Kurg A, Tonisson N, Georgiou I, Shumaker J, Tollett J, Metspalu A. Arrayed primer extension: solid-phase four-color DNA resequencing and mutation detection technology. Genet Test 2000;4:1–7.
215. Grupe A, Germer S, Usuka J, et al. In silico mapping of complex disease-related traits in mice. Science 2001;292:1915–1918.
216. Patil N, Berno AJ, Hinds DA, et al. Blocks of limited haplotype diversity revealed by high-resolution scanning of human chromosome 21. Science 2001;294:1719–1723.
217. Dubchak I, Brudno M, Loots GG, et al. Active conservation of noncoding sequences revealed by three-way species comparisons. Genome Res 2000;10: 1304–1306.

218. Loots GG, Locksley RM, Blankespoor CM, et al. Identification of a coordinate regulator of interleukins 4, 13, and 5 by cross-species sequence comparisons. Science 2000;288:136–140.
219. Symula DJ, Frazer KA, Ueda Y, et al. Functional screening of an asthma QTL in YAC transgenic mice. Nat Genet 1999;23:241–244.
220. Lacy DA, Wang ZE, Symula DJ, et al. Faithful expression of the human 5q31 cytokine cluster in transgenic mice. J Immunol 2000;164:4569–4574.
221. Chen Y, Zhao YH, Wu R. In silico cloning of mouse Muc5b gene and upregulation of its expression in mouse asthma model. Am J Respir Crit Care Med 2001;164:1059–1066.
222. Temann UA, Ray P, Flavell RA. Pulmonary overexpression of IL-9 induces Th2 cytokine expression, leading to immune pathology. J Clin Invest 2002;109:29–39.
223. O'Neal WK, Hasty P, McCray PB, Jr, et al. A severe phenotype in mice with a duplication of exon 3 in the cystic fibrosis locus. Hum Mol Genet 1993;2:1561–1569.
224. Hasty P, O'Neal WK, Liu KQ, et al. Severe phenotype in mice with termination mutation in exon 2 of cystic fibrosis gene. Somat Cell Mol Genet 1995;21:177–187.
225. Cohn L, Homer RJ, Niu N, Bottomly K. T helper 1 cells and interferon gamma regulate allergic airway inflammation and mucus production. J Exp Med 1999;190:1309–1318.
226. Coyle AJ, Tsuyuki S, Bertrand C, et al. Mice lacking the IFN-gamma receptor have impaired ability to resolve a lung eosinophilic inflammatory response associated with a prolonged capacity of T cells to exhibit a Th2 cytokine profile. J Immunol 1996;156:2680–2685.
227. Seymour BW, Gershwin LJ, Coffman RL. Aerosol-induced immunoglobulin (Ig)-E unresponsiveness to ovalbumin does not require CD8+ or T cell receptor (TCR)-gamma/delta+ T cells or interferon (IFN)-gamma in a murine model of allergen sensitization. J Exp Med 1998;187:721–731.
228. Brusselle GG, Kips JC, Tavernier JH, et al. Attenuation of allergic airway inflammation in IL-4 deficient mice. Clin Exp Allergy 1994;24:73–80.
229. Cohn L, Tepper JS, Bottomly K. IL-4-independent induction of airway hyperresponsiveness by Th2, but not Th1, cells. J Immunol 1998;161:3813–3816.
230. Hogan SP, Mould A, Kikutani H, Ramsay AJ, Foster PS. Aeroallergen-induced eosinophilic inflammation, lung damage, and airways hyperreactivity in mice can occur independently of IL-4 and allergen-specific immunoglobulins. J Clin Invest 1997;99:1329–1339.
231. Rankin JA, Picarella DE, Geba GP, et al. Phenotypic and physiologic characterization of transgenic mice expressing interleukin 4 in the lung: lymphocytic and eosinophilic inflammation without airway hyperreactivity. Proc Natl Acad Sci USA 1996;93:7821–7825.
232. Trifilieff A, Fujitani Y, Coyle AJ, Kopf M, Bertrand C. IL-5 deficiency abolishes aspects of airway remodelling in a murine model of lung inflammation. Clin Exp Allergy 2001;31:934–942.

233. Coyle AJ, Kohler G, Tsuyuki S, Brombacher F, Kopf M. Eosinophils are not required to induce airway hyperresponsiveness after nematode infection. Eur J Immunol 1998;28:2640–2647.

234. Lee JJ, McGarry MP, Farmer SC, et al. Interleukin-5 expression in the lung epithelium of transgenic mice leads to pulmonary changes pathognomonic of asthma. J Exp Med 1997;185:2143–2156.

235. Wang J, Homer RJ, Chen Q, Elias JA. Endogenous and exogenous IL-6 inhibit aeroallergen-induced Th2 inflammation. J Immunol 2000;165:4051–4061.

236. DiCosmo BF, Geba GP, Picarella D, et al. Airway epithelial cell expression of interleukin-6 in transgenic mice. Uncoupling of airway inflammation and bronchial hyperreactivity. J Clin Invest 1994;94:2028–2035.

237. De Sanctis GT, MacLean JA, Qin S, et al. Interleukin-8 receptor modulates IgE production and B-cell expansion and trafficking in allergen-induced pulmonary inflammation. J Clin Invest 1999;103:507–515.

238. Makela MJ, Kanehiro A, Borish L, et al. IL-10 is necessary for the expression of airway hyperresponsiveness but not pulmonary inflammation after allergic sensitization. Proc Natl Acad Sci USA 2000;97:6007–6012.

239. Hogan SP, Foster PS, Tan X, Ramsay AJ. Mucosal IL-12 gene delivery inhibits allergic airways disease and restores local antiviral immunity. Eur J Immunol 1998;28:413–423.

240. Webb DC, McKenzie AN, Koskinen AM, Yang M, Mattes J, Foster PS. Integrated signals between IL-13, IL-4, and IL-5 regulate airways hyperreactivity. J Immunol 2000;165:108–113.

241. Mattes J, Yang M, Siqueira A, et al. IL-13 induces airways hyperreactivity independently of the IL-4R alpha chain in the allergic lung. J Immunol 2001; 167:1683–1692.

242. Walter DM, Wong CP, DeKruyff RH, Berry GJ, Levy S, Umetsu DT. Il-18 gene transfer by adenovirus prevents the development of and reverses established allergen-induced airway hyperreactivity. J Immunol 2001;166:6392–6398.

243. Zhang DH, Yang L, Cohn L, et al. Inhibition of allergic inflammation in a murine model of asthma by expression of a dominant-negative mutant of GATA-3. Immunity 1999;11:473–482.

244. Finotto S, De Sanctis GT, Lehr HA, et al. Treatment of allergic airway inflammation and hyperresponsiveness by antisense-induced local blockade of GATA-3 expression. J Exp Med 2001;193:1247–1260.

245. Finotto S, Neurath MF, Glickman JN, et al. Development of spontaneous airway changes consistent with human asthma in mice lacking T-bet. Science 2002;295:336–338.

246. Kuperman D, Schofield B, Wills-Karp M, Grusby MJ. Signal transducer and activator of transcription factor 6 (Stat6)-deficient mice are protected from antigen-induced airway hyperresponsiveness and mucus production. J Exp Med 1998;187:939–948.

247. Akimoto T, Numata F, Tamura M, et al. Abrogation of bronchial eosinophilic inflammation and airway hyperreactivity in signal transducers and activators of transcription (STAT)6-deficient mice. J Exp Med 1998;187:1537–1542.

248. Mehlhop PD, van de Rijn M, Goldberg AB, et al. Allergen-induced bronchial hyperreactivity and eosinophilic inflammation occur in the absence of IgE in a mouse model of asthma. Proc Natl Acad Sci USA 1997;94:1344–1349.

249. Hatfield CA, Brashler JR, Winterrowd GE, et al. Intercellular adhesion molecule-1-deficient mice have antibody responses but impaired leukocyte recruitment. Am J Physiol 1997;273:L513–L523.

250. Humbles AA, Lu B, Nilsson CA, et al. A role for the C3a anaphylatoxin receptor in the effector phase of asthma. Nature 2000;406:998–1001.

251. Korsgren M, Erjefalt JS, Korsgren O, Sundler F, Persson CG. Allergic eosinophil-rich inflammation develops in lungs and airways of B cell-deficient mice. J Exp Med 1997;185:885–892.

252. Justice JP, Shibata Y, Sur S, Mustafa J, Fan M, Van Scott MR. IL-10 gene knockout attenuates allergen-induced airway hyperresponsiveness in C57BL/6 mice. Am J Physiol Lung Cell Mol Physiol 2001;280:L363–L368.

253. Takeda K, Hamelmann E, Joetham A, et al. Development of eosinophilic airway inflammation and airway hyperresponsiveness in mast cell-deficient mice. J Exp Med 1997;186:449–454.

7

Murine Models of Osteoporosis

Robert F. Klein

1. INTRODUCTION

Osteoporosis is a disease characterized by an inadequate amount and/or faulty structure of bone, which increases the susceptibility to fracture with minimal trauma. Osteoporotic fractures are most commonly observed among the elderly. Yet, the pathogenesis of osteoporosis starts early in life, leading some researchers to view osteoporosis as a pediatric disease *(1)*. Considerable past research has centered on the influence of reproductive, nutritional, and/or life-style factors on the development of osteoporosis. With the advent of new molecular genetic approaches, the focus of research has recently shifted toward genetic factors. Genetic epidemiological studies provide convincing descriptive data including population and ethnic differences, studies of familial aggregation, familial transmission patterns, and comparisons of twin concordance rates that tell a significant part of how the vulnerability to developing osteoporosis is inherited *(2,3)*. Almost certainly, the development of osteoporosis will be found to involve a complex interplay between both genetic and environmental factors that are difficult to control in complex populations.

Susceptibility to osteoporosis appears to involve the interaction of multiple environmental and genetic factors *(4)*. It has been argued that fracture is the most relevant trait for a genetic analysis of osteoporosis *(5)*. However, any fracture event is the result of a number of elements including the amount and quality of bone, as well as nonskeletal factors, such as muscle mass and neurological coordination *(6–8)*. Consequently, most investigators have adopted alternative strategies employing surrogate phenotypes for genetic studies of osteoporosis. Studies that resolve the global phenotype of fragility fracture into relevant intermediate traits, such as density and geometry, are likely to yield more mechanistic insights not only into the regulation of skeletal strength but also into the overall processes of skeletal development.

From: *Computational Genetics and Genomics*
Edited by: G. Peltz © Humana Press Inc., Totowa, NJ

The load-bearing capacity of a skeletal element is determined by both its intrinsic material properties (density) and the total amount (size) and spatial distribution (shape) of the bone tissue. Low bone mineral density (BMD), independent of other factors, such as falls and aging, is the strongest known determinant of osteoporotic fracture risk *(6,7,9)*. However, osteoporotic fractures are also more likely in subjects with smaller bone size *(10–12)*. Studies of stress fractures in young, healthy adults indicate that diaphyseal dimensions (even after correction for body weight) are significantly smaller in fracture cases *(13–15)*. Bone morphology is strongly driven by gender, physical activity, and dietary and genetic factors *(16,17)*. Skeletal structural phenotypes behave as quantitative (polygenic) traits with continuous variation. The continuous variation is the consequence of the additive effects of genes (alleles) at multiple genetic loci that influence skeletal development. Discrete skeletal phenotypes are not generally discernible by studying the frequency distributions. Polygenic inheritance for skeletal traits makes sense, because bone development is known to be influenced by multiple biochemical, mechanical, and physiological systems, each of which may have its own genetic inputs. The challenge is to characterize these multiple genetic inputs *(5)*. Quantitative traits pose new problems for gene cloning experiments. The deoxyribonucleic acid (DNA) sequence variants that are responsible for them are unlikely to be immediately recognizable. In contrast to many qualitative traits, in which a discrete phenotypic difference is often the consequence of an inactivating mutation, the allelic variation responsible for quantitative traits probably has a subtler basis.

There are two general approaches to the genetic basis of individuality in complex traits: candidate gene analysis and quantitative trait locus (QTL) analysis. Candidate gene analysis seeks to test the association between a particular genetic variant (i.e., allele) and a specific trait. If the variant is more frequent in subjects with the trait than those without it, one can infer that either there is a causal relationship between the genetic variant and the trait or the variant is in linkage disequilibrium with a responsible gene residing near the locus in question. Although a straightforward enterprise, osteoporosis researchers employing candidate gene analysis face a dilemma. Given the complexity of skeletal physiology, there are likely to be an incredibly large number of candidate genes responsible for the acquisition and maintenance of bone mass. Analysis of each one of these candidates, in isolation of the others, is likely to be prohibitive and difficult to interpret statistically and biologically *(18,19)*. In contrast, QTL analysis involves a true search for genes at different chromosomal locations without any assumptions about the candidacy of particular genes or genomic regions. A QTL is defined as a site

specific genes. The obvious requirement for a reasonably detailed knowledge of basic genomic structure currently limits the choice for genetic animal models of osteoporosis to mice, rats, and nonhuman primates.

Mice and rats are by far the most commonly used animals in bone research. Both mice and rats reach peak bone mass early in their lifespan and then undergo bone loss with aging *(39–43)*. Following ovariectomy, a reduction in bone mass and strength occurs, which can be prevented by estrogen replacement *(44–49)*. The SAMP6 (senescence-accelerated mouse/prone) mouse has low peak bone mass and develops fractures in middle and old age *(50–57)*. It is the only experimental animal model with documented fragility fractures of aging. Histomorphometric studies of primates and humans yield very similar values *(58)*. The nonhuman primate has both growing and adult skeletal phases. Peak bone mass occurs around age 9 yr in cynomologus macaques *(59)* and around 10–11 yr in rhesus monkeys *(60,61)*. Nonhuman primates experience decreased bone mass after ovariectomy *(62–64)*, but the response to estrogen replacement has not been well characterized. Nonhuman primates experience bone loss with age *(65,66)*, but older animals also develop osteoarthritis with spinal osteophyte formation *(67–69)* that can obscure the accurate radiographic assessment of spinal bone mass *(70)*. The extreme requirements for housing and care of nonhuman primates limit their use to a relatively small number of facilities.

Of the three currently available options, the mouse is arguably the model of choice because of the following:

1. Mice are much cheaper to house and easier to handle.
2. Mouse genetic resources are quite extensive.
3. Once candidate genes are identified, the ability to manipulate them in mice and to unambiguously deduce their role in disease is unparalleled *(71,72)*.

Moreover, gene targeting has reached new heights in mice but is barely on the horizon in other animals. With gene targeting, perhaps, as the ultimate arbiter for establishing cause-and-effect relationships between a candidate gene and osteoporosis susceptibility, the mouse is apt to remain the primary experimental model system for the foreseeable future *(72)*. However, nonhuman primates maintained in controlled environments are excellent subjects for extended family pedigree analysis *(73,74)*, the most powerful method of establishing genetic linkage to phenotypic traits *(18)*. Combining mouse and nonhuman primate studies to dissect the genetic regulation of bone mass may offer the most expeditious way of identifying relevant hypotheses that are likely to prove fruitful for future exploration in humans.

3. CURRENT RESEARCH

3.1. Inbred Strains

A strain of a species is inbred when virtually every genetic locus is homozygous. What this means is that all individuals within an inbred strain share a set of characteristics that uniquely define them compared to other strains. Typically, inbred strains are derived from 20 or more consecutive generations that have been brother-sister mated; the strain can then be maintained with this same pattern of propagation. Individual animals within an inbred strain are as identical as monozygotic twins. There are several qualities of inbred strains that make them especially valuable for research. The first is their long-term relative genetic stability. This is important because it allows researchers to build on previous investigations. Genetic change can occur only as a result of mutation within an inbred strain. A second important quality of inbred animals is their homozygosity, because inbred strains will breed true. Once the characteristics of a strain are known, they can be reproduced repeatedly, allowing for replicate experimentation, as well as for studies by other investigators. The influence of genotype on a particular characteristic can be investigated by placing mice from several inbred strains in a common environment. Observed differences must then be, within limits, the consequence of genetic factors. By reversing this strategy, and placing mice from a single inbred strain in a variety of environments, it is possible to estimate the importance of environmental influences on a parameter of interest. Thus, inbred animals can be used to determine whether genetic variation in the expression of a characteristic exists, as well as the environmental malleability of the characteristic. Experiments with inbred strains also have some limitations. Although strain differences are easily demonstrated, it is often very difficult to attach much meaning to these differences, because the genes and gene products involved are usually unknown. Because comparisons of mice from two or more strains do not usually provide any information about the nature of the genetic differences, crosses between genotypes must be used to analyze patterns of genetic influence. Additionally, when using an inbred strain to investigate any type of phenomenon, it is important to be aware that the observations may be relevant only to that strain. Because an inbred strain differs from all others, there will be characteristics unique to it. It is therefore important to use more than one strain to confirm that any observation obtained pertains to the species and not just to the strain studied.

Inbred mice of different strains exhibit marked differences in parameters of skeletal integrity. Kaye and Kusy *(75)* examined bone tissue from five inbred mouse strains (A/J, BALB/CByJ, C57BL/6J, DBA/2J, and PL/J).

Although body weight was similar in all five strains, tibial bone mass, composition, and biomechanical strength varied considerably. Using peripheral quantitative computed tomography, Beamer et al. *(76)* surveyed female mice from 11 inbred strains. This seminal study found that phenotypically normal inbred strains of mice possess remarkable differences in total femoral BMD that were detectable as early as 2 mo of age. Although these genetically distinct strains of mice were raised in the same controlled environment, the observed differences are, in all likelihood, the result of genetic variation. As mentioned earlier, bone strength is a complex phenotype that includes bone density, size, and shape, as well as other anthropomorphic variables. A subsequent analysis of three of those inbred strains (C57BL/6J, DBA/2J, and C3H/HeJ) found additional evidence for genetic regulation of long bone size and shape, as well as BMD *(77)*. In a study of 10 inbred strains of mice, Li et al. *(78)* found heritability estimates for humeral breaking strength to be moderately high at 0.68 and multiregression analysis showed that forearm BMD, forelimb grip strength, and forearm bone size were the three major determinants of bone strength-explaining 61% of the variation in bone breaking strength. A recent detailed examination of two inbred strains of mice with very different femoral peak bone densities (C57BL/6J and C3H/HeJ) suggested that bone strength in an inbred strain can differ considerably by site *(79)*. C3H/HeJ mice possessed thicker femoral and vertebral cortices compared with C57BL/6J mice. However, C3H/HeJ mice had fewer trabeculae in the vertebral bodies, and vertebral bone strength was reduced in the C3H/HeJ compared to the C57BL/6J, suggesting the presence of distinct genetic determinants that regulate the trabecular vs cortical compartments of bone. These preliminary investigations clearly indicate substantial genetic regulation of skeletal traits in mice. Modern genetic methods, such as selective breeding and QTL analysis, can exploit these heritable strain differences to find and more directly evaluate the genetic linkage of osteoporosis-related traits (*see* Subheading 3.4). Furthermore, modern computational methods are now being developed that can scan a murine single nucleotide polymorphism (SNP) database and, only on the basis of known inbred strain phenotypes and genotypes, rapidly identify the chromosomal regions that most likely contribute to a given complex trait *(80)*.

3.2. Single Gene Mutations

As described in Subheading 3.1., the study of inbred strains usually provides very little information about specific mechanisms of gene action. The analysis of single mutant vs normal genes is often a more effective approach. Comparisons between homozygous mutant mice and their "normal" homozygous wild-type and heterozygous litter mates may provide considerable information on cellular mechanisms critical for discrete aspects of bone biology *(81,82)*. Mouse enthusiasts have been breeding mice for centuries, thus maintaining spontaneous mutations. More than 140 spontaneous mutations affecting mouse bone morphology have been summarized by Green *(83)*. For example, the short ear *(se/se)* mutation (the result of a disruption of the bone morphogenetic protein-5) is associated with a number of skeletal defects, including reductions in long bone length and width and the size of several vertebral processes, the absence of several small sesamoid bones and a pair of ribs, and impaired fracture healing *(84–87)*. There is also an expanding list of induced mutations in mice that cause recognizable skeletal pathology. Several lines of mice with mutations in type 1 collagen genes develop a phenotype of skeletal fragility with extensive fractures of long bones and ribs *(88–91)*, and mice that are deficient in certain extracellular noncollagenous matrix components, such as biglycan and osteopontin, have been shown to have decreased bone mass after birth *(92,93)*. Mutations of a number of genes necessary for normal osteoclast development and/or function have been shown to result in abnormal skeletal development in mice *(94–98)*. Such studies of both naturally occurring and engineered (transgenic) mutant mice have clearly extended our current knowledge of skeletal development *(99)*. It can be anticipated that future work with such models will not only further expand our understanding of the role of known regulators on skeletal development but also may identify new genes with unexpected roles in skeletal biology.

3.3. Recombinant Inbred Strains

Independently inbred strains of mice frequently exhibit numerous phenotypic differences reflecting the substantial allelic variability that can exist between laboratory strains. These differences have been accentuated further by the introduction of recombinant inbred (RI) strains, which are derived by systematic inbreeding starting from a cross between two inbred strains known to differ at some characteristic of interest (Fig. 1). They are called RI strains because the parental chromosomes are recombined several times per chromosome during their development, resulting in a unique pattern of recombinations of the two initial parental genomes in each RI strain. The starting points are two inbred genotypes that are used to produce a group of F1 hybrids. Brother–sister pairs of F1 hybrids are mated to create an F2 generation, in which all genes now segregate independently. Following the production of an F2 generation from this interstrain cross, 20 or more different brother–sister pairs of F2 individuals are mated. In each subsequent

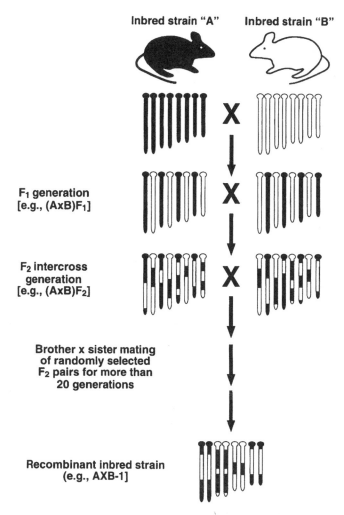

Fig. 1. Generation of recombinant inbred strains. Only four of the 19 autosome pairs from parental inbred strains "A" and "B" and the assortment of chromosomes in the subsequent crosses derived from these strains, are shown. F1 hybrids are genetically identical to each other but individuals in the subsequent F2 generation are not because of recombination events. Recombinant inbred strains also harbor recombinations but are homozygous at all loci as a result of the extensive inbreeding involved in their production.

generation, only a single male and female from each pair are mated. After 20 generations, one has many inbred lines that differ from each other because of random differences in gene segregation, a process begun with the F2. All the RI lines contain only those genes that were present in one or another of the parental strains. RI lines have been very useful in genetic mapping of traits that differ between inbred strains.

The RI strains were originally developed as a tool for detecting and mapping major gene loci *(100)*. Over the years, the RI strains have been characterized in respect to many genetic markers with known locations on different chromosomes. The influence of a single major gene on a given trait can be inferred when RI strain means for the trait are found to fall in a bimodal distribution (i.e., all the RI strains with one allele are in one phenotypic group, and all those with the other allele are in the other group). Comparison of the strain distribution pattern (SDP) for that trait can be made with the SDPs for known marker loci previously mapped to a particular chromosome region. A close match in SDPs between the unknown locus and a marker locus would thus allow provisional mapping to a chromosome region of the latter *(100,101)*. Recent advances in statistics have succeeded in tailoring this experimental approach to a broader range of phenotypes, including continuously distributed traits without apparent major gene effects *(102–104)*.

The first panel of RI strains to be used for exploration of skeletal traits was the BXD panel, derived from a cross between C57BL/6J and DBA/2J progenitors *(105,106)*. Peak whole-body areal BMD values differed by approx 20% among individual RI strains—indicating the presence of strong genetic influences. When the pattern of differences in peak whole body BMD in the BXD (C57BL/6 × DBA/2) strains was integrated with a large database of genetic markers previously defined in the RI BXD strains, chromosome map sites (QTLs) for BMD were generated. Interestingly, separate analyses of male and female RI strain sets provisionally identified two chromosomal loci associated with peak BMD that were shared between genders, pointing out that in some cases common genetic mechanisms influence skeletal development. However, the majority of the provisional loci were associated with peak BMD in one, but not both genders, suggesting the presence of gender-specific determinants of BMD. Using a similar approach, Shimizu et al. recently examined cortical thickness index in adult male mice from the AKR/J strain and the 13 senescence-accelerated mouse (SAM) strains, which are considered to be a series of RI strains derived from the AKR/J strain and other unspecified strains *(107)*. These investigators found substantial variation in cortical thickness index (50%) among the SAM RI strain set and found evidence for polygenic inheritance of this skeletal trait. As an initial exploration of the genetic determinants of bone strength, Turner et al. examined female mice from 12 BXH RI strains of mice derived from C57BL/6J and C3H/HeJ progenitor strains *(108)*. Biomechanical properties measured across the BXH RI panel showed greater variability than either B6 or C3H progenitors, indicating that combinations of genes play an important role in determining bone strength. Furthermore, vertebral strength was not correlated consistently with femoral strength among the BXH RI strains, suggesting that genetic regulation of bone strength may be site-specific.

An especially important feature of the RI method is the fixed nature of the genotypes of each of the RI strains. This means that any new hypothesis about a physiological mechanism underlying a trait can be assessed by making only observations on the new variable and relating the outcome to the database already established *(109)*. For example, epidemiological studies have clearly demonstrated that body weight is a very strong predictor of BMD *(110–113)*. However, the mechanism underlying the strong association of weight with BMD is poorly understood. The coincidence of increased body weight with increased BMD could stem from environmental factors, such as complementary nutritional effects on body composition and skeletal mass, or the association could largely be the result of mechanical loading *(114)*. In addition to environmental causes, body weight and BMD may be modulated by linked genes or perhaps even the same genes. In the previously described BXD RI experiment *(105)*, four genetic loci for body weight were identified. All of these loci had been previously identified by Keightley et al. *(115)* in a prior analysis of mouse lines divergently selected for body weight from a base population derived from C57BL/6J and DBA/2J parental strains. Interestingly, one locus that was linked to body weight was also strongly linked to inherited variation in BMD. These findings raised the intriguing possibility that body weight and peak BMD may be influenced by linked genes or perhaps by common genes with pleiotropic effects. Furthermore, they demonstrate the increasing value of an RI series as data, both about phenotypes and genotypes, are gathered from all of the laboratories utilizing them.

There are two additional aspects of the RI approach that deserve comment. First, only a few inbred strains are represented in the existing RI sets (e.g., the BXD RI set is the largest, and it currently is composed of only 36 separate strains), and it is not easy to construct new sets. Inasmuch as the strain means are the units of analysis, the statistical power of the RI method is directly related to the number of RI strains within a given set. Thus, genetic associations only above a certain impact size will be discernible with this experimental method. For osteoporosis research purposes, this limitation is a modest one because the current objective is simply to identify any relevant genetic associations in either animal models or humans. A second, perhaps more serious, disadvantage of the RI method is that some genetic correlations of marker and phenotype are likely to be fortuitous. Because of the large number of statistical tests performed (e.g., more than 1500 informative genetic markers have been genotyped in the BXD RI strains), the type 1 error rate relative to a single correlation similarly increases. One way to reduce the chance of such errors is to increase the required significance level and consider only those correlations that are significant at a very high probability *(116)*. However, in choosing this level of stringency, one risks not considering QTLs that may be important (i.e., type 2 error). A useful compromise is to use a moderately stringent α level and regard correlational analysis in RI strains as a preliminary screen for genetic associations to be confirmed using other techniques, such as verification in an F2 population *(117)*.

Another genetic tool, similar to the RI method, is a panel of recombinant congenic strains. These strains differ from RI strains because two additional backcrosses are made to a recipient strain to achieve progeny that carry 12.5% of genes from the donor strain (rather than the 50% present in RI strains). The intent of this strategy is to isolate small assemblages of genes in individual inbred strains. Using a set of 24 HcB/Dem recombinant congenic strains (derived from donor C57BL/10ScSnA and recipient C3H/DiSnA strains), Yershov et al. *(118)* have identified seven different QTLs that influence bone strength and/or various parameters of skeletal geometry.

3.4. QTL Analysis

For a number of reasons, the laboratory mouse has proven to be an especially powerful tool for the identification and mapping of QTLs affecting complex polygenic traits *(119)*. First, there is a wide range of phenotypic variation in genetically characterized animals *(120)*, which is a prerequisite for QTL analysis. Second, factors, such as short generation interval, ability to make designed matings and raise very large populations relatively inexpensively, and capacity to control or experimentally alter environmental factors, enable QTL experiments in mice to have increased power, precision, and flexibility. Third, the mouse has an extensively developed and well-organized molecular marker map, consisting of more than 6500 easily typed polymerase chain reaction (PCR) based microsatellite markers *(121)* that exhibit allelic variation between lines. And fourth, the mouse is an anchor species in comparative genome maps representing homology among mammalian species *(122)*. Once a chromosomal region harboring a murine QTL is identified, candidate chromosomal regions in humans, in which homologous QTLs may reside, will be immediately apparent. Based on these attributes, research groups have successfully used mice in QTL detection studies for a number of quantitative traits, including obesity *(123)*, body weight *(115)*, and drug-seeking behavior *(124)*.

Osteoporosis researchers are just now embarking on QTL analyses in large populations of mice in the hopes of obtaining a more complete picture of the polygenic control of bone mass and an improved understanding of the complex interactions and physiological mechanisms involved. The basic strategy of such QTL mapping experiments is outlined in Fig. 2.

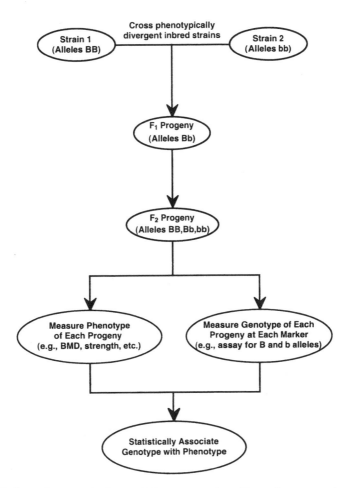

Fig. 2. Steps in quantitative trait locus mapping. To perform quantitative trait locus (QTL) analysis, two different inbred strains are first crossed to produce genetically heterogeneous F2 progeny. All of the progeny undergo phenotype assessment, and following this, DNA samples are obtained to allow genotyping of each individual at multiple marker loci distributed throughout the genome. Statistical associations of markers and phenotypes are then performed to identify putative QTLs underlying the trait(s) of interest. BMD, bone mineral density.

The procedure, as applied to the detection of BMD QTLs, involves cross-ing one inbred mouse strain that has low BMD with another mouse strain that has high BMD. The resulting F1 offspring usually exhibit BMD val-ues between those of the parental strains. The next step is to intercross the F1 mice with one another to create a second filial generation (F2). Because of recombination between the parental alleles and segregation of these alle-les in the offspring, the variation in BMD within the population of F2 mice can exceed that of the parental strains. By genotyping the F2 generation of mice and correlating genotype with phenotype, it is possible to identify regions of the genome (QTL) that segregate with BMD and hence show evidence of linkage to BMD. The most recent QTL mapping efforts have primarily utilized microsatellite markers, also known as simple sequence length polymorphisms, which are highly polymorphic, naturally occurring variations in the number of repetitive base pair sequences *(19,23,24)*. These are readily genotyped by PCR amplification using oligonucleotide primer pairs specific to each markers followed by resolution of PCR prod-ucts (alleles) on standard agarose or denaturing polyacrylamide genes *(23,24)*. This development has greatly facilitated the genotyping of large numbers of individuals in a genetically heterogeneous F2 population to determine which alleles each animal possesses at many marker loci. In the mouse, there are presently more than 15,000 PCR-based microsatellite markers available, each with known chromosomal location that can be used in a genome-wide search *(27)*.

Several recent studies have illustrated that QTL analysis can be success-fully applied to skeletal phenotypes, and importantly, some QTLs have been independently confirmed. Results from these complementary studies should begin to define the landscape of the genetic regulation of BMD and help par-tition this quantitative trait into separate genetic components amenable for more detailed evaluation. Table 1 summarizes data from several sets of genetically heterogeneous F2 populations including: C57BL/6J vs Castaneus/EiJ *(125)*, C57BL/6J vs C3H/HeJ *(126)*, C57BL/6J vs DBA/2J *(106,117,127)*, SAMP6 vs SAMP2 *(128)*, SAMR1 vs SAMP6 *(129)*, and AKR/J vs SAMP6 *(129)*. It is apparent that QTL analyses of diverse skeletal phenotypes (whole-body BMD, femoral cortical thickness, and vertebral and total femoral BMD) in genetically heterogeneous murine populations derived from disparate inbred strains have succeeded in identifying common chromosomal regions that strongly influence bone mass. Although the most parsimonious explanation for the concordance of findings between the vari-ous murine models is the presence of a single important gene at the same chromosomal site *(129)*, much higher resolution fine-mapping will be

Table 1
Bone Mineral Density QTLs Identified in Various
Laboratory Mouse Populations

Chromosome	Position	Skeletal site	F2 cross	References
1	Distal	S, F, WB	B6XD2, B6XCast, B6XC3H	*117,125,126*
2	Proximal	S	AKRXSAMP6, SAMR1XSAMP6	*129*
2	Mid	WB	B6XD2	*117*
2	Distal	F	B6XD2	*127*
3	Proximal	F	B6XD2	*127*
4	Mid	S, F, WB	B6XD2, B6XC3H	*117,126*
5	Mid	F	B6XCast	*125*
6	Mid	F	B6XC3H, B6XD2	*126,127*
7	Proximal	S, F, WB	B6XD2, SAMR1XSAMP6	*106,129*
7	Distal	S	B6XC3H	*126*
9	Mid	S	B6XC3H	*126*
11	Mid	S, F, WB	B6XD2, B6XC3H, SAMP6XSAMP2, AKRXSAMP6	*117,126,128,129*
12	Proximal	F	B6XC3H	*126*
13	Proximal	S, F, WB	B6XD2, B6XCast, B6XC3H, SAMP6XSAMP2, AKRXSAMP6	*80,125,126, 128,129*
13	Mid	S, F	B6XC3H	*126*
14	Mid	S, F	B6XC3H	*126*
15	Proximal	F	B6XD2, B6XCast	*125,127*
15	Distal	F	B6XD2	*127*
16	Proximal	S, F	B6XC3H, SAMR1XSAMP6	*126,129*
18	Proximal	S, F	B6XC3H	*126*

S, spinal; F, femoral; WB, whole body.

needed to exclude the possibility of multiple strain-specific, closely linked loci within a given common QTL region.

Genotyping intercross progeny for an average-sized QTL mapping experiment has traditionally required many months and thousands of individual genotyping reactions. An alternative source of naturally occurring variations is SNPs. Current databases contain allele information across many common inbred strains for thousands of SNPs at defined locations in the mouse genome. Recently, the genome of pooled DNA samples obtained from inter-cross progeny was analyzed by two different genotyping methods *(80)*. The traditional method of genotyping individual DNA samples with a panel of microsatellite markers was directly compared to a streamlined approach in which allele frequencies of a panel of SNPs were determined by allele-specific kinetic PCR in pooled DNA samples. Both methods identified the exact same linkage regions, but SNP-based genotyping of pooled samples required about 20-fold fewer PCR reactions and was performed much more quickly than the traditional method. Such strategies promise to reduce the frustrations and overcome some of the difficulties (e.g., cost) associated with QTL analysis in murine complex disease models.

4. FUTURE DIRECTIONS

The primary objective of QTL analysis is the identification of the chromo-somal position of genes influencing osteoporosis-related traits. However, the ultimate goals of complex trait analysis—to identify coding sequences and to understand their biological roles at a molecular level—remain the major challenge. Cloning the gene underlying a QTL requires refining the position of the QTL at much higher resolution than does initial detection of the QTL. As an example, for positional cloning to be feasible, the size of the candidate region must be reduced to less than approx 1 Mb (~0.5 cM), which on aver-age is expected to contain about 10–15 genes in the mouse *(130)*. Interval analysis of F2 mapping data has generally resulted in fairly large chromoso-mal assignments for each of the BMD-related QTLs (10–30 cM or 100–500 possible genes). This is because the phenotypes of individual animals are easily swayed by the influence of unlinked or environmental noise *(72)*. Positional cloning of human disease genes has demonstrated that even when the position of a gene has been defined within 1 or 2 million bp and all the DNA sequences within that region have been isolated, identification of the relevant gene can still be a formidable task. Fortunately, new experimental strategies for fine QTL mapping, development of transgenic technologies, and more traditional approaches employing congenic strains, promise to eventually bridge the gap between cloning and disease.

QTL fine-mapping involves careful analysis of recombinants within an interval previously found to contain the gene, a concept termed genetic chro-mosome dissection. Although genetic chromosome dissection was first intro-duced by *Drosophila* geneticists *(131)*, this experimental approach has been successfully adapted to animal models *(132–134)*. For a compilation of the various experimental designs currently available, the reader is referred to an excellent recent review by Darvasi in which several options for attaining 1-cM map resolution in the mouse are described *(135)*. One of these approaches, termed RI segregation testing, takes advantage of the fixed recombination between parental alleles that exist in RI strains *(100)*. This strategy employs a RI strain that possesses a crossover (recombination point) within the QTL of interest to generate two F2 populations—one with each parental strain. By using linkage analysis to determine within which of the two genetically heterogeneous populations phenotype segregates with genotype, the QTL can be mapped either above or below the recombination point, and successive iterations of this strategy can be used to narrow the QTL to a smaller chromosomal region (Fig. 3). Once the QTL has been resolved to such a narrow region, an examination of candidate genes within that region can take place. This approach has recently been successfully employed to substantially narrow two BMD-related chromosomal regions and, in the process, eliminated a number of candidate genes *(117)*.

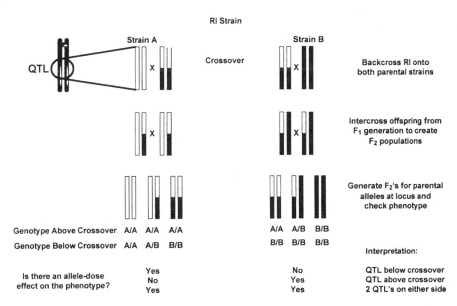

Fig. 3. The recombinant inbred (RI) segregation test strategy. A RI strain that possesses a recombination or crossover point in the region of a quantitative trait locus (QTL) is used to generate two F2 populations-one with each parental strain. Analysis of the two populations will detect the population on which the QTL is segregating and accordingly locate the QTL above or below the recombination point.

Transgenic technology creates a very effective tool for analyzing the physiological roles of specific genes. A transgenic animal contains a segment of exogenous genetic material stably incorporated into its genome, resulting in a new trait that can be transmitted to further generations. Two widely used methods introduce exogenous genetic material into the genome:

1. Microinjection of one-cell fertilized embryos.
2. Genetic manipulation of embryonic stem (ES) cells.

In contrast to traditional "gain-of-function" mutations, typically created by microinjection of the gene of interest into the one-celled zygote, gene targeting via homologous recombination in pluripotential ES cells allows one to precisely modify the gene of interest *(136)*. Employing ES methodology, investigators have generated site-specific deletions ("knockouts"), insertions ("knockins"), gene duplications, gene rearrangements, and point mutations. In addition to facilitating the study of known candidate genes, molecular complementation (transfer of specific genes) of selected phenotypes is a potentially important tool for gene identification. The recent success of transgenic technologies employing yeast artificial chromosomes (YAC transgenics) holds great promise for studying QTLs that influence a developmentally restricted phenotype which requires the transfer of both the locus and the long-range regulatory element(s) responsible for normal temporal or regional expression of the gene *(137)*. Traditionally, the mouse has been considered the optimal animal model for conducting transgenic and gene-targeting experiments. Although investigators have succeeded in creating transgenic rats *(138)*, the considerable time and expense involved limit the feasibility of widespread use of this animal model. Furthermore, gene-targeting technology to "knockout" endogenous genes is currently feasible only in the mouse.

Classical transmission genetics can also be used to transfer a gene of interest from a donor strain or mutant onto the genetic background of an inbred strain. Using this approach, one is able to transfer regions containing risk or protective QTLs, or even multiple QTLs, onto appropriate background strains. Such congenic strains are produced by repeated backcrossing to the background inbred strain and genotypic selection of the desired allele at a marker or markers at each backcross generation *(100,139,140)*. After seven backcross generations, the congenic and background strains can be expected to be about 98% genetically identical except for the transferred (introgressed) chromosomal region *(140)*. The primary advantage of the congenics is that the influence of an individual QTL on any trait can be tested using the congenic vs background strain comparison at any level from the molecular to the physiological. Any differences found would strongly implicate a QTL in the introgressed chromosomal region as the cause of the differences. When there are several congenic strains for a given QTL, their differing sites of recombination can aid in attaining higher resolution mapping of the QTL with respect to neighboring markers. The near elimination of "genetic noise" because of unlinked loci greatly aids the search for candidate genes associated with each QTL and for studies of differential gene expression *(141)*. Ultimately, congenic strains will provide an invaluable resource for further defining specific aspects of genetic architecture (e.g., mode of inheritance, gene order, and gene–gene and gene–environment interactions, and so on) and for in-depth studies of the mechanisms by which they affect skeletal development.

A number of groups have now reported the generation and initial characterization of congenic strains bearing BMD-relevant QTLs. Shimizu et al. constructed a congenic strain P6.P2-Pbd2b, which carried a single genomic interval from chromosome 13 of SAMP2 on a SAMP6-derived osteoporotic background *(142)*. This congenic strain had a higher bone density (~10%) than the background strain. Orwoll et al. are currently developing a congenic strain for a BMD QTL on chromosome 2 and have found that mice carrying the *C57BL/6* allele on a DBA/2 background exhibit reduced BMD (~5%) compared to the background strain *(106)*. Moreover, the effect of the QTL on BMD was observed only in female mice, just as had been predicted from previous F2 studies *(106)*. Congenics can also offer insight into the mechanisms involved in peak bone mass acquisition. Bouxsein et al. recently constructed congenic mice carrying a genomic interval from chromosome 6 of C3H/HeJ on a C57BL/6J-derived background *(143)*. The chromosome 6 region contained a QTL known to strongly influence serum insulin-like growth factor-I (IGF-I) levels. As expected, congenic mice had 11–21% lower serum IGF-I levels at 16 wk of age compared with B6, but importantly, these mice also exhibited reduced femoral and vertebral BMD, implicating a role of IGF-I variation in normal skeletal development. Finally, it may be possible to combine the mapping data present in congenic strains with expression analysis (e.g., complementary DNA microarray analysis) to identify, without bias about potential roles, putative target genes underlying a given QTL. Gu et al. *(144)* generated a congenic strain, B6.CAST-1T, in which the chromosomal fragment containing a femoral BMD QTL had been transferred from the Castaneus to the C57BL/6 (B6) background. The congenic mice had significantly higher bone density than the B6 mice. Preliminary complementary DNA microarray analysis demonstrated approx 60% of 8734 gene accessions on murine GEM I chips (Incyte Genomics,

Palo Alto, CA) were expressed in the femur of B6 mice. Interestingly, expression levels of genes related to bone formation were lower in congenic than in B6 mice, and expression levels of genes that might have negative regulatory action on bone resorption were higher in congenic than in B6 mice. Together, these findings suggest that the congenic mice might have a lower bone turnover rate than B6 mice and raise the possibility that the high bone density in the congenic mice could be caused by reduced bone resorption rather than increased bone formation.

5. CONCLUSIONS

Peak bone mass is a major determinant of risk of osteoporotic fracture. However, BMD is a complex trait whose expression is complicated by environmental influences and polygenic inheritance. The number, locations, and effects of the individual genes contributing to natural variation in this trait are all unknown. Experimental animal models furnish a means to largely circumvent confounding environmental factors, and the availability of dense genetic maps based on molecular markers now provides the opportunity to resolve quantitative genetic variation in individual regions of the genome (QTLs) influencing a given trait. Animals are easily bred to provide the sample sizes needed. Inbred strains are homozygous at all loci. Therefore, all members of any inbred strain are genetically identical, eliminating the problem of genetic heterogeneity. Phenotypes can be carefully measured and laboratory conditions held uniform to reduce phenotypic variation.

The systematic analysis of inbred strain databases is beginning to reveal important aspects of the genetic regulation of bone mass acquisition and maintenance. The recent advances in genetic analysis of complex traits, such as QTL mapping of genetically heterogeneous intercross populations, are especially promising. A major strength of this approach is that it enables the provisional identification of candidate genes in the absence of any prior hypothesis about the mechanism by which the phenotype is expressed. The identification of those chromosomal regions, in which marker allelic and trait variation significantly covary, is now a straightforward (although large-scale) enterprise. QTL mapping offers an attractive interface between forward and reverse genetics. Molecular cloning has shown that almost all genes in mice have homologs in humans and vice-versa *(145)*. Thus, identification and mapping of genes in the mouse offers immediate hope for extrapolation to the human genome. For the future, more molecularly based techniques are likely to be on the leading edge of progress. As candidate genes are identified as having important skeletal functions, the tools of molecular biology will allow the genetic diversity underlying their expression and function to be more fully examined. Discoveries made with animal models can often set the stage for skeletal research in human subjects to augment the results from animals and confirm their relevance to our own species. Perhaps the most versatile aspect of animal model systems is in their use as a proving ground for hypotheses regarding the genetic, as well as the epigenetic, basis of osteoporosis. Old ideas regarding disease mechanisms can now be rigorously tested in vivo, and what is more important, provocative new concepts can emerge.

ACKNOWLEDGMENTS

This work was supported by funds from the National Institutes of Health (AR 44659) and the Medical Research Service of the Veterans Affairs.

REFERENCES

1. Matkovic V. Osteoporosis as a pediatric disease: role of calcium and heredity. J Rheumatol 1992;33(Suppl):54–59.
2. Stewart TL, Ralston SH. Role of genetic factors in the pathogenesis of osteoporosis. J Endocrinol 2000;166:235–245.
3. Rizzoli R, Bonjour JP, Ferrari SL. Osteoporosis, genetics and hormones. J Mol Endocrinol 2001;26:79–94.
4. Eisman JA. Genetics of osteoporosis. Endocr Rev 1999;20:788–804.
5. Deng H-W, Chen W-M, Recker S, et al. Genetic determination of Colles' fracture and differential bone mass in women with and without Colles' fracture. J Bone Miner Res 2000;15:1243–1252.
6. Hui SL, Slemenda CW, Johnston CCJ. Age and bone mass as predictors of fracture in a prospective study. J Clin Invest 1988;81:1804–1809.
7. Cummings SR, Black DM, Nevitt MC, et al. Appendicular bone density and age predict hip fracture in women. JAMA 1990;263:665–668.
8. Nguyen T, Sambrook P, Kelly P, et al. Prediction of osteoporotic fractures by postural instability and bone density. BMJ 1993;307:1111–1115.
9. Nguyen T, Sambrook P, Kelly P, et al. Prediction of osteoporotic fractures by postural instability and bone density. Br Med J 1993;307:1111–1115.
10. Bradney M, Karlsson MK, Duan Y, Stuckey S, Bass S, Seeman E. Heterogeneity in the growth of the axial and appendicular skeleton in boys: implications for the pathogenesis of bone fragility in men. J Bone Miner Res 2000;15: 1871–1878.
11. Vega E, Ghiringhelli G, Mautalen C, Rey Valzacch IG, Scaglia H, Zylberstein C. Bone mineral density and bone size in men with primary osteoporosis and vertebral fractures. Calcif Tissue Int 1998;62:465–469.
12. Seeman E. The structural basis of bone fragility in men. Bone 1999;25: 143–147.

13. Beck T, Ruff C, Mourtada F, et al. DXA derived structural geometry for stress fracture prediction in male U.S. Marine Corps recruits. J Bone Miner Res 1996;11:645–653.

14. Crossley K, Bennell KL, Wrigley T, Oakes BW. Ground reaction forces, bone characteristics, and tibial stress fracture in male runners. Med Sci Sports Exerc 1999:1088–1093.

15. Beck T, Ruff CB, Shaffer RA, Betsinger K, Trone DW, Brodine S. Stress fracture in military recruits: gender differences in muscle and bone susceptibility factors. Bone 2000;27:437–444.

16. Bonjour J-P, Rizzoli R. Bone acquisition in adolescence. In: Marcus R, Feldman D, Kelsey J, eds. Osteoporosis. San Diego: Academic, 1996:465–476.

17. Seeman E. Sexual dimorphism in skeletal size, density, and strength. J Clin Endocrinol Metab 2001;86:4576–4584.

18. Lander ES, Schork NJ. Genetic dissection of complex traits. Science 1994;265:2037–2048.

19. Risch N, Merikangas K. The future of genetic studies of complex human disease. Science 1996;272:1516–1517.

20. Lander ES, Botstein D. Mapping mendelian factors underlying quantitative traits using RFLP linkage maps. Genetics 1989;121:185–199.

21. Dietrich W, Katz H, Lincoln SE, et al. A genetic map of the mouse suitable for typing intraspecific crosses. Genetics 1992;131:423–447.

22. Dietrich WF, Miller JC, Steen RG, et al. A genetic map of the mouse with 4,006 simple sequence length polymorphisms. Nature Genet 1994;7:220–245.

23. Weeks DE, Lathrop GM. Polygenic disease: methods for mapping complex disease traits. Trends Genet 1995;11:513–519.

24. Schork N, Chakravarti A. A nonmathematical overview of modern gene mapping techniques applied to human diseases. In: Mockrin S, ed. Molecular genetics and gene therapy of cardiovascular disease. New York: Marcel Dekker, 1996:79–109.

25. Botstein D, White R, Skolnick M, Davis R. Construction of a genetic linkage map in man using restriction fragment length polymorphisms. Am J Hum Genet 1980;32:314–331.

26. Riordan JR, Rommens JM, Kerem Z-S, et al. Identification of the cystic fibrosis gene: cloning and characterization of complementary DNA. Science 1989;245:1066–1073.

27. Wallace M, Marchuk D, Andersen L, et al. Type 1 neurofibromatosis gene: identification of large transcript disrupted in three NF1 patients. Science 1990;249:181–186.

28. Lander ES, Botstein D. Mapping complex genetic traits in humans: new strategies using a complete RFLP linkage map. Cold Spring Harb Symp Quant Biol 1986;51:46–61.

29. Schork NJ. Genetically complex cardiovascular traits: origins, problems, and potential solutions. Hypertension 1997;29:145–149.

30. Schork NJ. Extended multipoint identity-by-descent analysis of human quantitative traits: efficiency, power, and modeling considerations. Am J Hum Genet 1993;53:1306–1319.

31. Schork NJ, Xu X. Sibpairs versus pedigrees: what are the advantages? Diabetes Rev 1996;5:1–7.
32. Schork NJ, Nath SP, Lindpaintner K, Jacob HJ. Extensions of quantitative trait locus mapping in experimental organisms. Hypertension 1996;28:1104–1111.
33. Kruglyak L, Lander ES. High-resolution genetic mapping of complex traits. Am J Hum Genet 1995;56:1212–1223.
34. Flint J, Corley R. Do animal models have a place in the genetic analysis of quantitative human beavioural traits? J Mol Med 1996;74:515–521.
35. Turner RT, Maran A, Lotinun S, et al. Animal models for osteoporosis. Rev Endocr Metab Disord 2001;2:117–127.
36. Miller SC, Bowman BM, Jee WSS. Available animal models of osteopenia-small and large. Bone 1995;17(Suppl):117S–123S.
37. Kimmel DB. Animal models for in vivo experimentation in osteoporosis research. In: Marcus R, ed. Osteoporosis. San Diego: Academic, 1996:671–690.
38. Aerssens J, Boonen S, Lowet G, Dequeker J. Interspecies differences in bone composition, density, and quality: potential implications for in vivo bone research. Endocrinol 1998;139:663–670.
39. Bar-Shira-Maymon B, Coleman R, Cohen A, Steinhagen-Thiessen E, Slibermann M. Age-related loss in lumbar vertebrae of CW-1 female mice: a histomorphometric study. Calcif Tissue Int 1989;44:36–45.
40. Weiss A, Arbell I, Steinhagen-Thiessen E, Silbermann M. Structural changes in aging bone: osteopenia in the proximal femurs of female mice. Bone 1991;12:165–172.
41. Kimmel DB. Quantitative histologic changes in the proximal tibial epiphyseal growth cartilage of aged female rats. Cells Mater 1992;1(Suppl):101–105.
42. Schapira D, Laton-Miller R, Barzilai D, Silbermann M. The rat as a model for studies of the aging skeleton. Cell Mater 1992;1(Suppl):181–188.
43. Li XJ, Jee WJS, Ke HZ, Mori S, Akamine T. Age-related changes of cancellous and cortical bone histomorphometry in female Sprague-Dawley rats. Cell Mater 1992;1(Suppl):25–37.
44. Suzuki HK. Effects of estradiol-17-β-n-valerate on endosteal ossification and linear growth in the mouse femur. Endocrinol 1958;60:743–747.
45. Edwards MW, Bain SD, Bailey MC, Lantry MM, Howard GA. 17-β-estradiol stimulation of endosteal bone formation in the ovariectomized mouse: an animal model for the evaluation of bone-targeted estrogens. Bone 1992;13:29–34.
46. Donahue LR, Rosen CJ, Beamer WG. Reduced bone density in hypogonadal mice. J Bone Miner Res 1994;9(Suppl 1):S193.
47. Kalu DN. The ovariectomized rat as a model of postmenopausal osteopenia. Bone Miner 1991;15:175–191.
48. Wronski TJ. The ovariectomized rat as an animal model for postmenopausal bone loss. Cell Mater 1992;1(Suppl):69–74.
49. Mosekilde L, Danielsen CC, Knudsen UB. The effect of aging and ovariectomy on the vertebral bone mass and biomechanical properties of mature rats. Bone 1993;14:1–6.

50. Matsushita M, Tsuboyama T, Kasai R, et al. Age-related changes in the senescence-accelerated mouse (SAM). Am J Pathol 1986;125:276–283.

51. Tsuboyama T, Takahashi K, Matsushita M, et al. Decreased endosteal formation during cortical bone modeling in SAM-P/6 mice with a low peak bone mass. Bone Miner 1989;7:1–12.

52. Tsuboyama T, Matsushita M, Okumura H, Yamamuro T, Hanada K, Takeda T. Modification of strain-specific femoral bone density by bone marrow chimerism in mice: a study on the spontaneously osteoporotic mouse (SAM-P/6). Bone 1989;10:269–277.

53. Takahashi K, Tsuboyama T, Matsushita M, et al. Modification of strain-specific femoral bone density by bone marrow-derived factors administered neonatally: a study on the spontaneously osteoporotic mouse (SAM-P/6). Bone Miner 1994;23:57–64.

54. Takahashi K, Tsuboyama T, Matsushita M, et al. Effective intervention of low peak bone mass and modeling in the spontaneous murine model of senile osteoporosis, SAM-P/6, by calcium supplement and hormone treatment. Bone 1994;15:209–215.

55. Tsuboyama T, Takahashi K, Yamamuro T, Hosokawa M, Takeda T. Cross-mating study on bone mass in the spontaneously osteoporotic mouse (SAM-P/6). Bone Miner 1993;23:57–64.

56. Jilka RL, Weinstein RS, Takahashi K, Parfitt MA, Manolagos SC. Linkage of decreased bone mass with impaired osteoblastogenesis in a murine model of accelerated senescence. J Clin Invest 1996;97:1732–1740.

57. Weinstein RS, Jilka RL, Parfitt AM, Manolagos SC. The effects of androgen deficiency on murine bone remodeling and bone mineral density are mediated via cells of the osteoblastic lineage. Endocrinol 1997;138:4013–4021.

58. Schnitzler CM, Ripamonti U, Mesquita JM. Histomorphometry of iliac crest trabecular bone in adult male baboons in captivity. Calcif Tissue Int 1993;52:447–454.

59. Jayo MJ, Jerome CP, Lees CJ, Rankin SE, Weaver DS. Bone mass in female cynomolgus macaques: a cross-sectional and longitudinal study by age. Calcif Tissue Int 1994;54:231–236.

60. Pope NS, Gould KG, Anderson DC, Mann DR. Effects of age and sex on bone density in the rhesus monkey. Bone 1989;10:109–112.

61. Jayo MJ, Rankin SE, Weaver DS, Carlson CS, Clarkson TB. Accuracy and precision of lumbar bone mineral content by DXA in live female monkeys. Calcif Tissue Int 1991;49:438–440.

62. Jerome C, Kimmel DB, McAlister JA, Weaver DS. Effects of ovariectomy on iliac trabecular bone in baboons (*Papio anubis*). Calcif Tissue Int 1986;39:206–208.

63. Miller C, Weaver D. Bone loss in ovariectomized monkeys. Calcif Tissue Int 1986;38:62–65.

64. Lundon K, Dumitriu M, Grynpas M. The long-term effect of ovariectomy on the quality and quantitiy of cancellous bone in young macaques. Bone Miner 1994;24:135–149.

65. Aufdemorte TB, Fox WC, Miller D, Buffum K, Holt GR, Carey KD. A nonhuman primate model for the study of osteoporosis and oral bone loss. Bone 1993;14:581–586.
66. Grynpas MD, Huckell CB, Reichs KJ, Derousseau CJ, Greenwood C, Kessler MJ. Effect of age and osteoarthritis on bone mineral in rhesus monkey vertebrae. J Bone Miner Res 1993;8:909–917.
67. Carlson CS, Loeser RF, Jayo MJ, Weaver DS, Adams MR, Jerome CP. Osteoarthritis in cynomolgus macaques: a primate model of naturally occuring disease. J Orthop Res 1994;12:331–339.
68. Kimmel DB, Lane NE, Kammerer CM, Stegman MR, Rice KS, Recker RR. Spinal pathology in adult baboons. J Bone Miner Res 1993;8(Suppl 1):S279.
69. Hughes KP, Kimmel DB, Kammerer CM, Stegman MR, Rice KS, Recker RR. Vertebral morphometry in adult female baboons. J Bone Miner Res 1994; 9(Suppl 1):S209.
70. Orwoll ES, Oviatt SK, Mann T. The impact of osteophytic and vascular calcifications on vertebral mineral density measurements in men. J Clin Endocrinol Metab 1990;70:1202–1207.
71. Paigen K. A miracle enough: the power of mice. Nature Med 1995;1:215–220.
72. Frankel WN. Taking stock of complex trait genetics in mice. Trends Genet 1995;11:471–477.
73. VandeBerg JL, Williams-Blangero S. Advantages and limitations of nonhuman primates as animal models in genetic research on complex diseases. J Med Primatol 1997;26:113–119.
74. Rogers J, Hixson JE. Insights from model systems: baboons as an animal model for genetic studies of common human disease. Am J Hum Genet 1997;61:489–493.
75. Kaye M, Kusy RP. Genetic lineage, bone mass, and physical activity. Bone 1995;17:131–135.
76. Beamer WG, Donahue LR, Rosen CJ, Baylink DJ. Genetic variability in adult bone density among inbred strains of mice. Bone 1996;18:397–403.
77. Akhter MP, Iwaniec UT, Covey MA, Cullen DM, Kimmel DB, Recker RR. Genetic variations in bone density, histomorphometry, and strength in mice. Calcif Tissue Int 2000;67:337–344.
78. Li X, Mohan S, Gu W, Wergedal J, Baylink DJ. Quantitative assessment of forearm muscle size, forelimb grip strength, forearm bone mineral density, and forearm bone size in determining humerus breaking strength in 10 inbred strains of mice. Calcif Tissue Int 2001;68:365–369.
79. Turner CH, Hsieh YF, Müller R, et al. Genetic regulation of cortical and trabecular bone strength and microstructure in inbred strains of mice. J Bone Miner Res 2000;15:1126–1131.
80. Grupe A, Germer S, Usuka J, et al. *In silico* mapping of complex disease-related traits in mice. Science 2001;292:1915–1918.
81. McLean W, Olsen BR. Mouse models of abnormal skeletal development and homeostasis. Trends Genet 2001;17:S38–S43.

82. Priemel M, Schilling AF, Haberland M, Pogoda P, Rueger JM, Amling M. Osteopenic mice: animal models of the aging skeleton. J Musculoskelet Neuron Interact 2002;2:212–218.

83. Green MC. Catalogue of mutant genes and polymorphic loci. In: Searle M, ed. Genetic variants and strains of the laboratory mouse. Oxford, UK: Oxford University Press, 1989:12–403.

84. Green MC. Further morphological effects of the short-ear gene in the house mouse. J Morphol 1951;88:1–22.

85. Green MC. Effects of the short-ear gene in the mouse on cartilage formation in healing bone fractures. J Exp Zool 1958;137:75–88.

86. Mikiç B, van der Meulen MC, Kingsley DM, Carter DR. Long bone geometry and strength in adult BMP-5 deficient mice. Bone 1995;16:445–454.

87. Kingsley DM, Bland AE, Grubber JM, et al. The mouse short ear skeletal morphogenesis locus is associated with defects in a bone morphogenetic member of the TGF beta superfamily. Cell 1992;71:399–410.

88. Lohler J, Timpl R, Jaenisch R. Embryonic lethal mutation in mouse collagen I gene causes rupture of blood vessels and is associated with erythropoietic and mesenchymal cell death. Cell 1984;38:597–607.

89. Bonadio J, Saunders TL, Tsai E, et al. A transgenic mouse model of osteogenesis imperfecta type I. Proc Natl Acad Sci USA 1990;87:7145–7149.

90. Khillan JS, Olsen AS, Kontsaari S, Sokolov B, Prockop DJ. Transgenic mice that express a mini-gene version of the human gene for type I procollagen (COL1A1) develop a phenotype resembling a lethal form of osteogenesis imperfecta. J Biol Chem 1991;266:23,373–23,379.

91. Pereira RF, Hume EL, Halford KW, Prockop DJ. Bone fragility in transgenic mice expressing a mutated gene for type I procollagen (COL1A1) parallels the age-dependent phenotype of human osteogenesis imperfecta. J Bone Miner Res 1995;10:1837–1843.

92. Xu T, Bianco P, Fisher LW, et al. Targeted disruption of the bglycan gene leads to an osteoporosis-like phenotype in mice. Nat Genet 1998;20:78–82.

93. Delany AM, Amling M, Priemel M, Howe C, Baron R, Canalis E. Osteopenia and decreased bone formation in osteonectin-deficient mice. J Clin Invest 2000;105:915–923.

94. Yoshida H, Hayashi S, Kunisada T, et al. The murine mutation osteopetrosis is in the coding region of the macrophage colony stimulating factor gene. Nature 1990;345:442–444.

95. Soriano P, Montgomery C, Geske R, Bradley A. Targeted disruption of the c-src proto-oncogene leads to osteopetrosis in mice. Cell 1991;64:693–702.

96. Wang Z, Ovitt C, Grigoriadis AE, et al. Bone and hematopoietic defects in mice lacking c-fos. Nature 1992;360:741–745.

97. Hodgkinson CA, Moore KJ, Nakayama A, et al. Mutations at the mouse microphthalmia locus are associated with defects in a gene encoding a novel basic-helix-loop-helix-zipper protein. Cell 1993;74:395–404.

98. Bucay N, Sarosi I, Dunstan CR, et al. Osteoprotegerin-deficient mice develop early onset osteoporosis and arterial calcification. Genes Dev 1998;12:1260–1268.

99. Gunther T, Schinke T. Mouse genetics have uncovered new paradigms in bone biology. Trends Endocrinol Metab 2000;11:189–193.

100. Bailey DW. Recombinant inbred strains and bilineal congenic strains. In: Foster HL, Small JD, Fox JG, eds. The mouse in biomedical research, VolI. New York City: Academic, 1981:223–239.

101. Taylor BA. Recombinant inbred strains: use in gene mapping. In: Morse HC, ed. Origins of inbred mice. New York City: Academic, 1978:423–438.

102. Gora Maslak G, McClearn GE, Crabbe JC, Phillips TJ, Belknap JK, Plomin R. Use of recombinant inbred strains to identify quantitative trait loci in psychopharmacology. Psychopharmacology (Berl) 1991;104:413–424.

103. Plomin R, McClearn GE, Gora Maslak G, Neiderhiser JM. Use of recombinant inbred strains to detect quantitative trait loci associated with behavior. Behav Genet 1991;21:99–116.

104. Plomin R, McClearn GE. Quantitative trait loci (QTL) analyses and alcohol-related behaviors. Behav Genet 1993;23:197–211.

105. Klein RF, Mitchell SR, Phillips TJ, Belknap JK, Orwoll ES. Quantitative trait loci affecting peak bone mineral density in mice. J Bone Miner Res 1998;13: 1648–1656.

106. Orwoll ES, Belknap JK, Klein RF. Gender specificity in the genetic determinants of peak bone mass. J Bone Miner Res 2001;16:1962–1971.

107. Takeda K, Hosokawa M, Higuchi K. Senescence-accelerated mouse (SAM): a novel murine model of accelerated senescence. J Am Geriatr Soc 1991;39: 911–919.

108. Turner CH, Hsieh YF, Muller R, et al. Variation in bone biomechanical properties, microstructure, and density in BXH recombinant inbred mice. J Bone Miner Res 2001;16:206–213.

109. McClearn GE. Prospects for quantitative trait locus methodology in gerontology. Exp Gerontol 1997;32:49–54.

110. Liel Y, Edwards J, Shary J, Spicer KM, Gordon L, Bell NH. The effects of race and body habitus on bone mineral density of the radius, hip, and spine in premenopausal women. J Clin Endocrinol Metab 1988;66:1247–1250.

111. Slemenda CW, Hui SL, Longcope C, Wellman H, Johnson CC. Predictors of bone mass in perimenopausal women. A prospective study of clinical data using photon absorptiometry. Ann Intern Med 1990;112:96–101.

112. Bauer DC, Browner WS, Cauley JA, Orwoll ES, Scott JC, Black Dm. Factors associated with appendicular bone mass in older women: the study of osteoporotic fractures Research Group. Ann Intern Med 1993;118: 657–665.

113. Orwoll ES, Bauer DC, Vogt TM, Fox KM. Axial bone mass in older women. Ann Intern Med 1996;124:187–196.

114. Glauber HS, Vollmer WM, Nevitt MC, Ensrud KE, Orwoll ES. Body weight versus body fat distribution, adiposity, and frame size as predictors of bone density. J Clin Endocrinol Metab 1995;80:1118–1123.

115. Keightley PD, Hardge T, May L, Bulfield G. A genetic map of quantitative trait loci for body weight in the mouse. Genetics 1996;142:227–235.

116. Belknap JK, Mitchell SR, O'Toole LA, Helms ML, Crabbe JC. Type I and type II error rates for quantitative trait loci (QTL) mapping studies using recombinant inbred mouse strains. Behav Genet 1996;26:149–160.

117. Klein RF, Carlos AS, Vartanian KA, et al. Confirmation and fine mapping of chromosomal regions influencing peak bone mass in mice. J Bone Miner Res 2001;16:1953–1961.

118. Yershov Y, Baldini TH, Villagomez S, et al. Bone strength and related traits in HcB/Dem recombinant congenic mice. J Bone Miner Res 2001;16:992–1003.

119. Moore KJ, Nagle DL. Complex trait analysis in the mouse: the strengths, the limitations and the promise yet to come. Annu Rev Genet 2000;34:653–686.

120. Lyon MF, Searle AG. Genetic variants and strains of the laboratory mouse. New York: Oxford Univesity Press, 1989.

121. Dietrich WF, Miller J, Steen R, et al. A comprehensive genetic map of the mouse genome. Nature 1996;380:149–152.

122. Andersson L, Archibald A, Ashburner M, et al. Comparative geome organization of vertebrates. Mammal Genome 1996;7:717–734.

123. West DB, Goudey Lefevre J, York B, Truett GE. Dietary obesity linked to genetic loci on chromosomes 9 and 15 in a polygenic mouse model. J Clin Invest 1994;94:1410–1416.

124. Crabbe JC, Belknap JK, Buck KJ. Genetic animal models of alcohol and drug abuse. Science 1994;264:1715–1723.

125. Beamer WG, Shultz KL, Churchill GA, et al. Quantitative trait loci for bone density in C57BL/6J and CAST/EiJ inbred mice. Mamm Genome 1999;10:1043–1049.

126. Beamer WG, Shultz KL, Donahue LR, et al. Quantitative trait loci for femoral and lumbar vertebral bone mineral density in C57BL/6J and C3H/HeJ inbred strains of mice. J Bone Miner Res 2001;16:1195–1206.

127. Drake TA, Schadt E, Hannani K, et al. Genetic loci determining bone density in mice with diet-induced atherosclerosis. Physiol Genomics 2001;5:205–215.

128. Shimizu M, Higuchi K, Bennett B, et al. Identification of peak bone mass QTL in a spontaneously osteoporotic mouse strain. Mamm Genome 1999;10:81–87.

129. Benes H, Weinstein RS, Zheng W, et al. Chromosomal mapping of osteopenia-associated quantitative trait loci using closely related mouse strains. J Bone Miner Res 2000;15:626–633.

130. Rikke BA, Johnson TE. Towards the cloning of genes underlying murine QTLs. Mamm Genome 1998;9:963–968.

131. Breese EL, Mather K. The organization of polygenic activity within a chromosome in *Drosophila*: 1. Hair characters. Heredity 1957;11:373–395.

132. Darvasi A. Interval-specific congenic strains (ISCS): an experimental design for mapping a QTL into a 1-centimorgan interval. Mamm Genome 1997;8:163–167.

133. Jacob HJ, Lindpaintner K, Lincoln SE, et al. Genetic mapping of a gene causing hypertension in the stroke-prone spontaneously hypertensive rat. Cell 1991;67:213–224.

134. Rapp JP, Deng AY. Detection and positional cloning of blood pressure quantitative trait loci: is it possible? Hypertension 1995;25:1121–1128.

135. Darvasi A. Experimental strategies for the genetic dissection of complex traits in animal models. Nat Genet 1998;18:19–24.

136. Moreadith RW, Radford NB. Gene targeting in embryonic stem cells: the new physiology and metabolism. J Mol Med 1997;75:208–216.

137. Porcu S, Kitamura M, Witkowska E, et al. The human beta globin locus introduced by YAC transfer exhibits a specific and reproducible pattern of developmental regulation in transgenic mice. Blood 1997;90:4602–4609.

138. Mullins JJ, Peters J, Ganten D. Fulminant hypertension in transgenic rats harbouring the mouse Ren-2 gene. Nature 1990;234:541–544.

139. Dudek BC, Underwood K. Selective breeding, congenic strains, and other classical genetic approaches to the analysis of alcohol-related polygenic pleotropisms. Behav Genet 1993;23:179–190.

140. Flaherty L. Congenic strains. In: Foster HL, Small JD, Fox JG, eds. The mouse in biomedical research. Volume I: History, genetics, and wild mice. New York: Academic, 1981:215–222.

141. Lisitsyn NA, Segre JA, Kusumi K, et al. Direct isolation of polymorphic markers linked to a trait by genetically directed representational difference analysis. Nature Genet 1994;6:57–63.

142. Shimizu M, Higuchi K, Kasai S, et al. Chromosome 13 locus, Pbd2, regulates bone density in mice. J Bone Miner Res 2001;16:1972–1982.

143. Bouxsein ML, Rosen CJ, Turner CH, et al. Generation of a new congenic mouse strain to test the relationships among serum insulin-like growth factor I, bone mineral density, and skeletal morphology in vivo. J Bone Miner Res 2002;17:570–579.

144. Gu W, Li X, Lau KH, et al. Gene expression between a congenic strain that contains a quantitative trait locus of high bone density from CAST/EiJ and its wild-type strain C57BL/6J. Funct Integr Genomics 2002 2002;1:375–386.

145. Silver LM, Nadeau JH, Goodfellow PN. Encyclopedia of the mouse genome. IV. Mamm Genome 1994;6:S1–S295.

8

Murine Models of Substance and Alcohol Dependence

Unraveling Genetic Complexities

Kim Cronise and John C. Crabbe

1. GENETICS AND COMPLEX DISEASE

Most behavioral traits operate on a phenotypic and genetic continuum, i.e., the phenotypic output is quantitative based on the genetic input. No one gene is either necessary or sufficient to account for the observed phenotype; rather, a collection of genes is responsible. This phenotypic and genetic complexity is particularly evident in psychological disorders. For instance, first-degree relatives of schizophrenics have a 9% risk for a diagnosis, whereas the risk drops to 2% for a third-degree relative *(1)*. These findings suggest that many genes contribute, and as the proportion of shared genes increases among relatives, so does the likelihood of shared diagnosis. Regardless of commonalities among genotypes, phenotypic expression may vary significantly in the frequency and severity of symptoms. This further supports the contention that several genes contribute to the trait, each with small effects.

This chapter has three objectives. First, we will discuss briefly the phenotypic and genetic complexities of disease. Second, we will discuss some of the methods used to address disease risk and pathophysiology with genetic animal models. Finally, we will discuss some specific examples of genetic influence on complex traits and include consideration of the subtleties of interpreting data from animal models, suggesting how their use may be improved in the future. We have chosen substance dependence and alcoholism as an example of complex disease because there is a rich history of genetic animal model research addressing these disorders.

From: *Computational Genetics and Genomics*
Edited by: G. Peltz © Humana Press Inc., Totowa, NJ

2. COMPLEXITIES ASSOCIATED WITH SUBSTANCE DEPENDENCE

The general criteria for a diagnosis of substance dependence are broadly similar across sources. The American Psychological Association Diagnostic and Statistical Manual IV, Text Revision (DSM-IV TR) defines substance dependence as comprising three key diagnostic features: tolerance (i.e., requiring higher drug doses to achieve the same drug effect), withdrawal (i.e., the experience of physical and psychological symptoms when the drug is discontinued, thought to reflect a state of physical dependence), and compulsive drug taking *(2)*. The website for the National Institute of Health National Institute on Alcohol Abuse and Alcoholism (www.niaaa.nih.gov) identifies four key diagnostic features by further differentiating compulsive drug taking into craving for the drug vs persistence of self-administration in the face of adverse medical consequences and loss of control over drug taking. Loss of control can be inferred from the intrusion of drug-related behavior into work and personal relationships. Similarly, tolerance and withdrawal are also further differentiated by some clinicians and researchers. Both features are actually syndromes of symptoms rather than discrete indicators. For example, withdrawal is indicated by any number of symptoms including, but not limited to nausea, sleeplessness, anxiety, depression, or seizures. Thus, the diagnosis of drug or alcohol dependence constitutes a complex behavioral phenotype. Each individual displays a unique collection of traits, and the genotypes that underlie risk for each individual symptom may or may not be similar. This behavioral and genetic diversity makes assessment of dependence and its etiology a complicated task.

Comorbidity is the co-occurrence of two or more disease processes that may or may not be biologically related. For substance dependence, the rates of comorbidity are high, and this further complicates the task of behavioral and genetic assessment. For instance, in a British sample, rates of other comorbid psychiatric diagnoses were 22% for nicotine dependence, 30% for alcohol dependence, and 45% for other drug dependence *(3)*. Specifically, the incidence of major depression in alcoholics is as high as 42.2% *(4)*. Such diagnostic complexities also exist for most other psychiatric disorders, so comorbidity makes diagnosis and isolation of genetic etiologies for each disorder even more difficult *(5)*.

The nature of the relationship between two disorders may provide insight into the genetic contributions to each condition. If each disease process is a risk factor for the other, the genes involved in one may affect risk for the other disorder as well. Pleiotropism is defined as the influence of a gene on multiple phenotypes and is presumed to underlie shared genetic risk. Although co-occurrence of multiple phenotypes may aid identification of common genetic origins, it should be noted that the two disorders might be transmitted separately and independently. For instance, although substance dependence and depression are both hereditary and often comorbid, alcoholics are not more likely to beget depressed individuals unless there is a family history of depression as well *(6–8)*. This suggests that some genes may affect risk for both diagnoses, whereas others separately increase risk for one or the other. These distinctions may be difficult to tease apart genetically.

3. ANIMAL MODELS FOR SUBSTANCE-DEPENDENCE DISORDERS

Many variables may influence the assessment of a disorder in humans. A partial list includes age, race, sex, nutrition, family background, socioeconomic status, and other environmental variables. Human populations cannot be assigned to experimental treatment groups, so genetic risk factors must be teased out of the complex, interactive contribution of environmental variables. Modeling disease in animals is a particularly attractive alternative for genetic studies as animals with known genotypes can be studied under relatively controlled environmental conditions. However, certain caveats for and limitations to interpretation of data from animal models should be recognized. In order to be useful, an animal model must meet the criteria of both face and construct validity. Face validity requires the animal model to be as nearly identical as possible both behaviorally and physiologically to the human phenotype, whereas construct validity requires that the phenotype the model claims to represent is, in fact, what it represents. For instance, rodent models have been developed for most of the key features of substance abuse and alcoholism described earlier. However, it is not as easy to model some features as it is to model others. Although drug tolerance can be modeled straightforwardly using a variety of behavioral drug responses, the squandering of emotional or work-related rewards that accompanies loss of control over drug taking is less easy to visualize in a mouse's behavior. Therefore, it is difficult to claim that any single animal model is sufficient to represent a complex human phenotype.

In attempts to address these complexities, partial animal models have been targeted to individual components of the larger disease phenotypes. Each partial model creates a more simplified model system. Partial models often focus on particular phenotypes that suggest vulnerability to a disorder or on those that are the most robust phenotypes for a disorder. This is variously called the candidate symptom or endophenotype approach. It has been noted that one of the scales used to assess novelty seeking, the sensation-seeking scale, is considered a very good indicator of concomitant substance abuse *(9)*. Additionally, patients with a history of substance abuse have been shown to demonstrate higher levels of impulsivity *(10)*, and Cloninger *(10)* cites novelty seeking and impulsivity as two associated traits in characterizing one subtype (type 2) of alcoholics. Furthermore, in schizophrenic patients, sensation seeking may be a factor that prompts drug abuse *(12)*. Therefore, sensation seeking or impulsivity may be an endophenotype worthy of investigation in an animal model of substance abuse. Mice can be trained to withhold responding to a tone that signals a food reward, and inability to wait has been used as a model of impulsivity *(13)*. Before considering some specific phenotypes relevant for substance abuse that have been modeled in rodents, we first describe three basic methods applied to genetic animal model research.

3.1. Inbred Strains

Rodent matings are easily arranged in a laboratory setting. Mating parent and offspring, or sibling pairs, for approx 20 generations creates an inbred strain. Inbreeding eliminates all variability in genotypes and produces animals that are homozygous at every gene. These animals are virtually identical, like monozygotic twins, barring any relevant spontaneous mutations. The use of inbred strains is an excellent means to detect genetically influenced differences. If animals from several strains are all tested under nearly identical environmental conditions, any differences among strains derive principally from genetic sources, whereas individual differences among members of a single strain must be nongenetic in origin.

To date, there are approx 100 inbred mouse strains available for use in assessing the range of genetic influences on a particular phenotype. Because of one famous early use of inbreds in psychopharmacology *(14)*, hundreds of studies have used inbred strains to demonstrate genetic influences on alcohol and drug self-administration, sensitivity and tolerance to various effects of alcohol and drugs, and drug withdrawal (for review, *see* refs. *15–17*). Inbred strains are genetically stable across laboratories and time, which has allowed researchers to accumulate much knowledge about drug responses in a few common inbred strains of mice. If the pattern of strain differences for two different traits is very similar, it may be inferred that some genes exert important pleiotropic effects on both traits, i.e., that the traits are genetically correlated.

3.2. Selected Lines

Selective breeding can be applied to any phenotype that is genetically influenced. Typically, a phenotype of interest is identified, and animals that are high and low responders for that trait are bred. As generations of artificial selection are applied in the laboratory, the oppositely selected lines differ more and more in the trait, and the populations can achieve very extreme behavioral differences. Response to selection occurs because the genes influencing high response become more and more common in the population selected for high response and more rare in the low response line. Because it can take years to create a fully selected line, it is important to define the phenotype of interest very carefully. Selected lines have an advantage over inbred strains because primarily, the genes relevant for a particular trait are selected and fixed, whereas animals otherwise remain genetically unique, like individual (non-twinned) humans. When selected lines are found to differ on traits other than that used for their creation, there is a strong inference that the selected genes affected these correlated responses through pleiotropic influences.

3.3. Targeted Mutations

Both inbred strains and selectively bred lines are based on naturally occurring polymorphisms at many genes. As such, they differ at many genes, probably thousands, and which genes are responsible for the behavioral differences is unknown. They can, however, be used to search for the source of the genetic differences, as we shall see in Subheadings 4.1. and 4.2. (and *see also* Chapter 9). The third basic way to create animal models for studying complex disease differs fundamentally in that the individual genes are chosen for study *a priori* based on knowledge of the biological underpinnings of the phenotype. The entry-level manipulation of this sort is to create a null mutant, or "knockout," mouse in which a particular gene is altered in the germ line of the mouse (alternatively, an overexpression mutation can be introduced). The use of targeted mutations (which include knockin, transgenic overexpression, and many other variants) can be a good tool for the investigation of the genetic etiology of disease. However, findings from these studies should be interpreted with caution. The cautions are familiar to neurobiologists who have used any other sort of lesion to disrupt a pathway implicated in a response. Even if negative results are seen in a targeted mutagenesis study, this does not necessarily mean that the gene of interest is not involved in the phenotype. Because the mutations are present (and the gene's product absent) throughout development, compensatory responses in unknown biological systems may have masked any contribution of the mutant gene. However, new techniques are being enlisted that utilize second-generation mutagenesis technology, such as inducible knockouts and knockins, expressed in restricted tissue types, and other innovations in gene targeting. Although these have not yet been extensively used for studies of

In humans, the opiate antagonist, naltrexone, has been somewhat successful in the treatment of alcoholism *(28)*. It is thought that by blocking opioid action, the reinforcing effects of alcohol are reduced, thereby decreasing subsequent alcohol consumption. A link between opiates and dopamine for the reinforcing effects of alcohol has been demonstrated in rats. The administration of opiate antagonists has been shown to reduce dopamine release in the nucleus accumbens of the mesolimbic dopaminergic system and subsequently reduce alcohol reward *(29)*. Consistent with these contentions, Hall et al. demonstrated a reduction in voluntary alcohol consumption and a reduction in the reward properties of alcohol in μ-opioid receptor knockout mice *(30)*. Ethanol drinking has a large effect on brain-regional messenger ribonucleic acid (mRNA) levels for μ and δ opioid receptors in both B6 and D2 mice, although the strains do not differ *(31)*. However, proenkephalin and proopiomelanocortin mRNA levels were higher in B6 than in D2 mice in several brain regions *(32)*. Using both animal models and human subjects, Gianoulakis and her group have documented substantial differences in opioid peptide levels and activity between genetically susceptible groups. For example, Dai et al. recently reported that subjects with a family history positive for alcoholism had higher baseline levels of β-endorphin than those with a negative family history, and that stress elevated β-endorphin levels more in the low-risk subjects *(33)*.

Both alcoholic and depressed patients show reduced serotonin levels *(34,35)*. Whereas the D2 and μ-opioid receptors may be involved in initiating alcohol consumption, the 5-HT$_{1B}$ receptor may be involved in inhibiting consumption. Crabbe et al. *(36)* demonstrated that mice lacking 5-HT$_{1B}$ receptors showed elevated alcohol consumption levels, although subsequent studies have been less consistent and offer a good object lesson in the difficulties surrounding interpretation of knockout experiments *(37)*. Collectively, these results suggest a role for the D2, μ-opioid, and the 5-HT$_{1B}$ receptor genes in alcohol-seeking behavior and demonstrate the usefulness of targeted mutagenesis in furthering our understanding of how genes affect phenotypic expression.

Beginning in the late 1940s, several selective breeding projects in rats have provided genetic animal models very fruitful in generating information about the neurobiology underlying preference drinking (for review, *see* ref. *17*). Grahame et al. began selectively breeding mice for alcohol preference and avoidance, resulting in the high alcohol preference (HAP) and low alcohol preference (LAP) lines of mice that differ markedly in alcohol consumption *(38)*. Subsequent studies have shown that HAP mice may develop greater sensitization to the locomotor stimulant effects of ethanol than LAP mice, and that the lines did not differ in development of acute functional tolerance to ethanol *(39,40)*. Interestingly, the lines did not differ markedly in sensitivity to develop an alcohol-conditioned place preference, another measure of ethanol reinforcement *(41)*. It will be very useful to compare the genomes of HAP and LAP mice. For example, one would predict that they will differ in the frequencies of some genes located within the QTL regions previously mapped for ethanol preference.

4.2. Alcohol Withdrawal

The development of drug dependence produces functional changes in the brain such that the subsequent removal of the drug results in a rebound display of symptoms, one of the key features of substance dependence. Handling induced convulsions during withdrawal are a quantifiable trait in mice. After acute or chronic exposure to alcohol, animals are lifted by the tail and scored based on the severity of the observed convulsion. In 1973, Goldstein demonstrated via selective breeding that chronic withdrawal severity is a heritable trait *(42)*. Since that time a number of studies with inbred strains and selected lines have been conducted and more than 20 inbred strains have been assessed for differences in withdrawal susceptibility following chronic alcohol exposure. Among these strains, the B6 and D2 strains show notable differences in withdrawal severity, with the D2 strain demonstrating severe alcohol withdrawal convulsions *(43,44,45)*. An important note is that genetic differences in withdrawal severity can also be seen during acute withdrawal following a single, highdose administration of alcohol *(46,47)*.

In the early 1980s, a large-scale selection study was initiated *(48)*. Withdrawal Seizure-Prone (WSP) and Withdrawal Seizure-Resistant (WSR) mice differed markedly in the severity of alcohol withdrawal-induced convulsions. These lines have been shown to differ in withdrawal susceptibility to other central nervous system depressant drugs, such as barbiturates and benzodiazepines *(49,50)*, which suggests that some genes influencing ethanol withdrawal convulsion severity have pleiotropic effects on withdrawal from similar classes of drugs. Furthermore, they underscore the genetic complexity of drug withdrawal, because genes influencing ethanol withdrawal convulsions do not have pleiotropic effects on certain traits modeling other features of alcoholism, such as tolerance and initial sensitivity.

Although comparisons of behavioral differences between selectively bred lines can identify patterns of genetically correlated and uncorrelated traits, they are unable to identify the responsible genes. However, in other studies, candidate genes have been explored. Because γ-amino butyric acid (GABA) is the most ubiquitous inhibitory neurotransmitter and is known to play a role in epilepsy and the inhibition of seizure activity, investigation of the role of GABA in alcohol withdrawal convulsions seemed a plausible choice. Studies have demonstrated that there are substantial differences between the two selected lines in mRNA expression for genes encoding certain subunits of the $GABA_A$ receptor. Decreases in the expression of α_1, α_3, and α_6 subunits, and increases in the γ_2 subunit, are seen in the WSP but not the WSR line in response to either acute or chronic alcohol administration *(51,52)*.

Focusing on specific GABA receptor subunit genes offers evidence of the convergence of information from gene expression and QTL analyses. A number of QTLs have been mapped for acute withdrawal to alcohol. Buck et al. examined acute withdrawal in three populations derived from B6 and D2 inbred strains-BXD-recombinant inbred strains, a B6D2F2 intercross, and lines of mice selectively bred from the B6D2F2 population for high and low alcohol withdrawal *(53)*. Their analysis initially indicated five possible QTLs (on chromosomes 1, 2, 4, and 11) that appeared to influence withdrawal liability. The QTL on chromosome 11 encompasses a region of DNA that includes genes that encode the γ_2, α_1, α_2, and α_6 subunits (as well as many other genes). Furthermore, inbred strains that differ significantly in withdrawal severities show significant allelic variation in the α_6 receptor subunit gene *(54)*, and when chronically treated with ethanol, the D2 strain showed greater increases in β_2 subunit expression in cerebellum than the B6 strain, in which regulation by ethanol was more complex *(55)*. These data are consistent with, but are insufficient to prove, the fact that the basis for the chromosome 11 QTL effect on withdrawal is a polymorphism in one or more of the $GABA_A$ receptor subunit genes. Several studies with mice bearing null mutations for $GABA_A$ receptor subunits are reviewed by Dowling et al (*see* Chapter 9). The chromosome 11 QTL was also mapped in similar studies of acute pentobarbital withdrawal *(56)*. Evidence for the involvement of $GABA_A$ receptor genes in both alcohol and pentobarbital withdrawal has been reviewed *(57)*.

An interesting outcome of studies of ethanol withdrawal has been that the genetic contributions to acute and chronic withdrawal are not entirely overlapping. Acute withdrawal is monitored 4 to 10 h after a single high-dose alcohol injection, whereas chronic withdrawal is monitored after exposure to alcohol vapor continuously for several days, or feeding animals a liquid diet containing alcohol for many days. QTLs for chronic withdrawal after vapor inhalation have also been mapped in BXD recombinant inbred mice *(58)*. Significant associations were found on chromosomes 1 and 19 and provisional associations on chromosomes 1, 4, and 13 *(59)*. Thus, QTL regions were mapped for both acute and chronic withdrawal on chromosomes 1 and 4, but new QTLs, unique to chronic withdrawal, were seen on chromosomes 13 and 19, and the strong associations with the *GABA* gene-rich area of chromosome 11 seen for acute withdrawal were absent for chronic withdrawal. For the QTL regions on 1 and 4 that overlap between acute and chronic withdrawal, it may be the case that a single gene accounts for both, but this is not yet proven. Finally, when chronic ethanol withdrawal severity was mapped in genotypes extending beyond the B6- and D2-derived populations, additional findings emerged. Bergeson et al. used a large F2 cross between inbred strains derived from the WSP and WSR selected lines, as well as the cross of another pair of similarly selected lines in a genome-wide search for QTLs *(60)*. They found significant QTLs, on chromosomes 1, 4, 8, 11, and 14. Thus, in this cross, the chromosome 11 QTL appeared also to influence chronic ethanol withdrawal. Furthermore, tests for interactions among QTLs showed that the chromosome 13 QTL also emerged but only when certain genotypes were present at the chromosome 11 QTL.

As noted in preceding paragraphs of this Subheading, both inbred strains and selected lines have demonstrated some correspondence of genetic contribution to withdrawal from alcohol, pentobarbital, and diazepam. Progress toward the identification of the gene or genes responsible for a particular QTL involves narrowing the interval on a chromosome containing the effective DNA (*see* Chapter 9). For both acute and chronic alcohol and acute pentobarbital withdrawal, the same QTL region on chromosome 4 was identified *(53,56,58,60)*. Recently, this locus was narrowed from 200 possible candidate genes to fewer than 15 *(61)*. Evidence from specialized congenic strains derived from B6 and D2 crosses, as well as comparisons of standard inbred strains, has provided compelling evidence that the responsible gene may be a multiple PDZ–domain zinc finger protein gene called *Mpdz*.

Subsequent analyses comparing other chromosome 4 congenics with their background revealed that an interval of only 1.8 Mb contained the QTL. Within this interval, there were only three known and three novel (predicted) genes. Five could be confirmed, but of these five, only *Mpdz* showed genotype-dependent differences in coding sequence and differential expression between B6 and D2. Furthermore, Mpdz was differentially expressed between congenic and background strains, and lower expression of *Mpdz* was correlated with higher withdrawal severity from ethanol and pentobarbital across five inbred strains *(62)*. In summary, no data currently available can exclude Mpdz as the gene responsible for the chromosome 4 QTL effect on withdrawal.

Finally, expression-profiling studies with B6 and D2 mice have compared expression of 7634 genes in B6 and D2 mouse hippocampi during acute and chronic alcohol withdrawal *(63)*. Twice the number of genes (2% vs 1%) were affected by chronic withdrawal in D2 mice than in B6 mice. Clusters of genes differentially expressed identified the Janus kinase/signal transducer and activator of transcription and mitogen-activated protein kinase cellular signaling pathways as potential mediators of differential cellular neuroadaptation during alcohol withdrawal. The *Mpdz* gene was also differentially regulated in these arrays.

4.3. Preference and Withdrawal—Are There Common Genetic Influences?

Studies reviewed in the previous Subheadings 4.1. and 4.2. show that genetic animal models have provided substantial evidence for genetic contributions to both alcohol dependence and the voluntary self-administration of alcohol. For each trait, advances in genomics have allowed recent progress toward identifying the specific genes responsible. Are these related traits or are the responsible genes entirely different? Evidence from the two most often studied strains, B6 and D2, are suggestive of a genetic relationship. B6 mice prefer alcohol in comparison to the D2 (and most other) strains, and the D2 strain consistently demonstrates more severe withdrawal than the B6 strain. This apparent negative genetic relationship could be caused by the pleiotropic influence of some genes that act both to enhance withdrawal severity and to limit alcohol self-administration (or vice-versa). However, an important caveat is that the "correlation" is built entirely from two genetic data points. If a third strain were included, it might show both high consumption and high withdrawal, which would undermine the evidence for pleiotropism.

In 1998, Metten et al. took the available literature on genetic differences in preference and withdrawal and conducted a meta-analysis to determine whether genotypes that show higher preference for alcohol do, in fact, consistently demonstrate lower withdrawal scores than strains that do not prefer alcohol *(64)*. Across the 20-odd recombinant inbred strains from B6 and D2, the negative correlation held. It also held in the High-Alcohol Withdrawal and Low-Alcohol Withdrawal lines selectively bred from B6D2F2 for acute withdrawal (Low-Alcohol Withdrawal mice showed higher preference) and in the high and low ethanol preference lines also bred from the B6D2F2 (high ethanol preference lines showed lower withdrawal; *64*). The negative correlation also held for individual B6D2F2 mice tested for both traits *(65)*. Even when the analysis was extended to include genotypes that have alleles other than those derived from B6 and D2 inbreds, the negative genetic relationship endures. Fifteen standard inbred mouse strains differ widely in withdrawal severity *(45)* and preference *(19)*, and these two traits were negatively genetically correlated *(64, 66)*. Earlier studies with the WSP and WSR mice had shown that WSR (the low withdrawal lines) drank more than WSP *(67)*.

This pattern of results clearly shows that there is a negative genetic relationship between the severity of withdrawal convulsions following ethanol and the propensity to drink alcohol solutions. Yet, one issue that has not been addressed is the physiological relationship between these two behaviors. It is possible that a set of genes influences both behavioral tendencies but through independent mechanisms. A more intriguing possibility is that postingestional consequences affect alcohol preference. This hypothesis ventures that animals who self-administer large amounts of alcohol do so because they do not suffer adverse physiological symptoms during withdrawal. The phenomenon of conditioned taste aversion shows clearly that animals intoxicated with a large alcohol injection will show a subsequent aversion for a flavored solution that was paired with the alcohol injection *(66)*. For this to "explain" the current pattern of strain differences in withdrawal, however, it is necessary to suppose that over evolutionary time, access to alcohol and experience with withdrawal symptoms following self-administration of large quantities has led high withdrawal genotypes to avoid alcohol. There is currently no evidence for or against this hypothesis. In all the studies to date (with the exception of the B6D2F2 mice), naive animals were studied for a single trait-withdrawal or preference drinking. The B6D2F2 mice were tested for both traits, but with an interval between, precluding the possibility of drinking to ameliorate withdrawal.

An interesting finding has been that inbred strains that show High-Alcohol Withdrawal and Low-Alcohol Preference also show high sensitivity to alcohol-conditioned taste aversion *(66)*. This is consistent with the mechanistic relationship just postulated between drinking and withdrawal. Similarly, strains lower in ability to inhibit rewarded responding had high-alcohol preference *(13)*. Such attempts to piece back together more complex phenotypes from essentially pairwise genetic relationships represent a first step toward reassembling more complex genetic animal models. Along these lines, our group has begun to explore multivariate analyses of data from inbred mouse strains. Mice from 15 standard inbred strains were tested for locomotor and thermal responses to multiple doses of ethanol, pentobarbital, diazepam, or morphine. In other studies already mentioned, voluntary oral self-administration and severity of withdrawal were assessed. Multidimensional scaling analyses, which force a two-factor solution to such complex data sets, revealed three major clusters of genetically correlated responses. Sensitivity to the thermal and locomotor effects of ethanol, pentobarbital, and diazepam, and consumption of pentobarbital and diazepam, formed one cluster. Sensitivity to all effects of morphine, including morphine drinking, formed a second cluster, which included alcohol drinking. The third cluster represented withdrawal severity from alcohol, pentobarbital, and diazepam. Consistent with the negative genetic correlations between alcohol withdrawal and drinking, as well as the postulated role of endogenous opioid peptides in alcohol dependence liability discussed in Subheading 4.1., the latter two clusters were negatively correlated in the analysis *(68, 68a)*.

5. FUTURE DIRECTIONS

The use of inbred strains, selected lines, and genetically engineered mice has contributed significantly to identifying the genetic and neurobiological bases of alcoholism and addiction. Substantial progress is being made toward the identification of individual genes that influence particular traits. Thus far, such progress has necessarily depended on the application of reductionism, i.e., employing partial genetic models that capture only part of the complex human traits. As the example of withdrawal, drinking, response inhibition, and endogenous opioids suggests, we are beginning to move toward the ability to synthesize information about genetic influences. More traits relevant for the addictions need to be modeled, particularly in mice, in which the power of the genetic analyses is greatest.

However, the relationships between genes and behaviors are not one to one. In addition to contributions of genes considered individually, there are interactions among genes as well. Gene action is said to be epistatic when the effect of one gene masks or potentiates the effect of another gene. An excellent example of an epistatic interaction has been reported for pentobarbital withdrawal. Hood et al. demonstrated that the presence of particular alleles at a QTL on chromosome 11 were effective in elevating withdrawal but only if the mice also had specific alleles at a second QTL on chromosome 1 *(69)*. Similarly, Bergeson et al. found that the effect of a QTL on chromosome 13 depended on genotype at the chromosome 11 QTL *(60)*. They also found significant epistatic interactions between QTLs on chromosomes 4 and 8 and 8 and 14. It is likely that epistasis occurs for all complex psychological disorders and that the importance of epistatic interactions increase with the addition of comorbid disorders. The interaction of the chromosome 11 and 13 QTLs is especially interesting, as the most highly associated marker for chromosome 13 is in fact a candidate gene, which synthesizes steroid 5-α reductase 1 *(Srd5a1)*. This steroid enzyme is important in the synthesis of neurosteroids (e.g., allopregnanolone), a class of endogenous compounds that modulate $GABA_A$ receptors. When administered allopregnanolone, WSP mice are more sensitive than WSR mice to the anticonvulsant effects *(70)*, and they also show greater acute withdrawal from an acute dose of allopregnanolone *(71)*. Thus, the emergence of a significant interaction between the chromosome 11 and 13 QTLs may reflect the physiological interaction of these candidate gene products. As more candidate genes are identified, the ability to study their independent and epistatic effects in animal models will increase, along with the difficulties attendant to the increased statistical power needed to detect such interactions.

Discussions of genetic influence are only meaningful in the context of the environment in which they are measured. An obvious environmental factor is development-genes expressed at early developmental stages are not the same as those expressed during adulthood. For the more permanent genetic animal models (standard inbred strains, selected lines), there is a paucity of information about the role of environmental milieu in affecting genetic differences. Cabib et al. recently altered the environment of B6 and D2 mice with a brief period of food shortage *(72)*. This manipulation blocked an amphetamine-conditioned place preference in D2, but not B6, mice, showing that the gene–behavior link can be moderated by experience. The generality of such a finding across multiple mouse strains is, of course, open to question as the results were derived from only two genotypes. In fact, the environmental conditions that can affect strain-specific behavior may not even be identifiable. In a study including eight strains, all environmental and procedural conditions that could easily be rendered identical in three laboratories were controlled, and the strains were tested for several simple behaviors. Some behaviors (e.g., alcohol preference drinking) yielded strain patterns that were nearly invariant across laboratories, but for other behaviors (e.g., exploration of an elevated plus maze), different laboratories found rather different patterns of strain differences. It is unknown what the environmental mediators of these effects were, but it is clear that a given genotype's behavior may be quite different in various environmental circumstances *(73)*. These issues are not without consequence for human studies. Rose et al. report that urban vs rural living settings modulates the influence of genetic risk on alcohol use in Finnish adolescents *(74)*.

The refinement of phenotypes in various animal models will be extremely important as well. There is a natural tendency for investigators to anthropomorphize the responses of animals in behavioral assays. Indeed, the ability to do this is central to the validity of any such assay. Nonetheless, the perspectives of mouse and man differ, and different assays that seem to be assessing quite similar functions to the experimenter may be tapping different mouse dimensions. A recent study with inbred strains used a common measure of alcohol intoxication, the rotarod. When strain sensitivities to alcohol were compared between the accelerating and fixed-speed variants of this test, they were found to be completely unrelated under some conditions of testing, even though the apparatus was identical *(75)*. The only reasonable solution for such environmental sensitivity of genetic influences is to employ a broad range of assessment tools before drawing conclusions about a genotype's characteristic responses.

In summary, recent advances in the use of animal models are making it possible to address some of the complexities associated with substance abuse disorders. However, it is important to remember that there are limitations to these studies, some of which were discussed here. It is also important to remember that identification of the genetic basis in the animal model is not the final endpoint—the ultimate goal is to use the genetic animal models to in turn identify the underlying genetics of the human condition. What is relevant in the animal model may or may not be relevant in the clinical realm. Nonetheless, as the sophistication of genetic animal model experiments increases, the potential for application to pharmacogenetic analyses to develop novel therapeutics will come closer to being realized.

ACKNOWLEDGMENTS

Preparation of this chapter was supported by grants from the Department of Veterans Affairs and National Institutes of Health Grants AA10760, AA12714, AA05828, AA13519, AA07468, DA05228, and DA10913.

REFERENCES

1. McGuffin P, Owen MJ, Farmer AE. Genetic basis of schizophrenia. Lancet 1995;346:678–682.
2. American Psychiatric Association. DSM-IV TR: diagnostic and statistic manual of mental disorders, 4th ed [Text revision]. Washington, DC: American Psychiatric, 2000.
3. Farrell M, Howes S, Bebbington P, et al. Nicotine, alcohol and drug dependence and psychiatric comorbidity. Results of a national household survey. Br J Psychiatry 2001;179:432–437.
4. Schuckit MA, Tipp JE, Bucholz KK, et al. The life-time rates of three major mood disorders and four major anxiety disorders in alcoholics and controls. Addiction 1997;92:1289–1304.

5. Crabbe JC. Genetic contributions to addiction. Annu Rev Psychol 2002;53: 435–462.
6. Cloninger CR, Reich T, Wetzel R. Alcoholism and affective disorders: familial associations and genetic models. In: Cloninger CR, Reich T, Wetzel R, eds. Alcoholism and affective disorders: clinical, genetic and biochemical studies. New York, NY: Spectrum Publications, 1979:57–86.
7. Merikangas KR, Gelernter CS. Comorbidity for alcoholism and depression. Psychiatr Clin North Am 1990;13:613–632.
8. Schuckit MA. Genetic and clinical implications of alcoholism and affective disorder. Am J Psychiatry 1986;143:140–147.
9. Jaffe LT, Archer RP. The prediction of drug use among college students from MMPI, MCMI, and sensation seeking scales. J Pers Assess 1987; 51:243–253.
10. Allen TJ, Moeller FG, Rhoades HM, Cherek DR. Impulsivity and history of drug dependence. Drug Alcohol Depend 1998;50:137–145.
11. Cloninger CR. Neurogenetic adaptive mechanisms in alcoholism. Science 1987;236:410–416.
12. Dervaux A, Bayle FJ, Laqueille X, et al. Is substance abuse in schizophrenia related to impulsivity, sensation seeking, or anhedonia? Am J Psychiatry 2001;158:492–494.
13. Logue SF, Swartz RJ, Wehner JM. Genetic correlation between performance on an appetitive-signaled nosepoke task and voluntary ethanol consumption. Alcohol Clin Exp Res 1998;22:1912–1920.
14. McClearn GE, Rodgers DA. Differences in alcohol preference among inbred strains of mice. Q J Stud Alcohol 1959;20:691–695.
15. Crabbe JC, Harris RA. The genetic basis of alcohol and drug actions. Crabbe JC and Harris RA, eds. New York, NY: Plenum, 1991.
16. Phillips TJ. Behavior genetics of drug sensitization. Crit Rev Neurobiol 1997;11:21–23.
17. McBride WJ, Li TK. Animal models of alcoholism: neurobiology of high alcohol drinking behavior in rodents. Crit Rev Neurobiol 1998;12:339–369.
18. Rodgers DA. Factors underlying differences in alcohol preference in inbred strains of mice. In: Kissin B, Begleiter H, eds. The biology of alcoholism. New York: Plenum, 1972:107–130.
19. Belknap JK, Crabbe JC, Young ER. Voluntary consumption of ethanol in 15 inbred mouse strains. Psychopharmacology 1993;112:503–510.
20. Belknap JK, Atkins AL. The replicability of QTLs for murine alcohol preference drinking behavior across eight independent studies. Mamm Genome 2001;12:893–899.
21. Belknap JK, Richards SP, O'Toole LA, Helms ML, Phillips TJ. Short term selective breeding as a tool for QTL mapping: ethanol preference drinking. Behav Genet 1997;27:55–66.
22. Whatley VJ, Johnson TE, Erwin VG. Identification and confirmation of quantitative trait loci regulating alcohol consumption in congenic strains of mice. Alcohol Clin Exp Res 1999;23:1262–1271.

23. Brodie MS, Pesold C, Appel SB. Ethanol directly excites dopaminergic ventral tegmental area reward neurons. Alcohol Clin Exp Res 1999;23:1848–1852.

24. Imperato A, DiChiara G. Preferential stimulation of dopamine release in the nucleus accumbens of freely moving rats by ethanol. J Pharmacol and Exp Ther 1986;239:219–228.

25. Milner PM. Brain-stimulation reward: a review. Can J Psychol 1991;45:1–36.

26. Phillips TJ, Crabbe JC, Metten P, Belknap JK. Localization of genes affecting alcohol drinking in mice. Alcohol Clin Exp Res 1994;18:931–941.

27. Phillips TJ, Brown KJ, Burkhart-Kasch S, et al. Alcohol preference and sensitivity are markedly reduced in mice lacking dopamine D2 receptors. Nat Neurosci 1998;1:610–615.

28. Streeton C, Whelan G. Naltrexone, a relapse prevention maintenance treatment of alcohol dependence: a meta-analysis of randomized controlled trials. Alcohol Alcohol 2001;36:544–552.

29. Benjamin D, Grant ER, Pohorecky LA. Naltrexone reverses ethanol-induced dopamine release in the nucleus accumbens in awake, freely moving rats. Brain Res 1993;621:137–140.

30. Hall FS, Sora I, Uhl GR. Ethanol consumption and reward are decreased in mu–opiate receptor knockout mice. Psychopharmacology 2001;154:43–49.

31. Winkler A, Búzás B, Siems W-E, Heder G, Cox BM. Effect of ethanol drinking on the gene expression of opioid receptors, enkephalinase, and angiotensis-converting enzyme in two inbred mouse strains. Alcohol Clin Exp Res 1998;22:1262–1271.

32. Jamensky NT, Gianoulakis C. Comparison of the proopiomelanocortin and proenkephalin opioid peptide systems in brain regions of the alcohol-preferring C57BL/6 and alcohol-avoiding DBA/2 mice. Alcohol 1999; 18:177–187.

33. Dai X, Thavundayil J, Gianoulakis C. Differences in the responses of the pituitary beta-endorphin and cardiovascular system to ethanol and stress as a function of family history. Alcohol Clin Exp Res 2002;26:1171–1180.

34. Coppen A, Wood K. Adrenergic and serotonergic mechanisms in depression and their response to amitriptyline. Ciba Found Symp 1979;74:157–166.

35. LeMarquand D, Pihl RO, Benkelfat C. Serotonin and alcohol intake, abuse, and dependence: findings of animal studies. Biol Psychiatry 1994;36:326–337.

36. Crabbe JC, Phillips TJ, Feller DJ, et al. Elevated alcohol consumption in null mutant mice lacking 5-HT$_{1B}$ serotonin receptors. Nat Genet 1996;14:98–101.

37. Phillips TJ, Hen R, Crabbe JC. Complications associated with genetic background effects in research using knockout mice. Psychopharmacology 1999;147:5–7.

38. Grahame NJ, Li TK, Lumeng L. Selective breeding for high and low alcohol preference in mice. Behav Genet 1999;29:47–57.

39. Chester JA, Grahame NJ, Li TK, Lumeng L, Frochlich JC. Effects of acamprosate on sensitization to the locomotor-stimulant effects of alcohol in mice selectively bred for high and low alcohol preference. Behav Pharmacol 2001;12:535–543.

40. Grahame NJ, Rodd-Henricks K, Li TK, Lumeng L. Ethanol locomotor sensitization, but not tolerance correlates with selection for alcohol preference in high- and low-alcohol preferring mice. Psychopharmacology 2000;151:252–260.

41. Grahame NJ, Chester JA, Rodd-Henricks K, Li TK, Lumeng L. Alcohol place preference conditioning in high- and low-alcohol preferring selected lines of mice. Pharmacol Biochem Behav 2001;68:805–814.

42. Goldstein DB. Inherited differences in intensity of alcohol withdrawal reactions in mice. Nature 1973;245:154–156.

43. Goldstein DB, Kakihana R. Alcohol withdrawal reactions and reserpine effects in inbred strains of mice. Life Sci 1974;15:415–425.

44. Griffiths PJ, Littleton JM. Concentrations of free amino acids in brains of mice of different strains during the physical syndrome of withdrawal from ethanol. Br J Exp Pathol 1977;58:391–399.

45. Crabbe JC, Young ER, Kosobud A. Genetic correlations with ethanol withdrawal severity. Pharmacol Biochem Behav 1983;18(Suppl 1):541–547.

46. Crabbe JC, Merrill CD, Belknap JK. Acute dependence on depressant drugs is determined by common genes in mice. J Pharmacol Exp Ther 1991; 257:2:663–667.

47. Metten P, Crabbe JC.Common genetic determinants of severity of acute withdrawal from ethanol, pentobarbital and diazepam in inbred mice. Behav Pharmacol 1994;5:533–547.

48. Crabbe JC, Kosobud A, Young ER,Tam BR, McSwigan JD. Bidirectional selection for susceptibility to ethanol withdrawal seizures in *Mus musculus*. Behav Genet 1985;15:521–536.

49. Belknap JK, Danielson PW, Lamé M, Crabbe JC. Ethanol and barbiturate withdrawal convulsions are extensively codetermined in mice. Alcohol 1988;5:167–171.

50. Belknap JK, Crabbe JC, Laursen SE. Ethanol and diazepam withdrawal convulsions are extensively codetermined in WSP and WSR mice. Life Sci 1989;44:2075–2080.

51. Buck KJ, McQuilken SJ, Harris RA. Chronic alcohol treatment alters brain levels of γ-aminobutyric acid$_A$ receptor subunit mRNAs: relationship to genetic differences in ethanol withdrawal seizure severity. J Neurochem 1991;57:2100–2105.

52. Keir WJ, Morrow AL. Differential expression of GABA$_A$ receptor subunit mRNAs in ethanol-naïve withdrawal seizure resistant (WSR) vs. withdrawal seizure prone (WSP) mouse brain. Brain Res Mol Brain Res 1994; 25:200–208.

53. Buck KJ, Metten P, Belknap JK, Crabbe JC. Quantitative trait loci involved in genetic predisposition to acute alcohol withdrawal in mice. J Neurosci 1997;17:3946–3955.

54. Hood HM, Buck KJ. Allelic variation in the GABA A receptor gamma2 subunit is associated with genetic susceptibility to ethanol-induced motor incoordination and hypothermia, conditioned taste aversion, and withdrawal in BXD/Ty recombinant inbred mice. Alcohol Clin Exp Res 2000;24:1327–1334.

55. Reilly MT, Buck KJ. GABA$_A$ receptor γ2 subunit mRNA content is differentially regulated in ethanol-dependent DBA/2J and C57BL/6J mice. Neurochem Int 2000;37:443–452.

56. Buck KJ, Metten P, Belknap JK, Crabbe JC. Quantitative trait loci affecting risk for pentobarbital withdrawal map near alcohol withdrawal loci on mouse chromosomes 1, 4, and 11. Mamm Genome 1999;10:431–437.

57. Buck KJ, Finn DA. Genetic factors in addiction: QTL mapping and candidate gene studies implicate GABAergic genes in alcohol and barbiturate withdrawal in mice. Addiction 2001;96:139–149.

58. Crabbe JC. Provisional mapping of quantitative trait loci for chronic ethanol withdrawal severity in BXD recombinant inbred mice. J Pharmacol Exp Ther 1998;286:263–271.

59. Buck KJ, Rademacher BLS, Metten P, Crabbe JC. Mapping murine loci for physical dependence on ethanol. Psychopharmacology 2002;160:398–407.

60. Bergeson SE, Warren RK, Crabbe JC, Metten P, Erwin VG, Belknap JK. Chromosomal loci influencing chronic alcohol withdrawal severity. Mamm Genome 2003;14:454–463.

61. Fehr C, Shirley RL, Belknap JK, Crabbe JC, Buck KJ. Congenic mapping of alcohol and pentobarbital withdrawal liability loci to a <1 centimorgan interval of murine chromosome 4: Identification of *Mpdz* as a candidate gene. J Neurosci 2002;22:3730–3738.

62. Shirley RL, Walter NA, Reilly MT, Fehr C, Buck KJ. Mdpz is a quantitative trait gene for drug withdrawal seizures. Nat Neurosci 2004;7:699–700.

63. Daniels GM, Buck KJ. Expression profiling identifies strain-specific changes associated with ethanol withdrawal in mice. Genes Brain Behav 2002;1:35–45.

64. Metten P, Phillips TJ, Crabbe JC, et al. High genetic susceptibility to ethanol withdrawal predicts low ethanol consumption. Mamm Genome 1998;9:983–990.

65. Tarantino LM, McClearn GE, Rodriguez LA, Plomin R. Confirmation of quantitative trait loci for alcohol preference in mice. Alcohol Clin Exp Res 1998;22:1099–1105.

66. Broadbent J, Muccino KJ, Cunningham CL. Ethanol-induced conditioned taste aversion in 15 inbred mouse strains. Behav Neurosci 2002;116:138–148.

67. Kosobud AE, Bodor AS, Crabbe JC. Voluntary consumption of ethanol in WSP, WSC and WSR selectively bred mouse lines. Pharmacol Biochem Behav 1988;29:601–607.

68. Crabbe JC, Belknap JK, Buck KJ. Genetic animal models of alcohol and drug abuse. Science 1994;264:1715–1723.

68a. Belknap JK, Metten P, Crabbe JC. Genetic codetermination of drug abuse liability: multivariate analyses of mouse inbred strain responses to ethanol, morphine, diazepam and pentobarbital, submitted.

69. Hood HM, Belknap JK, Crabbe JC, Buck KJ. Genomewide search for epistasis in a complex trait: pentobarbital withdrawal convulsions in mice. Behav Genet 2001;31:93–100.

70. Finn DA, Roberts AJ Crabbe JC. Neuroactive steroid sensitivity in Withdrawal Seizure-Prone and -Resistant mice. Alcohol Clin Exp Res 1995;19:410–415.

71. Reilly MT, Crabbe JC, Rustay NR, Finn DA. Acute neuroactive steroid withdrawal in withdrawal seizure-prone and withdrawal seizure-resistant mice. Pharmacol Biochem Behav 2000;67:709–717.

72. Cabib S, Orsini C, LeMoal M, Piazza PV. Abolition and reversal of strain differences in behavioral responses to drugs of abuse after a brief experience. Science 2000;289:463–465.

73. Crabbe JC, Wahlsten D, Dudek BC. Genetics of mouse behavior: interactions with laboratory environment. Science 1999;284:1670–1672.

74. Rose RJ, Dick DM, Viken RJ, Kaprio J. Gene-environment interaction in patterns of adolescent drinking: regional residency moderates longitudinal influences on alcohol use. Alcohol Clin Exp Res 2001;25:637–643.

75. Rustay NR, Wahlsten D, Crabbe JC. Assessment of genetic susceptibility to ethanol intoxication in mice, Proc Natl Acad Sci USA 2003;100:2917–2922.

9

Murine Models of Alcoholism

From QTL to Gene

Chris Downing, Beth Bennett, and Thomas E. Johnson

1. INTRODUCTION

Most behavioral responses to alcohol are known to be influenced by genetic factors. Human twin and adoption studies consistently show that susceptibility to alcohol abuse is heritable *(1)*. The mode of inheritance is unknown, but is certainly polygenic and multifactorial, with a substantial environmental effect *(1,2)*. Despite much research, the genes and causal pathways determining susceptibility to alcohol abuse and dependence remain relatively unknown. Identifying genes that mediate alcoholism will improve strategies for diagnosis, treatment, and ultimately prevention.

Although the *Diagnostic and Statistical Manual of Mental Disorders* does not define alcoholism *per se*, it identifies a number of behaviors that constitute substance abuse and dependence *(3)*. A brief summary of these criteria is presented in Table 1. Because of ethical concerns, and because it is a complex and heterogeneous disorder, the genetic basis of alcoholism is difficult to study in humans. Murine models offer many advantages for elucidating the genetic architecture underlying alcohol susceptibility. In addition to the high degree of synteny and functional homology between mouse and human genomes, transgenic and knockout technologies in mice allow functional analysis of single genes that are not possible in most other organisms. The use of a well-characterized animal system allows simplification of complex behaviors by producing models that are relevant to the human condition.

Several behavioral phenotypes in mice have been used to model human alcoholism, including alcohol consumption or preference, sedative–hypnotic sensitivity, physical dependence and withdrawal, psychomotor activation, ataxia, hypothermia, and conditioned place preference (CPP). Each of these

From: *Computational Genetics and Genomics*
Edited by: G. Peltz © Humana Press Inc., Totowa, NJ

Table 1
DSM-IV Criteria for Substance Abuse and Dependence

Substance abuse
A maladaptive pattern of substance use leading to clinically significant impairment, as manifested by one or more of the following, occurring within a—12-mo period:
  a. Recurrent substance use resulting in a failure of major obligations-home, work, and so on.
  b. Recurrent substance use in situations in which it is physically hazardous.
  c. Recurrent legal problems related to the substance.
  d. Continued use despite having persistent social or interpersonal problems related to the substance.

Substance dependence
A maladaptive pattern of substance use, leading to clinically significant impairment, as manifested by three or more of the following, occurring at any time in a 12-mo period:
  a. Tolerance, either a need for increased amounts of the substance to achieve intoxication, or a diminished effect with continued use of the same amount of the substance.
  b. Withdrawal—each substance has a characteristic withdrawal syndrome.
  c. The substance is taken in larger amounts over a longer period than was intended.
  d. Persistent, unsuccessful attempts to cut down or control the substance use.
  e. Much time spent in activities necessary to obtain the substance.
  f. Social, occupational, or recreational activities are given up or reduced because of substance abuse.
  g. Substance use is continued despite knowledge of having a persistent physical or psychological problems caused by the substance.

DSM-IV, *Diagnostic and Statistical Manual of Mental Disorders, 4th ed.*

phenotypes (Table 2; refs. *4–12*) is believed to be clinically relevant and may play a role in susceptibility to alcoholism. Our own work has focused on the sedative–hypnotic properties of alcohol, which reflect one form of initial sensitivity. Schuckit and colleagues have shown that, in humans, initial sensitivity to alcohol is a reliable predictor of alcohol-related problems *(13,14)*. Sons of alcoholics had less intense reactions to alcohol as measured by subjective self-reports, body sway indices, changes in level of several hormones, and electrophysiological changes. Follow-up evaluations 10 yr later showed that a low level of response to alcohol was associated with a fourfold greater likelihood of future alcoholism *(13–15)*. Although initial sensitivity has been shown to be an important factor in susceptibility to abuse alcohol, the

Table 2
Behavioral Responses to Alcohol Investigated in Mice

Phenotype	Description
Loss of righting reflex	Measured by injecting a mouse with a high (3.3–5.1 g/kg) dose of alcohol. The mouse is placed on its back in a V-shaped trough. When the mouse can right itself three times within 60 s, it has regained the righting reflex.[a] Alternatively, mice are placed in cylindric restrainer, which is rotated every 2–3 s. Mice lose the righting reflex if they cannot right themselves from a supine position within 5 s.[b]
Consumption or preference	Reflects the rewarding or reinforcing properties of drugs (alcohol). Mice are typically given a choice between bottles containing water or alcohol (6–10%). Consumption is reported as gram/kilogram alcohol consumed, whereas preference is a ratio of alcohol to total fluid consumed.[c] In some paradigms, mice are first forced to drink ethanol for 2–3 d, and then given a choice between water and ethanol.[d]
Dependence and withdrawal	Dependence is usually achieved by maintaining mice on ethanol vapor for a number of days in an inhalation chamber. Withdrawal is measured as handling-induced convulsions.[e]
Psychomotor activation	Believed to be a measure of the rewarding or reinforcing properties of alcohol. Animals are injected with a low dose of alcohol (1.5–2 g/kg) and activity is assessed, usually in automated activity monitors.[f]
Ataxia	An index of motor coordination. Mice are injected with alcohol, then placed on a rotarod or wooden dowel,[g] or placed in a chamber with a metal grid floor (grid test).[h] These tests have been commonly used to assess tolerance.
Hypothermia	Measured as a temperature change following alcohol injection using a rectal probe.[a]

Table 2 (continued)

Phenotype	Description
Conditioned place preference (CPP)	Reflects rewarding or reinforcing properties. CPP is induced by first repeatedly pairing ethanol and saline injections with distinctive floors within a chamber. On the test day, mice are given access to both floors within the chamber. CPP is measured as the amount of time a mouse spends on the floor paired with ethanol.[i]

[a]Adapted from ref. *4.*
[b]Adapted from ref. *5.*
[c]Adapted from ref. *6.*
[d]Adapted from ref. *7.*
[e]Adapted from ref. *8.*
[f]Adapted from ref. *9.*
[g]Adapted from ref. *10.*
[h]Adapted from ref. *11.*
[i]Adapted from ref. *12.*

phenomena of tolerance (decreased sensitivity to a drug that develops with repeated exposure) and sensitization (an increase in drug sensitivity as a result of repeated exposure) also contribute to alcohol abuse and dependence. Determining the roles that each of these (initial sensitivity, tolerance, and sensitization) play, and how they interact to produce alcohol abuse and dependence, will be critical for formulating rational therapies in humans.

In this chapter, we outline a method for identifying genes mediating complex traits in mice (Fig. 1) and describe its use in mapping genes mediating alcohol-related behavioral responses. The first step is demonstrating genetic variation in the phenotype of interest, usually by detecting inbred strain differences or selective breeding. Next, quantitative trait locus (QTL) mapping is used to identify chromosomal regions influencing the phenotype. In murine research, initial mapping is often done in recombinant inbred strains (RI), with verification in the second filial (F2) or backcross (BC) populations or by creating congenic strains. The QTL region is then narrowed by using a variety of breeding schemes, including interval-specific congenic recombinant (ISCR) strains. These strategies can reduce the QTL interval to a point where candidate gene evaluation is feasible, ideally less than a centimorgan (cM). Bioinformatics are then used to investigate the deoxyribonucleic acid (DNA) sequence within this narrowed region and identify candidate genes. Strategies for demonstrating that a candidate gene underlies the QTL of interest include detecting DNA sequence variation, demonstrating

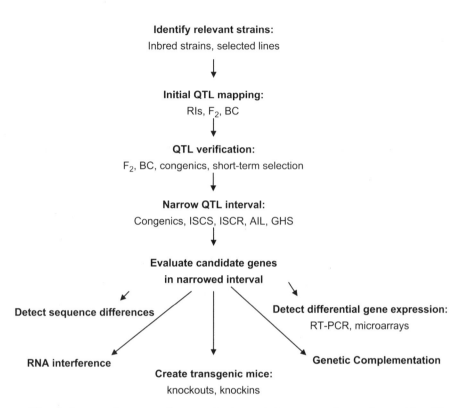

Fig. 1. A general strategy for quantitative trait locus mapping and gene identification using a murine model. QTL, quantitative trait locus; RIs, recombinant inbreds; F_2, second filial; BC, backcross; ISCS, interval-specific congenic strains; ISCR, interval-specific congenic recombinant; AIL, advanced intercross lines; GHS, genetically heterogeneous stock; RT-PCR, reverse transcription polymerase chain reaction.

differential gene expression, and functionally evaluating the effects of individual genes using transgenic (knockout and knockin) mice. We report here results from our laboratory and others, which have sought to identify genes that mediate alcohol-related behavioral traits. Although our research has focused on the sedative–hypnotic properties of alcohol, our discussion will include many different alcohol-mediated behaviors.

2. IDENTIFYING GENETIC INFLUENCES

2.1. Inbred Strains

Inbred strains are created by 20 or more generations of brother–sister mating, in which homozygosity is achieved at more than 99% of all loci *(16)*.

Thus, all mice within a given inbred strain are essentially genetically identical (isogenic). When such strains are reared and assessed under uniform conditions, phenotypic differences among strains demonstrate a genetic influence; phenotypic variation within an inbred strain is, by definition, the result of environmental effects. One of the primary strengths of inbred strains is the accumulated database of phenotypic and genotypic observations across time and in different laboratories. Recently, it has been proposed that such inbred strain phenotypic differences, in conjunction with a single nucleotide polymorphism (SNP) database, can be used to identify QTLs *(17)*. Traditionally, however, inbred strains have been used to demonstrate genetic variation, to estimate genetic correlations among phenotypes (which implies shared genetic control), and to identify strains for potential crosses that would maximize successful QTL detection.

Inbred strain differences have been reported for a number of alcohol-related behavioral measures, including sedative–hypnotic sensitivity, consumption or preference, dependence and withdrawal, locomotor activation, ataxia, hypothermia, and CPP (Table 3; refs. *11,18–23*). Table 3 is not meant to be all inclusive (*see* ref. *6*) but to show the range of genetic variation observed among the more commonly used inbred strains. It is important to note that widely varying results have been reported for many alcohol phenotypes in inbred mice. These discrepancies are most likely owing to differences in dose of ethanol, route of administration, and paradigm used, along with environmental influences. The most consistent results have been reported for the C57BL/6J (B6) and DBA/2J (D2) strains, the two most commonly used inbred strains of mice in alcohol research. These strains are highly polymorphic (www.jax.org) and differ significantly in a number of alcohol-related behavioral responses (Table 3). In general, B6 mice are high consumers, have less severe withdrawal reactions, show little ethanol-induced locomotor activation, and display marked ethanol-induced ataxia. In contrast, D2 mice are low consumers, have more severe withdrawal reactions, show high activation, and are less impaired in tests of ataxia. These two strains have been crossed to create RI lines and segregating populations, in which QTL mapping can be performed.

2.2. Selected Lines

In selective breeding, animals displaying extreme scores (high and low) for a given phenotype are chosen to propagate the next generation. In principle, selective breeding will identify all alleles in a population that increase a phenotype, and will increase the frequency of those alleles at all relevant loci in the high line; a parallel process occurs in the low line *(24)*. Selection

Table 3
Inbred Strain Differences in Several Alcohol-Related Behavioral Phenotypes

Strain	Hypnotic sensitivity[a]	Consumption/ Preference[b]	Dependence/ Withdrawal[c]	Locomotor activation[d]	Ataxia[e]
C57BL/6	Inconsistent results: low, moderate, or high sensitivity (96.2 min)	High consumers (68%)	Mild withdrawal convulsions (11.20)	Low activation (3000 cm)	Severely impaired (2.22)
DBA/2	Inconsistent results: moderate or high sensitivity (72.2 min)	Low consumers (20%)	Severe withdrawal convulsions (36.75)	High activation (3700 cm)	Mildly impaired (1.29)
129	High sensitivity (140.4 min)	Low to moderate consumers (25%)	Severe withdrawal convulsions	Low activation (2460 cm)	Moderately impaired (1.97)
BALB	Moderate sensitivity (64.4 min)	Moderate consumers (29%)	Mild withdrawal convulsions (5.70)	High activation (6500 cm)	Moderately impaired (1.48)
C3H	Inconsistent results: very low or very high sensitivity (34.4 min)	Moderate consumers (29%)	Severe withdrawal convulsions (32.21)	Moderate to high activation (3600 cm)	Moderately impaired (1.84)

[a]Data are adapted from ref. *11*, expressed as duration of loss of righting reflex following a 4 g/kg dose of ethanol.

[b]Data are adapted from ref. *18*, expressed as the percent of total fluid intake from the ethanol-containing bottle in a two-bottle choice test.

[c]Data are adapted from ref. *19*, expressed as area under the curve for handling-induced convulsions, following chronic ethanol exposure.

[d]Data are adapted from ref. *20*, expressed as the total distance traveled in 30 min (cm) following injection of 2 g/kg ethanol.

[e]Data are adapted from ref. *11*, expressed as mean number of errors made in a 3-min grid test following injection of 2 g/kg ethanol.

pressure is not imposed on nonrelevant loci, so these loci will continue to segregate, unless they are fixed because of linkage to genes that are selected. Mouse selection studies begin with an outbred population or genetically heterogeneous stock (GHS) of mice, in order to ensure genetic variability on which selection pressure can act. Selected lines are important for two reasons: (a) they provide conclusive evidence for a genetic influence on a given phenotype, i.e., there is additive genetic variance and the trait is heritable;

Table 4
Selected Lines of Mice and Rats Used in Alcohol Research

Selected line	Phenotype	References
Long-sleep and Short-sleep mice	Duration of loss of the righting reflex following a 4.1 g/kg dose of ethanol	*4*
HOT and COLD mice	Temperature decrease following a 3 g/kg dose of ethanol	*24*
Withdrawal Seizure-Prone and-Resistant mice	Handling induced seizures following 3 d of forced ethanol inhalation	*26*
FAST and SLOW mice	Locomotor activation following a 1.5 or 2 g/kg dose of ethanol	*9*
High- and low-alcohol preference mice	Two bottle choice—consumption (g/kg) of 10% ethanol over 30 d	*27*
High- and Low-Acute Functional Tolerance mice	Difference in blood ethanol level at regain of ability to remain on a dowel following a g/kg dose of ethanol	*28*
Severe or mild ethanol withdrawal mice	Multimeasure index of withdrawal after liquid ethanol diet	*29*
Preferring and Nonpreferring rats	Preference for drinking 10% ethanol	*30*
High- and low-alcohol drinking rats	Preference for drinking 10% ethanol	*31*
Sardinian Preferring and Nonpreferring rats	Preference for drinking 10% ethanol	*32*
High- and low-alcohol sensitive rats	Duration of loss of the righting reflex	*33*

and (b) they allow the detection of correlated characteristics. Selected lines of mice and rats have been developed for a number of alcohol-related behavioral phenotypes, including hypnotic sensitivity, withdrawal, consumption, locomotor activation, hypothermia, and acute functional tolerance (Table 4; refs. *4,9,25–33*).

3. QTL DETECTION

3.1. RI Strains

It is common in murine research to use RI strains in the first stage of QTL mapping. RI strains are generated by crossing two inbred strains, and intercrossing these offspring to create an F2 population, where genetic segregation occurs. Subsequent inbreeding leads to, and fixes, unique recombinations of parental alleles in each RI strain. RI strains were originally created to test for single gene effects; if the RIs phenotypically resembled one parental strain or the other, with no intermediate phenotypes, the influence of a single gene could be inferred. RI strains can also be used to identify and position genes that have a smaller effect on the phenotype of interest. Creation of RIs results in a fourfold expansion of the genetic map *(34)*, further facilitating the mapping of QTLs. This is valuable because most behavioral phenotypes, including alcohol-susceptibility phenotypes, are complex, quantitative traits with a continuous distribution, and are likely influenced by multiple genes (QTLs), each with a small effect. In alcohol research, no RI strains have been used as extensively as the BXD RIs, derived from a cross between B6 and D2 mice.

One major advantage of using RIs for QTL mapping is that each datapoint is a strain mean (and variance), derived by assessing several animals for a given phenotype. Multiple phenotypic assessments of the same genotype effectively reduces environmental variance, which raises heritability and allows for a more accurate measurement of the genetic effect *(35,36)*. Another advantage of using RIs for QTL mapping is that, unlike segregating populations, RI strains need only be genotyped once for each marker. The subsequent strain distribution pattern is stable; other investigators simply assess the RIs for a given phenotype and correlate the phenotypic data with the existing strain distribution pattern.

There are also some drawbacks to using RIs for QTL mapping. First, if one wants new strains, there is a considerable amount of time and expense necessary to generate them (at least 22 generations). Second, only a few RI strains are currently available, which limits the power to detect and map QTLs. However, this may be changing, as the Williams laboratory is assaying thousands of markers in several RI strains that share B6 as a parental strain *(35)*. This collected RI set, termed BXN, consists of more than 100 strains, which will improve the utility and power of QTL mapping. The power of RIs for QTL mapping can also be significantly increased by using RI inter-cross or RI BC designs (RIX and RIB, respectively; ref. *35*). Third, RI analysis can only detect the additive component of QTLs, as there are no heterozygotes in which to observe dominance. Epistasis (gene–gene inter-actions) evaluation is limited to that detected in homozygotes (i.e., addi-tive by additive).

The principles behind QTL mapping with RIs are relatively straight-forward; mapping involves correlating genotype with phenotype. Animals from a number of RIs are scored or measured for the phenotype of interest and assayed for a number of genetic markers throughout the genome. Significant correlations between a marker and a phenotype indi-cate the presence of a linked QTL. Although early studies in mice used restriction fragment length polymorphisms *(37)* and other, less than ideal, markers, the polymerase chain reaction (PCR) and other recent DNA technologies have allowed repetitive sequences (microsatellites) to be used as markers for mapping. Microsatellite markers (also known as sim-ple sequence repeats) are quite abundant and highly polymorphic in the mouse *(38)*, with the dinucleotide repeats of the monoidotyrosine series a common choice in murine mapping. The detection and use of SNPs as genetic markers will provide a much denser genetic map than is currently available.

In our laboratory, we have used a multistage mapping strategy for identi-fying and localizing QTLs mediating hypnotic sensitivity to ethanol. In the first stage, RI strains were derived from a cross between long-sleep and short-sleep mice (LS and SS, respectively). LS and SS mice were selec-tively bred for sensitivity and resistance to the sedative–hypnotic effects of ethanol. Starting from a GHS of mice, animals were selected for differences in loss of righting reflex due to ethanol (LORE) following a 3.3–4.1 g/kg dose of ethanol (for a description of the selection procedure, *see* ref. *39*). After 15 generations of selection, SS mice had a mean LORE duration of 10 min, whereas LS mice had a mean LORE duration of more than 2 h *(40)*. Because differences in ethanol metabolism between LS and SS mice are small, their differential response to ethanol is believed to be mediated primarily by the central nervous system *(40–43)*. Heritability estimates for LORE range from 0.18 to 0.42, with seven to nine QTLs mediating the dif-ference between LS and SS, or inbred LS (ILS) and inbred SS (ISS) mice *(4,44–46)*. LORE has been characterized as a relatively simple additive genetic system, with little evidence for significant dominance or maternal effects, some suggestion of epistasis, and sex effects of small magnitude *(44–46)*. These observations suggested that mapping QTLs for LORE duration in populations derived from LS and SS mice should be successful.

RI strains were created at the Institute for Behavioral Genetics (IBG) by reciprocally crossing LS and SS mice. Six males and females from the first filial (F1) generation were brother–sister mated, and the F2 generation randomly brother–sister mated to create 40 LS × SS RI lines *(45)*. Initial QTL analysis in the 27 extant RI strains involved both single-point and interval mapping for LORE duration and blood ethanol concentration following a 4.1 g/kg dose of ethanol *(47,48)*. In single-point analysis, markers are correlated individually with phenotypic data. For each marker, one-way analyses of variance (ANOVA) were carried out with LORE or blood ethanol concentration as the dependent variable, and RI strains were grouped by allele type (LS-like or SS-like). A significant *F* test (a significant difference in LORE duration between the two marker classes at the $\alpha = 0.05$ level) was taken as evidence for a QTL linked to the marker. Eleven provisional QTLs for LORE duration were identified by point analysis, using 124 markers distributed throughout the mouse genome; these putative QTLs were located on chromosomes 1(3 QTLs), 2(2), 4(2), 9(2), 16, and 18 *(47,48)*. The strongest association for LORE was found at marker *D2Mit21*, which is located 80 cM from the centromere on chromosome 2. This QTL explained about 40% of the genotypic variance in LORE.

Although single-point analysis can detect putative QTLs, there are several drawbacks to this approach *(37)*: (a) if the QTL does not lie at the marker locus, its phenotypic effect may be underestimated, depending on the recombination fraction between the marker and the QTL; (b) if the QTL does not lie at the marker locus, substantially more progeny may be required for QTL detection; and (c) single-point analysis does not define the position of the QTL; it cannot distinguish between tight linkage to a small-effect QTL and loose linkage to a large-effect QTL.

Lander and Botstein *(37)* described an improved QTL mapping strategy, interval mapping, which overcomes some of the problems associated with single-point analysis. Interval mapping tests the hypothesis that a QTL affecting the trait lies between a pair of flanking markers. This procedure involves fitting a model (additive, dominant, recessive, or unconstrained) at a series of positions throughout the interval between two flanking markers; maximum-likelihood methods or linear regression can be used to estimate QTL position and effect size *(37,49)*. Compared with single-point analysis, interval mapping gives better estimates of phenotypic effects and QTL positions. Lander and Botstein *(37)* derived formulas for interval mapping that are applicable to both F2 and BC populations.

Fulker et al. *(50)* derived an algorithm for interval mapping in RIs based on linear regression. Using this approach, 12 provisional QTLs were detected which influenced LORE *(48)*. Table 5 shows a comparison of provisional QTLs identified by single-point analysis and interval mapping. Both single-point and interval mapping strongly support a QTL mediating LORE at 80 cM on chromosome 2 *(48)*. This QTL accounted for a 20-min difference in LORE between LS and SS lines. Using multiple regression, 62% of the genetic variance in LORE was explained by the three most significant QTLs on chromosomes 1 (45 cM), 2 (80 cM), and 6 (46 cM). In contrast, only 44% of the genetic variance in LORE duration was explained by these three QTLs using single-point analysis, illustrating one strength of interval mapping over single-point QTL analysis. A second major advantage is the more precise QTL localization.

Table 5
Detection of QTLs for Ethanol Sensitivity by Single-Point and Interval Mapping

	Single-point method			Interval method			
Marker (cM)	F	p value	Genetic variance explained (%)	Chromosome (cM position)	t^a	p value	Genetic variance explained (%)
D1Mit20 (24)	4.22	0.025	14.4	1 (45)	3.14	0.00022	25.4
D1Mit46 (42)	2.75	0.042	18.6	1 (99)	1.98	0.0297	10.4
D1Mit45 (58)	7.96	0.005	21.1	2 (80)	4.04	0.0002	37.1
D2Mit7 (26)	5.65	0.005	32.0	3 (74)	2.01	0.0300	13.8
D2Mit21 (80)	16.33	0.001	39.5	4 (56)	1.92	0.0337	9.3
D4Mit11 (55)	3.25	0.042	11.5	4 (74)	2.00	0.0282	10.4
D4Mit42 (75)	3.97	0.024	13.7	5 (72)	1.89	0.0395	9.3
D9Mit42 (5)	5.30	0.021	30.6	6 (46)	2.33	0.0164	19.7
D9Mit12 (50)	7.90	0.002	39.7	12 (43)	2.18	0.0195	12.6
D16Mit5 (32)	4.6	0.021	15.5	13 (25)	2.23	0.0187	15.9
D18Mit3 (16)	4.22	0.025	14.4	16 (41)	2.26	0.0165	13.6
				18 (16)	2.06	0.0253	11.0

[a]Position of maximal *t* value. Data are from reference *48*.

3.2. Segregating Populations

Although RIs are often employed in the preliminary stages of QTL mapping, they are generally not efficient at detecting QTLs because of the low power associated with the limited number of strains available. Consequently, most groups have opted to accept a higher number of false positives in mapping with RI strains. This means that these QTLs should be viewed as provisional and need to be verified, typically using segregating populations, such as an F2 intercross or BC. When two inbred strains are crossed, their offspring are known as the *first filial*, or F1, generation. Although offspring will be heterozygous at all loci for which the parental strains are polymorphic, every mouse in the F1 generation is genetically identical. Mice from the F1 generation can be intercrossed to create the *second filial*, or F2, generation. Alternatively, F1 mice can be mated back to either or both parental strains, in a design known as a BC. In both F2 and BC populations, genetic segregation takes place, thus allowing QTL mapping. The main advantage that segregating generations have over RI strains for QTL mapping is that sample size is not a limitation; therefore, the power to detect and localize QTLs, and estimate their effect size, is usually greater. In general, the F2 design is more powerful than the BC, except in the case where dominance is observed, where one of the BC matings (to the strain carrying the recessive allele) will yield more informative progeny.

Typically, inbred strains that differ for a trait of interest are crossed to produce segregating generations for QTL mapping. Alternatively, F2 and BC mice can be produced by crossing lines that were selectively bred for differences in the relevant phenotype. Or, one can inbreed mice that were selectively bred, and then cross these lines to create mapping populations. This latter situation creates an ideal QTL mapping population. Selective breeding and subsequent inbreeding creates parental strains that are fixed for alternate alleles at both QTL and marker loci, and all alleles should be in association (all alleles that increase a trait are fixed homozygous in one line, whereas all alleles that decrease a trait are fixed in the other line; ref. *16*). In contrast, whereas mice within a given inbred strain are homozygous at virtually all loci, fixation at any given locus is a chance occurrence; thus, inbred strains, although differing for the trait of interest, will likely have some alleles that increase the phenotype and some alleles that decrease the phenotype. The drawback to selective breeding and subsequent inbreeding is the many years necessary to create the mapping population.

In our laboratory, F2 mice were generated by crossing the ILS and ISS lines, which had been produced by inbreeding the LS and SS lines. At generation

30 of inbreeding, ILS females were crossed with ISS males (L/S), with the reciprocal crosses also made (S/L), to create an F1 population *(51)*. All four possible F1 crosses were made (L/S × L/S, L/S × S/L, S/L × L/S, and S/L × S/L) to produce F2-generation mice. Mice from the F2 generation (*n* = 1072) were then assessed for LORE duration following a 4.1 g/kg dose of ethanol. Mice were tested twice, on day one, and again 7–10 d later, with QTL mapping performed on the average of the two LORE measures. Selective genotyping was employed, with 92 of the longest- and 92 of the shortest-sleeping F2 mice assayed for the twelve provisional QTLs (flanking markers) identified in the RI study. Selective genotyping reduces the cost of QTL analysis by measuring a large number of mice for a given phenotype but only genotyping the phenotypic extremes. The logic behind selective genotyping, as discussed by Lander and Botstein *(37)*, is that some progeny contribute more linkage information than others, with the most informative progeny found in the phenotypic extremes. For example, progeny with phenotypic values greater than 1 standard deviation (SD) from the mean comprise only 33% of the distribution (population) but capture about 80% of the genetic variance.

We performed QTL mapping of the selectively genotyped extremes using the programs Mapmaker/EXP and Mapmaker/QTL. Mapmaker/EXP creates a genetic linkage map, whereas Mapmaker/QTL uses maximum likelihood methods for QTL detection *(37)*. Other QTL mapping programs exist, such as Mapmanager/QT and QTL Cartographer *(52,53)*, with the various programs differing in their methods of QTL detection and other options available. When selective genotyping is performed, linear regression methods cannot be used because phenotypic effects would be greatly overestimated because of biased selection of progeny. Maximum likelihood methods can be used when all progeny have been phenotyped, with genotypes from the nonextremes recorded as missing data *(37)*. A logarithm of the odds (lod) score is calculated as the test statistic. A lod score is the logarithm of the odds of linkage to a QTL divided by the odds of no linkage, given a particular dataset. This test statistic can be calculated at various points throughout the genome. The lod score follows a chi-square distribution, and can be converted into a chi-square statistic by multiplying by $2(\log_e 10) \approx 4.6$ *(54)*. Similarly, with the regression approach, a likelihood ratio statistic can be calculated using mean square$_{regression}$/mean square$_{residual}$, at any point throughout the genome *(49)*. Although beyond the scope of this chapter, several excellent papers have discussed (and argued) criteria to be used for declaring statistical significance of a linked QTL *(37,55–57)*.

Using a whole-genome scan, the Mapmaker programs, and selective genotyping, only two out of twelve provisional QTLs previously identified in the

LS × SS RI strains were confirmed in the F2 mice, those on chromosomes 1 and 2 *(51)*. These confirmed QTLs had maximum lod scores of 5.4 at 54 cM on chromosome 1, and 6.6 at 85 cM on chromosome 2. Another QTL on chromosome 18 was confirmed but at a lower level of certainty (lod = 1.8). Three new QTLs with lod scores of 3.4 or higher were also detected on chromosomes 8 (59 cM), 11 (49 cM), and 15 (46 cM). In addition, using the entire F2 population, a weak QTL influencing LORE was identified, closely linked to the *Tyr* locus on chromosome 7 *(58)*. Thus, from the initial RI analysis and subsequent F2 mapping, seven QTLs mediating LORE were identified, and have been named *Lore1–Lore7*, for LORE *(51)*. These seven QTLs accounted for 59% of the genetic variance in LORE.

4. QTL VERIFICATION

4.1. Short-Term Selection

One strategy for conforming a provisional QTL is short-term selection. Belknap et al. outlined the use of an F2 population derived from a cross between inbred strains (B6 and D2) that differed in alcohol preference as the foundation population for selective breeding *(59)*. The presence of only two alleles at each locus greatly facilitates marker genotyping and QTL analysis. Because the two possible parental alleles are at an initial frequency of 0.50 ($p = q = 0.50$), changes in allele frequency as a result of selection can easily be monitored. Furthermore, the response to selection is at or near maximal at intermediate allele frequencies *(16)*, which greatly increases the probability of producing extremely divergent high and low lines in only a few generations. This design was used to verify a QTL mediating alcohol preference on chromosome 3 *(59)*.

4.2. Segregating Congenics

Another method for quick confirmation of a QTL is what we have called "segregating congenics" *(60,61)*. This method is similar to short-term selection as described in Subheading 4.1. In our laboratory, segregating congenics were created for the five *Lore* QTLs with the largest effects (explaining >5% of the genetic variance), *Lore1–Lore5*. Segregating congenics *(60,61)* are homozygous for the QTL of interest but unfixed at other relevant loci. They are created by screening an intercross population for relevant markers flanking a QTL, which allows a single QTL to be made homozygous on an otherwise segregating genetic background. Thus, the segregating congenics are fixed for one QTL but will still segregate new combinations of unfixed QTLs. The increased genetic variance owing to the segregating loci will

congenics," refs. *63–65*), one can introgress a single QTL onto the recipient background and drastically reduce the number of BC generations needed to create the congenic mice.

4.4. QTL-Marker-Assisted Counter Selection

We also created congenic lines for *Lore1–Lore5* using a strategy we term "QTL-Marker-Assisted Counter Selection" *(66)*. This approach is an alternative to speed congenics that takes advantage of prior knowledge of map positions of major QTLs. In QTL-marker-assisted counter selection, one selects for donor genetic markers flanking a single QTL, whereas selecting against donor genetic markers at the other QTLs. In our laboratory, F1 mice produced from reciprocal crosses between ILS and ISS were backcrossed to both parental strains to produce the N2 generation. "N" refers to the generation of backcrossing; for example, N2 refers to the second generation of backcrossing. Three hundred and eight N2 mice were genotyped at pairs of markers flanking each of the five *Lore* regions, with markers (based on Mouse Genome Database cM positions) chosen to enclose the 1-lod support interval for each *Lore* QTL (Fig. 3).

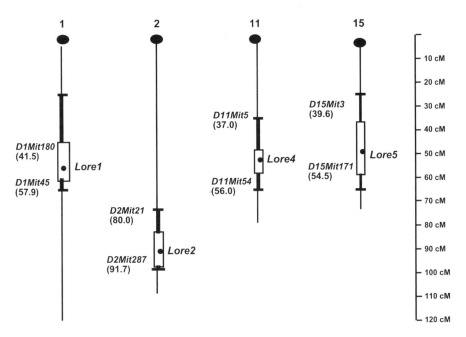

Fig. 3. Maximum likelihood positions for the *Lore* quantitative trait loci. The boxes indicate the 1-logarithm of the odds (lod) support intervals, whereas the bold vertical lines show the 2-lod support intervals. Markers and cM positions are shown to the left of each region. Data are adapted from ref. *44*.

Mice heterozygous and nonrecombinant over a given interval for a single *Lore*, while homozygous ISS or ILS at the other four *Lore* intervals were chosen as parents for the N3 generation and were backcrossed to ISS or ILS.

Congenics were constructed differently, depending on the recipient background. For mice with an ILS QTL on an ISS background (ISS.ILS), power analysis showed that it would take approx 30 mice to detect a heterozygote effect on an ISS background *(39)*. Therefore, we incorporated a phenotyping regimen into the ISS BC, beginning at the N4 generation, in order to monitor retention of the phenotype *(39,66)*. In contrast, power analysis showed that 200–300 mice would need to be tested in order to detect an effect of an ISS QTL on an ILS background (ILS.ISS). Consequently, no phenotyping was done on the ILS background until congenics were produced. At this time, we also conducted a dose–response analysis in order to determine the appropriate dosage so as to yield a measure of LORE with a standard deviation similar to ISS at 4.1 g/kg. A 2.5 g/kg dose gave the closest variance measure, and power analysis indicated it would be possible to detect the effect of an ISS allele on an ILS background by testing approx 30 mice. Subsequently, all ILS recipient congenics were tested at the 2.5 g/kg dose.

Both congenics, ILS.ISS and ISS.ILS, were backcrossed for 10 generations to create full congenics. As can be seen in Fig. 4, ISS QTL significantly decreased LORE by 20–30 min relative to ILS controls (2.5 g/kg), with the exception of lines 2C and 5D, in which only a few mice were tested. The expected values for each LORE congenic strain were derived from application of the MapMaker to the 1072 F2 mice in which the QTLs were identified *(47)*. An effect of *Lore3* could not be detected in any generation and those lines were discarded. Similarly, on the ISS background, the ILS QTL increased LORE. Comparing the congenic mice with heterozygotes and ISS homozygotes (Fig. 4) showed that *Lore2*, *Lore4*, and *Lore5* congenic strains exhibited the expected additive mode of inheritance, whereas the *Lore1* congenics showed a dominant pattern.

Fig. 4. (A) Mean length of sedation after intraperitoneal injection of 2.5 g/kg ethanol in inbred long-sleep/inbred short-sleep (ILS.ISS) congenics. Individual *Lore* (number) and subline (letter) are on the horizontal axis. Sample size is given at the top of the bar. The bar at the far right shows the phenotypic value for the ILS control. p values at the top of the panel indicate a one-tailed p for significance for the difference between that congenic subline and ILS (*$p < 0.05$, ** $p < 0.01$, *** $p < 0.001$). Observed values are represented in the black bars, whereas expected values, taken from MapMaker, are in gray. **(B)** Mean length of sedation after intraperitoneal

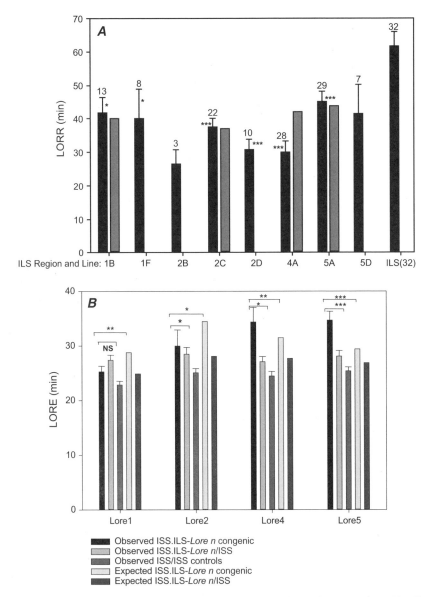

Fig. 4. (*Continued*) injection of 4.1 g/kg ethanol in ISS.ILS congenics. The first three bars (with standard errors) show loss of righting reflex due to ethanol (LORE) for congenic mice, mice heterozygous with ISS, and ISS homozygotes. The last two bars (no standard errors) show the expected LORE for ILS homozygotes and ISS.ILS congenic heterozygotes. The upper bracket shows the significance of the difference between the congenic strain and their ISS controls; lower brackets show the significance of the difference between congenics and heterozygotes (*$p < 0.05$, **$p < 0.01$, ***$p < 0.001$). Data are adapted from ref. *39*.

4.5. Additional Alcohol-Related QTLs

The use of RI strains, segregating populations, and congenics has identified and confirmed QTLs mediating many alcohol-related behavioral phenotypes. These QTLs have been summarized in Fig. 5 *(7,51,67–88)*. We will briefly review some of the more relevant findings. The most studied alcohol phenotype has been ethanol consumption or preference. Several QTLs have been identified which influence alcohol preference in mice; most have used mapping populations derived from B6 and D2 mice. These include two QTLs identified by Melo et al. *(68)*, on chromosomes 2 (male-specific; *Alcp1*) and 11 (female-specific; *Alcp2*). Peirce et al. *(69)* also identified two sex-specific QTLs mediating alcohol preference on chromosomes 3 (male-specific; *Alcp3*) and 1 (female-specific; *Alcp4*). Six QTLs were detected by Tarantino et al. *(70)*—three significant QTLs on chromosomes 1, 4, and 9, and three suggestive QTLs on chromosomes 2, 3, and 10, *Ap1q– Ap6q*. Congenic mice have been used to confirm the QTL on chromosome 2, and identify a new QTL on chromosome 1, *Alcp5 (7)*. A recent meta-analysis *(73)* of these and other alcohol-preference QTL studies has reported the strongest support for QTLs on chromosomes 1 (distal), 2 (proximal to mid), 3 (mid to distal), 4 (distal), 9 (proximal to mid), and 11 (mid). A QTL for alcohol consumption was also identified on chromosome 15, *Aaq1 (74)*.

Detected and verified QTLs influencing alcohol-related behaviors

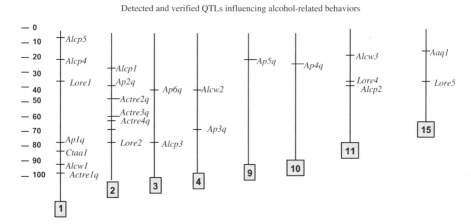

Fig. 5. Quantitative trait loci detected and verified for alcohol-related behaviors: *Alcp1–Alcp2* (alcohol preference; *see ref. 68). Alcp3–Alcp4, (see ref. 69). Alcp5, (see ref. 7). Ap1q–Ap6q* (alcohol preference; *see ref. 70). Aaq1* (alcohol acceptance; *see ref. 74). Lore1, 2, 4, 5* (loss of righting reflex owing to alcohol; *see ref. 51). Alcw1–Alcw3* (acute alcohol withdrawal; *see ref. 81). Actre1–Actre4* (activity response to alcohol; *see ref. 78). Ctaa1* (alcohol-conditioned taste aversion; *see refs. 85,86).

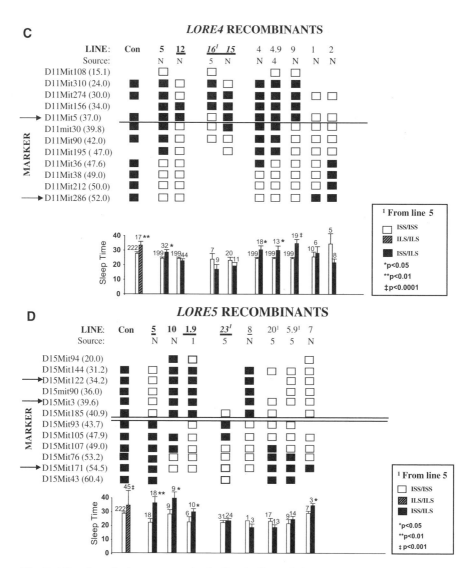

Fig. 7. (*Continued*) chromosome in the line indicated above. Results of progeny testing are shown in the histogram below each line; *p* values are shown in the legend. A significant difference between mice with the recombinant chromosome (ISS/ILS) and their homozygous littermates (ISS/ISS) indicates the ILS QTL was retained. The minimum interval containing the QTL is shown by the horizontal bold lines. The extent of the introgressed ILS region and the associated phenotype for the congenic strains are shown in the first line of each *Lore*. Bold lines show a significant phenotypic difference; underlined lines are being maintained but not tested, whereas italicized lines are still being tested. LORE, loss of righting reflex due to ethanol.

6. STRATEGIES FOR EVALUATING CANDIDATE GENES

Once mapping has identified and confirmed a QTL and fine-mapping has reduced the interval, identifying the relevant gene(s) or DNA sequence variants is still a daunting task. Historically, in the search for mouse QTLs, once fine-mapping has reduced a given region, the next step has been to evaluate candidate genes using bioinformatics, looking for obvious biological significance. However, whereas one may prioritize candidate genes based on *a priori* hypotheses or biological significance, often no candidate genes or too many candidate genes are immediately apparent. In addition, screening for polymorphisms in coding regions of candidate genes and demonstrating differential expression have been used to assess candidate gene likelihoods. Once candidate genes have been identified by showing DNA polymorphisms or differential expression, functional tests are still needed.

Few functional tests are available to the mouse geneticist for confirming a candidate gene as being the QTL of interest. The gold standard is to move the allele from one strain to another and show that the phenotype changes with the genotype. However, in mouse this is time-consuming, and is currently limited to the 129 and B6 embryonic stem cell lines. A more common approach in murine research has been the use of transgenic animals, in which a gene is overexpressed, or rendered nonfunctional (knockouts [KOs]). However, creating KOs, and interpreting results of KOs, can be problematic, as discussed in Subheading 6.3. Within the last couple of years, a new technique called RNA interference (RNAi) has been shown to be feasible in vivo in mice. Use of RNAi to functionally test candidate genes can overcome many of the problems associated with KOs.

6.1. Identifying DNA Sequence Differences

A necessity for a candidate gene being the QTL of interest is the existence of DNA sequence differences between the two parental strains from which the QTL mapping population was derived. DNA sequence differences in coding regions of a candidate gene may lead to amino acid changes and subsequent protein (functional) differences, whereas sequence differences in noncoding regions may lead to differential gene expression (*see* Subheading 6.2.). Thus, when one detects DNA polymorphisms in candidate genes, functional tests are necessary to determine the effect, if any, of the polymorphism.

Two general approaches for DNA sequencing are used: sequencing of complementary DNA or genomic DNA. When one is interested in sequencing coding regions of a candidate gene, typically RNA is extracted and reverse-transcribed into complementary DNA, which contains only coding regions (exons) and untranslated regions (UTRs). Alternatively, if one has found a candidate gene to be differentially expressed, and identification of the DNA polymorphism is desired, sequencing of nontranscribed, genomic DNA is necessary. Sequencing regulatory regions is not a trivial undertaking, depending on how large the candidate gene is. The genomic location and structure of eukaryotic regulatory regions is complex and not completely understood. Multiple transcription factors are required for gene expression. In mice, core promoter regions are usually located within 2 kb upstream of the transcription initiation site *(100)*. However, in addition to these core promoter elements, an increasing number of mammalian regulatory sequences have been identified in introns, exons, and 5′ and 3′ UTRs *(101)*. Furthermore, relevant regulatory regions (enhancer elements) may lie tens of thousands of basepairs from the transcription initiation site and are often difficult to identify. Thus, in order to detect a DNA polymorphism in a regulatory region, one may have to sequence approx 2 kb upstream of the transcription initiation site, introns, an exon or two, and enhancer elements, which may or may not have been identified for the candidate gene. With this much sequence, one is like to identify several SNPs; functional analysis of each individual SNP is expensive and time-consuming.

Few studies looking for coding region polymorphisms have been published for alcohol-related traits in mice. The Buck laboratory has identified a polymorphism between B6 and D2 mice in the γ-aminobutyric acid A (GABA$_A$)-γ$_2$ subunit gene (*Gabrg2*; a candidate gene for the *Alcw3* QTL), and correlated this polymorphism with alcohol-withdrawal severity *(102)*. This alteration involved a SNP at amino acid residue 11; an <u>ACT</u> codon in the D2 strain codes for a threonine residue, whereas a <u>GCT</u> codon in the B6 strain codes for an alanine residue. Their results indicated that the B6 allele is associated with greater withdrawal severity. In a follow-up study using mice from the BXD RI series, the polymorphism in the *Gabrg2* gene was also correlated with sensitivity to ethanol-conditioned taste aversion, ethanol-induced motor incoordination, and ethanol-induced hypothermia *(103)*. The Buck laboratory has also identified allelic variants in the *Mpdz* gene, a candidate gene for the *Alcw2* QTL, and correlated the variants with alcohol-withdrawal severity *(96)*. More recently, Xu et al. identified a SNP between B6 and D2 in the open reading frame of the *Cas1* gene, a candidate gene for ethanol-induced locomotor activation *(104)*. However, although some evidence supports the role of brain catalase in ethanol-induced locomotor activation, other evidence suggests that this polymorphism between B6 and D2 is not the previously identified QTL on mouse chromosome 2 *(104)*.

In relation to our own work, the Sikela laboratory *(105,106)* has detected coding region variants in a number of candidate genes throughout the four

Table 6 (continued)

Gene knocked out	Phenotype	References
Dopamine D_2 receptor	Reduced ethanol conditioned place preference (CPP). Decreased ethanol consumption and preference, reduced sensitivity to ethanol-induced locomotor activation. Increase in ethanol-induced locomotor activation (background dependent)	*142–144*
Dopamine D_3 receptor	No effect on ethanol CPP, ethanol consumption or preference	*145*
Dopamine D_4 receptor	Increased ethanol-induced locomotor activation	*146*
Protein Kinase C, γ isoform	Reduced ethanol-induced LORR; lack of tolerance to ethanol-induced LORR and hypothermia, but depended on genetic background; increased ethanol consumption; less sensitive to the anxiolytic effects of ethanol	*147–150*
Protein Kinase A	Increased ethanol consumption, reduced sensitivity to sedation (LORR)	*151*
m-neu1 (homolog of *Drosophila neuralized*)	Increased sensitivity to ethanol-induced ataxia (rotarod)	*152*
β-endorphin	Increased ethanol consumption	*153*
μ-opiate receptor	Decreased ethanol consumption and CPP	*154*
β-hydroxylase (synthesizes norepinephrine)	Reduced ethanol preference, delay in extinguishing ethanol-conditioned taste aversion, increased sedation and hypothermia	*155*
Monoamine oxidase A	No increase in ethanol consumption or preference, increased ethanol-induced LORR, reduced hypothermia	*156*
Angiotensin II	Decreased ethanol consumption and preference	*157*
DARPP-32	No difference in ethanol-conditioned taste aversion, greater locomotor activation, failure to acquire CPP	*158*

Table 6 (continued)

Gene knocked out	Phenotype	References
Homer2	Blunted ethanol reward (no ethanol CPP), reduced ehtnol consumption, increased ethanol-induced LORR, reduced sensitization to ethanol-induced locomotor activation	*159*
Fyn-kinase	No effect on ethanol consumption, ethanol-induced LORR. Increased ethanol-induced LORR, impaired acute tolerance to motor incoordinating effects of ethanol (stationary dowel), increased sensitivity to anxiolytic effects of ethanol (plus maze); males showed decreased preference for ethanol; no effects on ethanol-induced hypothermia, no effects on ethanol metabolism. Increased ethanol-induced LORR, no effect on ethanol consumption or ethanol CPP	*160–162*
Cannabinoid receptor	Reduced ethanol consumption. Absence of ethanol withdrawal symptoms (handling-induced convulsions), no differences in ethanol-induced ataxia (rotarod), no differences in acute sensitivity or tolerance to ethanol-induced hypothermia, no effect of foot-shock stress on alcohol preference (dramatic increase in wild-type). Decreased ethanol consumption and preference, increased sensitivity to sedative and hypothermic effects of ethanol, reduced sensitivity to locomotor activating effects of ethanol, increased sensitivity to alcohol-induced withdrawal	*163–165*
G protein-coupled inwardly rectifying potassium channel 2	Marked reduction of antinociceptive effects of ethanol (hot plate test). Reduced ethanol-induced CPP and conditioned taste aversion	*166,167*
Guanine nucleotide binding protein-α, stimulating	Increased sensitivity to sedative effects of ethanol, lack of within-session tolerance to ethanol-induced hypothermia	*168*
Dopamine transporter	Increased ethanol consumption in males, increased ethanol preference in females	*169*
Vesicular monoamine transporter	Increased ethanol consumption in males	*169*

have had particular neurotransmitter, receptor, or receptor subunit genes rendered nonfunctional. We will briefly review serotonin (5HT), GABA, and dopamine receptor KO mice, as these three neurotransmitter systems have all been implicated in the behavioral effects of alcohol.

Several mammalian 5HT-receptor types and subtypes have been identified. One subtype ($5HT_{1B}$ in mice, $5HT_{1D\beta}$ in humans) has received considerable attention in the alcohol field. Studies have reported the presence of a QTL influencing alcohol preference on mouse chromosome 9 near the *$5HT_{1B}$* gene *(73)*. When given the choice of ethanol or tap water, $5HT_{1B}$ KO mice consumed twice as much alcohol compared to wild-type (WT) 129/Sv-ter mice *(127)*. These mice were also less sensitive to ethanol-induced ataxia and showed no ethanol-CPP *(127,130)*. However, these results have been difficult to verify. Other studies have reported no increased ethanol consumption in *$5HT_{1B}$* KOs, although the genetic background on which the mutation is maintained is uncertain *(128,129,170)*. These differences are difficult to reconcile, but suggest that both genetic background and environmental factors play a significant role in determining ethanol intake in these KO mice.

GABA is the major inhibitory neurotransmitter in the mammalian brain. Many acute and chronic ethanol effects are thought to be mediated at the $GABA_A$ receptor complex *(171,172)*. As discussed in Subheadings 6.1. and 6.2., highly significant linkage for a QTL(s) influencing alcohol withdrawal was found on chromosome 11, near several $GABA_A$ subunit genes. Mice in which the α_6 subunit gene had been knocked out showed no differences (compared to wild-type) in ethanol-induced LORR, acute functional tolerance, or withdrawal severity *(133,134)*. Similarly, mice in which the γ_{2L} subunit gene has been rendered nonfunctional show no differences in many alcohol phenotypes, including withdrawal severity *(137)*. This suggests that these genes are not the alcohol withdrawal QTL. More recent studies that have used mice in which the α_1 subunit has been deleted have reported decreased ethanol-induced LORR (males only), decreased ethanol consumption, and increased ethanol-induced locomotor activation *(138–140)*.

Dopamine systems have also been implicated in the actions of most drugs of abuse, including alcohol. Dopamine receptors fall into two classes: D_1-like (D_1 and D_5) and D_2-like (D_2, D_3, and D_4). Rendering the D_1 or D_2 receptor genes nonfunctional reduces ethanol consumption/preference and ethanol-CPP, whereas knocking out the D_4 receptor gene increases ethanol-induced locomotor activation *(141–143,146)*. More recently a complex relationship between genetic background and ethanol-induced locomotor activation and sensitization has been demonstrated in D_2 KO mice *(144)*.

Several caveats must be kept in mind when using KO mice. First, the mutated gene is not expressed throughout development. Thus, any behavioral abnormalities may be the result of the missing gene product in general, or during key developmental processes throughout ontogeny. One way to deal with this situation is to use inducible KOs, in which a gene can be rendered nonfunctional in specific cell and tissue types at specific points in time. Although such technology exists *(173,174)*, no studies have yet reported the use of inducible KOs to study alcohol-related behaviors. Second, compensatory mechanisms may be activated when a gene is knocked out. More research on the redundancy of genes of interest will therefore be needed before one can rule out compensatory mechanisms in the expression of null mutant phenotypes.

A third consideration when using KO mice is the genetic background of the strain the mutation is maintained on. Although it has been shown for several alcohol-related phenotypes that genetic background influences the effects of a null mutation *(132,147,170)*, most studies have reported maintaining a mutant gene on a single genetic background, typically a mixed 129/B6 background. In order to fully elucidate the effects of a missing gene, one should examine the mutation on at least two different genetically defined backgrounds. A related problem occurs when backcrossing KO mice onto different backgrounds. In addition to the mutated gene, a small region of DNA surrounding the gene is also transferred in the BC. For historical and practical reasons, most KO mice have been created using embryonic stem cells derived from inbred 129 strains of mice, and are implanted into blastocysts of B6 females. Because 129 strains are often poor breeders, it is common to BC mice carrying the null mutation to a B6 background. When this is done, even after 10 or more generations of backcrossing, a segment (average of 20 cM after 10 generations) of 129 DNA surrounding the targeted allele will still remain. The possibility exists that any effects attributed to the null mutation may indeed be caused by other 129 alleles in the flanking region. Breeding strategies have been proposed to determine if the effects of a null mutation are resulting from that gene or flanking genes *(175,176)*.

6.4. Genetic Complementation

We have outlined a strategy that tests whether a mutant mouse gene corresponds to a QTL *(107)*, based on a strategy proposed by Long et al. using *Drosophila (177)*. An example of how this test might be applied to a gene KO derived from a 129-inbred strain is shown in Fig. 8. Heterozygous KOs are crossed with congenic donor and recipient strains. The phenotypic effect of the KO mutation is quantified among the progeny of both crosses. If the KO gene is not the same as the QTL gene and does not interact with the QTL gene, then within each cross, the offspring heterozygous for QTL would not be expected to affect the phenotypic difference between KO and WT off-spring (Fig. 8). Similarly, if the KO mutation affects the phenotype in the same way in both classes of progeny, it would mean that the KO gene and the QTL gene were acting independently, implying that they were not the same gene. However, if the effect of the KO gene is not the same in both progeny classes, it would mean that the KO mutation not only affects the phenotype but also interacts with the QTL. This latter situation would provide additional evidence that the KO gene is the same as the QTL gene. This test would not work for a completely recessive phenotype.

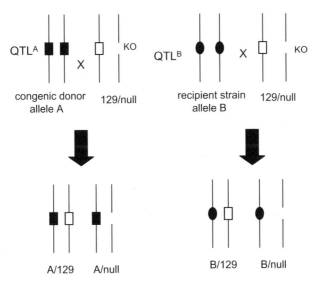

Fig. 8. A congenic test for genetic complementation (*see* ref. *107*). Heterozy-gous knockout (KO) mice are crossed with reciprocal congenics in which the quantitative trait locus (QTL) of interest lies within the differential chromosomal segment. Within each cross, offspring with or without the KO mutation are com-pared. If the QTL has been knocked out, the expectation is that the difference between the mutant and wild-type (WT) alleles opposite the A allele will not match the difference between the mutant and WT alleles opposite the B allele. The alterna-tive possibility (that the KO is *not* the gene responsible for the QTL) predicts that there will be only one phenotypic class of progeny from each of the crosses. Although not ideal, this test can provide additional support for the mutated gene being the QTL.

7. OTHER STRATEGIES

7.1. Genome-Wide Mutagenesis

Another approach has been the use of genome-wide mutagenesis, as opposed to targeted mutagenesis of a single gene. Using this strategy, a chemical mutagen (typically ethylnitrosourea) is injected into male mice that produces hundreds of single base pair germline mutations *(178)*. Male mice are then mated to wild-type females, and all offspring are screened for the phenotype of interest. These mutations are then mapped using methods similar to QTL analysis. One advantage of using genome-wide mutagenesis is that one can screen the entire genome for genes influencing a trait of interest (including monomorphic genes), as opposed to the more limited set of genes that are polymorphic between the two parental strains. However, there are several disadvantages to using genome-wide mutagenesis for identifying genes mediating complex traits. As discussed by Belknap et al. *(179)*: (a) for some traits, it may be very difficult to identify which animals have a mutation of interest; (b) identifying and mapping mutations is only a start towards an understanding of the phenotype of interest; (c) there are strong biases favoring mutation detection in some genes over others; (d) mutagenesis screens are designed to detect only mutations with large effects; and (e) most monomorphic genes may be so for a reason; inducing mutations in these genes often results in reduced fitness or lethality. Some of these criticisms have also been made with regard to QTL mapping *(180)*. It would seem prudent, therefore, to use genome-wide mutagenesis in conjunction with QTL analysis and targeted mutagenesis, as opposed to replacing QTL methods *(179,180)*. No studies yet exist which have used genome-wide mutagenesis to examine alcohol-related behaviors in mice.

7.2. RNA Interference

Given the inherent difficulties creating KO mice or conducting random mutagenesis studies, and the caveats one must consider in interpreting results from such studies, improved methods for manipulating genes are desired. One recent technology, RNAi, holds much promise for altering mRNA levels for a gene of interest without the confounds involved with the use of traditional KOs. RNAi involves introduction of short (21–23 nucleotides) RNA sequences complementary to the RNA of interest into an organism. This reduces or suppresses expression of the RNA by either RNA degradation or translational suppression *(181)*.

Although originally discovered in the nematode, RNAi has been observed in many organisms, including mammals. A recent study illustrates the potential of this new genetic tool in mice. Dileone et al. *(182)* constructed a short hairpin RNA complementary to a segment of the tyrosine hydroxylase (TH) gene and put the short hairpin RNA into an adeno-associated virus. Stereotaxic injections were used to deliver the adeno-associated virus to either the substantia nigra or ventral tegmental area. They observed a substantial decrease in TH levels in these brain regions approx 6 d later, with lower levels persisting for at least 50 d. The authors then correlated this reduction of TH with both an attenuated response to amphetamine and altered performance on the rotarod, a phenotype similar to neurotoxin-induced mouse models of Parkinson's disease. Thus, they demonstrated in vivo the ability to knock down the level of a gene of interest in specific brain regions for extended periods of time and documented resulting behavioral deficits. This technique takes less time than creating KO mice and eliminates issues such as spatial and temporal specificity, and genetic background effects. Although not yet perfected in vivo in mice, this technique has been heralded as perhaps the most important advance in biology in decades *(181)*. It seems likely that this technique will be used to test candidate genes in mice for alcohol-related phenotypes in the near future. This technique also holds great promise for gene therapy in humans *(183)*.

8. SUMMARY

Mice offer many advantages over humans in the genetic dissection of complex traits. Traditional mouse model systems, such as inbred strains, selected lines, RIs, and congenics, have laid the groundwork for investigating the genetic architecture of polygenic traits. Data obtained from these model systems, combined with advances in bioinformatics, and powerful new molecular tools, such as DNA microarrays and transgenic animals, have made possible expression and functional studies of candidate genes. Alcoholism is one such complex genetic disease, and various alcohol phenotypes have been modeled in mice. Genetic mapping has narrowed a few alcohol-QTL regions to the point where candidate gene evaluation is feasible, but many regions have yet to be fine-mapped and are quite large. Even when obvious candidate genes are known in these regions, it seems prudent to narrow the region as much as possible before exerting a great deal of time and effort evaluating candidate genes.

In mice, the gold standard for proving that a candidate gene is indeed one's QTL of interest is an allele-swapping or functional complementation test, where the allele of interest is moved from one strain to the other, showing that phenotype changes with genotype. To the best of our knowledge this has not been demonstrated for an alcohol-related QTL in mice. Short of this, it is likely that several lines of evidence will be necessary to demonstrate that a candidate gene is a QTL, including DNA sequence differences in coding regions, differential gene expression (which implies DNA sequence differences in regulatory regions or differential phosphorylation or methylation), use of transgenic mice to show that overexpression or deletion of a candidate gene affects the phenotype of interest, or a genetic complementation test where KOs are made heterozygous with the candidate allele and the phenotype subsequently assessed for complementation.

For candidate gene studies for alcohol-related behaviors in mice, only a few have identified DNA sequence variation in coding regions; even fewer have followed up with functional assays. Although several studies have shown differential expression of candidate genes in QTL regions, no study has shown the underlying molecular mechanism, i.e., DNA sequence differences in regulatory regions or differential phosphorylation or methylation. Although several studies have tested transgenic mice in which a candidate gene has been overexpressed or deleted, few of these have identified the underlying DNA sequence variant. Thus, with one possible exception, no candidate gene underlying an alcohol-related behavioral phenotype in mice has been conclusively demonstrated. The exception has been the work of the Buck laboratory, where, using several mouse models and behavioral tests, QTL mapping and fine-mapping, positional cloning, and sequence and expression analyses, has provided good evidence for the *Mpdz* gene as being a quantitative trait gene for physiological dependence and withdrawal from alcohol *(184)*. Given the improved QTL mapping programs now available and the recent advances in molecular genetics, it seems likely that good evidence for several other candidate genes for alcohol-related QTLs will be appearing shortly. The next step will be evaluating these candidate genes in human populations.

REFERENCES

1. Foroud T, Li TK. Genetics of alcoholism: a review of recent studies in human and animal models. Am J Addict 1999;8:261–278.
2. Schuckit MA. A clinical model of genetic influences in alcohol dependence. J Stud Alcohol 1994;55:5–17.
3. American Psychiatric Association. Diagnostic and statistical manual of mental disorders, 4th ed., Washington, DC: American Psychiatric Association, 1994.
4. McClearn GE, Kakihana R. Selective breeding for ethanol sensitivity: short-sleep and long-sleep mice. In: McClearn GE, Deitrich RA, Erwin VG, eds. Development of animal models as pharmacogenetic tools. Washington: NIAAA

Research Monograph No. 6, US Department of Health and Human Services, 1981:147–159.

5. Ponomarev I, Crabbe JC. A novel method to assess initial sensitivity and acute functional tolerance to hypnotic effects of ethanol. J Pharmacol Exp Ther 2002;302:257–263.

6. Phillips TJ, Crabbe JC. Behavioral studies of genetic differences in alcohol action. In: Crabbe JC, Harris RA, eds. The genetic basis of alcohol and drug actions. New York: Plenum, 1991:25–104.

7. Whatley VJ, Johnson TE, Erwin VG. Identification and confirmation of quantitative trait loci regulating alcohol consumption in congenic strains of mice. Alcohol Clin Exp Res 1999;23:1262–1271.

8. Kliethermes CL, Cronise K, Crabbe JC. Anxiety-like behavior in mice in two apparatuses during withdrawal from chronic ethanol vapor inhalation. Alcohol Clin Exp Res 2004;28:1012–1019.

9. Phillips TJ, Burkhart-Kasch S, Terdal ES, Crabbe JC. Response to selection for ethanol-induced locomotor activation: genetic analyses and selection response characterization. Psychopharmacology 1991;103:557–566.

10. Deitrich RA, Bludeau P, Erwin VG. Phenotypic and genotypic relationships between ethanol tolerance and sensitivity in mice selectively bred for initial sensitivity to ethanol (SS and LS) or development of acute tolerance (HAFT and LAFT). Alcohol Clin Exp Res 2000;24:595–604.

11. Crabbe JC. Sensitivity to ethanol in inbred mice: genotypic correlations among several behavioral responses. Behav Neurosci 1983;97:280–289.

12. Risinger FO, Cunningham CL, Blevins RA, Holloway FA. Place conditioning: what does it add to our understanding of ethanol reward? Alcohol Clin Exp Res 2002;26:1444–1452.

13. Schuckit MA. Reactions to alcohol in sons of alcoholics and controls. Alcohol Clin Exp Res 1988;12:465–470.

14. Schuckit MA. Low level of response to alcohol as a predictor of future alcoholism. Am J Psychiatry 1994;151:184–189.

15. Schuckit MA, Tsuang JW, Anthenelli RM, Tipp JE, Nurnberger JI, Jr. Alcohol challenges in young men from alcoholic pedigrees and control families: a report from the COGA project. J Stud Alcohol 1996;57:368–377.

16. Falconer DS, Mackay TF. Introduction to quantitative genetics, 4th ed., England: Longman, 1996.

17 Grupe A, Germer S, Usuka J, et al. In silico mapping of complex disease-related traits in mice. Science 2001;292:1915–1918.

18. Belknap JK, Crabbe JC, Young ER. Voluntary consumption of ethanol in 15 inbred mouse strains. Psychopharmacology 1993;112:503–510.

19. Crabbe JC, Young ER, Kosobud A. Genetic correlations with ethanol withdrawal severity. Pharmacol Biochem Behav 1983;18(Suppl):541–547.

20. Crabbe JC, Gallaher ES, Phillips TJ, Belknap JK. Genetic determinants of sensitivity to ethanol in inbred mice. Behav Neurosci 1994;108:186–195.

21. Crabbe JC, Janowsky JS, Young ER, Righter H. Handling induced convulsions in twenty inbred strains of mice. Subst Alcohol Actions/Misuse 1980;1: 149–153.

22. Crabbe JC. Genetic differences in locomotor activation in mice. Pharmacol Biochem Behav 1986;25:289–292.

23. Rodgers DA, McClearn GE. Mouse strain differences in preference for various concentrations of alcohol. Q J Stud Alcohol 1962;23:26–33.

24. McClearn GE. The tools of pharmacogenetics. In: Crabbe JC, Harris RA, eds. The genetic basis of alcohol and drug actions. New York: Plenum Press, 1991:1–23.

25. Crabbe JC, Kosobud A, Tam BR, Young ER, Deutsch CM. Genetic selection of mouse lines sensitive (COLD) and resistant (HOT) to acute ethanol hypothermia. Alcohol Drug Res 1987;7:163–174.

26. Crabbe JC, Phillips TJ. Selective breeding for alcohol withdrawal severity. Behav Genet 1993;23:171–177.

27. Grahame NJ, Li TK, Lumeng L. Selective breeding for high and low alcohol preference in mice. Behav Genet 1999;29:47–57.

28. Erwin VG, Deitrich RA. Genetic selection and characterization of mouse lines for acute functional tolerance to ethanol. J Pharmacol Exp Ther 1996; 279:1310–1317.

29. McClearn GE, Wilson JR, Petersen DR, Allen DL. Selective breeding in mice for severity of the ethanol withdrawal syndrome. Subst Alcohol Actions/ Misuse 1982;3:135–143.

30. Lumeng L, Waller MB, McBride WJ, Li TK. Different sensitivities to ethanol in alcohol-preferring and -nonpreferring rats. Pharmacol Biochem Behav 1982;16:125–130.

31. Li TK, Lumeng L, Doolittle DP, et al. Behavioral and neurochemical associations of alcohol-seeking behaviors. In: Kuriyama K, Takada A, Ishii H, eds. Biomedical and social aspects of alcohol and alcoholism. Amsterdam: Elsevier, 1988:435–438.

32. Fadda F, Mosca E, Colombo G, Gessa GL. Effect of spontaneous ingestion ethanol on brain dopamine metabolism. Life Sci 1989;44:281–287.

33. Spuhler KP, Deitrich RA, Baker RC. Selective breeding of rats differing in sensitivity to the hypnotic effects of acute ethanol administration. In: Deitrich RA, Pawlowski AA, eds. Initial sensitivity to alcohol. Washington, DC: National Institute on Alcohol Abuse and Alcoholism Research Monograph No. 20, 1990:87–102.

34. Bailey DW. Recombinant-inbred strains bilineal congenic strains. In: Foster HL, Small JD, Fox FG, eds. The mouse in biomedical research. New York: Academic Press, 1981:223–239.

35. Williams RW, Gu J, Qi S, Lu L. The genetic structure of recombinant inbred mice: High-resolution consensus maps for complex trait analysis. Genome Biol 2001;2:0046.1–0046.18.

36. Belknap JK. Effect of within-strain sample size on QTL detection and mapping using recombinant inbred mouse strains. Behav Genet 1998;28:29–38.

37. Lander ES, Botstein D. Mapping mendelian factors underlying quantitative traits using RFLP linkage maps. Genetics 1989;121:185–199.

38. Silver LM. Mouse genetics: concepts and applications. New York: Oxford University Press, 1995.

39. Bennett B, Beeson M, Gordon L, Johnson TE. Reciprocal congenics defining individual quantitative trait loci for sedative/hypnotic sensitivity to ethanol. Alcohol Clin Exp Res 2002;26:149–157.

40. Heston WDW, Erwin VG, Anderson SM, Robbins H. A comparison of the effects of alcohol in mice selectively bred for differences in ethanol sleep-time. Life Sci 1974;14:365–370.

41. Howerton TC, O'Connor MF, Collins AC. Differential effects of long-chain alcohols in long-and short-sleep mice. Psychopharmacology 1983; 79: 313–317.

42. Smolen TN, Smolen A. Blood and brain ethanol concentrations during absorption and distribution in long-sleep and short-sleep mice. Alcohol 1989; 6:33–38.

43. Phillips TJ, Gilliam DM, Dudek BC. An evaluation of the role of ethanol clearance rate in the differential response of long-sleep and short-sleep mice to ethanol. Alcohol 1984;l:373–378.

44. Dudek BC, Abbott ME. A biometrical genetic analysis of ethanol response in selectively bred long-sleep and short-sleep mice. Behav Genet 1984;14:1–19.

45. DeFries JC, Wilson JR, Erwin VG, Petersen DR. LS × SS recombinant inbred strains of mice: initial characterization. Alcohol Clin Exp Res 1989;13; 196–200.

46. Markel PD, DeFries JC, Johnson TE. Ethanol-induced anesthesia in inbred strains of long-sleep and short-sleep mice: a genetic analysis using repeated measures. Behav Genet 1995;25:67–73.

47. Markel PD, Johnson TE. Initial characterization of STS markers in the LS × SS series of recombinant inbred strains. Mamm Genome 1994;5:199–202.

48. Markel PD, Fulker DW, Bennett B, et al. Quantitative trait loci for ethanol sensitivity in the LS × SS recombinant inbred strains: interval mapping. Behav Genet 1996;26:447–458.

49. Haley CS, Knott SA. A simple regression method for mapping quantitative trait loci in line crosses using flanking markers. Heredity 1992;69:315–324.

50. Fulker DW, Markel PD, DeFries JC, Corley RP, Johnson, TE. Use of interval mapping to localize quantitative trait loci in recombinant inbred strains. Alcohol Clin Exp Res 1994;18:452.

51. Markel PD, Bennett B, Beeson M, Gordon L, Johnson TE. Confirmation of quantitative trait loci for ethanol sensitivity in long-sleep and short-sleep mice. Genome Res 1997;7:92–99.

52. Basten C, Weir BS, Zeng Z-B. QTL cartographer: a reference manual and tutorial for QTL mapping. Raleigh, NC: Department of Statistics, North Carolina State University, 1997.

53. Manly KF, Olson JM. Overview of QTL mapping software and introduction to MapManager QT. Mamm Genome 1999;10:327–334.

54. Lander E, Kruglyak L. Genetic dissection of complex traits: guidelines for interpreting and reporting linkage results. Nat Genet 1995;11:241–247.

55. Churchill GA, Doerge RW. Empirical threshold values for quantitative trait mapping. Genetics 1994;138:963–971.

56. Broman K. Review of statistical methods for QTL mapping in experimental crosses. Lab Anim 2001;30:44–52.
57. Doerge RW. Mapping and analysis of quantitative trait loci in experimental populations. Nat Rev Genet 2002;3:43–52.
58. Markel PD, Corley RP. A multivariate analysis of repeated measures: linkage of the albinism gene (*Tyr*) to a QTL influencing ethanol-induced anesthesia in laboratory mice. Psychiatr Genet 1994;4:205–210.
59. Belknap JK, Richards SP, O'Toole LA, Helms ML, Phillips TJ. Short-term selective breeding as a tool for QTL mapping: ethanol preference drinking in mice. Behav Genet 1997;27:55–66.
60. Dudek BC, Tritto T. Classical and neoclassical approaches to the genetic analysis of alcohol-related phenotypes. Alcohol Clin Exp Res 1995;19:802–810.
61. Bennett B, Beeson M, Gordon L, Johnson TE. Quick method for confirmation of quantitative trait loci. Alcohol Clin Exp Res 1997;21:767–772.
62. Flaherty L. Congenic strains. In: Foster HL, Small FD, Fox FG, eds. The mouse in biomedical research. New York: Academic, 1981:215–222.
63. Visscher PM. Speed congenics: accelerated genome recovery using genetic markers. Genet Res 1999;74:81–85.
64. Wakeland E, Morel L, Achey K, Yui M, Longmate J. Speed congenics: a classic technique in the fast lane. Immunol Today 1997;10:42–47.
65. Markel P, Shu P, Ebeling C, et al. Theoretical and empirical issues for marker-assisted breeding of congenic mouse strains. Nat Genet 1997;17:280–284.
66. Bennett B, Johnson TE. Development of congenics for hypnotic sensitivity to ethanol by QTL-marker-assisted counter selection. Mamm Genome 1998;9:969–974.
67. Phillips TJ, Crabbe JC, Metten P, Belknap JK. Localization of genes affecting alcohol drinking in mice. Alcohol Clin Exp Res 1994;18:931–941.
68. Melo JA, Shendure J, Pociask K, Silver LM. Identification of sex-specific quantitative trait loci controlling alcohol preference in C57BL/6 mice. Nat Genet 1996;13:147–153.
69. Peirce JL, Derr R, Shendure J, Kolata T, Silver LM. A major influence of sex-specific loci on alcohol preference in C57BL/6 and DBA/2 inbred mice. Mamm Genome 1998;9:942–948.
70. Tarantino LM, McClearn GE, Rodriguez LA, Plomin R. Confirmation of quantitative trait loci for alcohol preference in mice. Alcohol Clin Exp Res 1998;22:1099–1105.
71. Phillips TJ, Belknap JK, Buck KJ, Cunningham CL. Genes on mouse chromosomes 2 and 9 determine variation in ethanol consumption. Mamm Genome 1998;9:936–941.
72. Gill K, Desaulniers N, Desjardins P, Lake K. Alcohol preference in AXB/BXA recombinant inbred mice: gender differences and gender-specific quantitative trait loci. Mamm Genome 1998;9:929–935.
73. Belknap JK, Atkins AL. The replicability of QTLs for murine alcohol preference drinking behavior across eight independent studies. Mamm Genome 2001;12:893–899.

74. McClearn GE, Tarantino LM, Rodriguez LA, Jones BC, Blizard DA, Plomin R. Genotypic selection provides experimental confirmation for an alcohol consumption quantitative trait locus in mouse. Mol Psychiatry 1997; 2:486–489.

75. Hitzemann R, Cipp L, Demarest K, Mahjubi E, McCaughran J, Jr. Genetics of ethanol-induced locomotor activation: detection of QTLs in a C57BL/6J × DBA/2J F_2 intercross. Mamm Genome 1998;9:956–962.

76. Demarest K, McCaughran J, Jr, Mahjubi E, Cipp L, Hitzemann R. Identification of an acute ethanol response quantitative trait locus on mouse chromosome 2. J Neurosci 1999;15:549–561.

77. Hitzemann R, Demarest K, Koyner J, et al. Effect of genetic cross on the detection of quantitative trait loci and a novel approach to mapping QTLs. Pharmacol Biochem Behav 2000;67:767–772.

78. Demarest K, Koyner J, McCaughran J, Jr, Cipp L, Hitzemann R. Further characterization and high-resolution mapping of quantitative trait loci for ethanol-induced locomotor activity. Behav Genet 2001;31:79–91.

79. Erwin VG, Radcliffe RA, Gehle VM, Jones BC. Common quantitative trait loci for alcohol-related behaviors and central nervous system neurotensin measures: locomotor activation. J Pharmacol Exp Ther 1997;280:919–926.

80. Gill K, Boyle A, Lake K, Desaulniers N. Alcohol-induced locomotor activation in C57BL/6J, A/J, and AXB/BXA recombinant inbred mice: strain distribution patterns and quantitative trait loci analysis. Psychopharmacology 2000;150:412–421.

81. Buck KJ, Metten P, Belknap JK, Crabbe JC. Quantitative trait loci involved in genetic predisposition to acute alcohol withdrawal in mice. J Neurosci 1997;17:3946–3955.

82. Cunningham CL. Localization of genes influencing ethanol-induced conditioned place preference and locomotor activity in BXD recombinant inbred mice. Psychopharmacology 1995;120:28–41.

83. Crabbe JC, Belknap JK, Mitchell SR, Crawshaw LI. Quantitative trait loci mapping of genes that influence the sensitivity and tolerance to ethanol-induced hypothermia in BXD recombinant inbred mice. J Pharmacol Exp Ther 1994;269:184–192.

84. Crabbe JC, Phillips TJ, Gallaher EJ, Crawshaw LI, Mitchell SR. Common genetic determinants of the ataxic and hypothermic effects of ethanol in BXD/Ty recombinant inbred mice: genetic correlations and quantitative trait loci. J Pharmacol Exp Ther 1996;277:624–632.

85. Risinger FO, Cunningham CL. Ethanol-induced conditioned taste aversion in BXD recombinant inbred mice. Alcohol Clin Exp Res 1998;22:1234–1244.

86. Crabbe JC, Phillips TJ, Buck KJ, Cunningham CL, Belknap JK. Identifying genes for alcohol and drug sensitivity: recent progress and future directions. Trends Neurosci 1999;22:173–179.

87. Crabbe JC. Provisional mapping of quantitative trait loci for chronic ethanol withdrawal severity in BXD recombinant inbred mice. J Pharmacol Exp Ther 1998;286:263–271.

120. Tabakoff B, Bhave SV, Hoffman PL. Selective breeding, quantitative trait locus analysis, and gene arrays identify candidate genes for complex drug-related behaviors. J Neurosci 2003;23:4491-4498.

121. Treadwell JA, Singh SM. Microarray analysis of mouse brain gene expression following acute ethanol treatment. Neurochem Res 2004;29:357–369.

122. Engel SR, Lyons CR, Allan AM. 5-HT$_3$ receptor over-expression decreases ethanol self administration in transgenic mice. Psychopharmacology 1998; 140:243–248.

123. Sung K-W, Engel SR, Allan AM, Lovinger DM. 5-HT$_3$ receptor function and potentiation by alcohols in frontal cortex neurons from transgenic mice over-expressing the receptor. Neuropharmacology 2000;39:2346–2351.

124. Thiele TE, Marsh DJ, Ste. Marie L, Bernstein IL, Palmiter RD. Ethanol consumption and resistance are inversely related to neuropeptide Y levels. Nature 1998;396:366–369.

125. Rudolph U, Mohler H. Genetically modified animals in pharmacological research: future trends. Eur J Pharmacol 1999;375:327–337.

126. Babinet C, Cohen-Tannoudji M. Genome engineering via homologous recombination in mouse embryonic stem (ES) cells: an amazingly versatile tool for the study of mammalian biology. An Acad Bras Cienc 2001;73: 365–383.

127. Crabbe JC, Phillips TJ, Feller DJ, et al. Elevated alcohol consumption in null mutant mice lacking 5-HT$_{1B}$ serotonin receptors. Nat Genet 1996;14: 98–101.

128. Crabbe JC, Wahlsten D, Dudek BC. Genetics of mouse behavior: interactions with laboratory environment. Science 1999;284:1670–1672.

129. Bouwknecht JA, Hijzen TH, van der Gugten J, Maes RAA, Hen R, Olivier B. Ethanol intake is not elevated in male 5-HT$_{1B}$ receptor knockout mice. Eur J Pharmacol 2000;403:95–98.

130. Risinger FO, Bormann NM, Oakes RA. Reduced sensitivity to ethanol reward, but not ethanol aversion, in mice lacking 5-HT$_{1B}$ receptors. Alcohol Clin Exp Res 1996;20:1401–1405.

131. Kelai S, Aissi F, Lesch KP, Cohen-Salmon C, Hamon M, Lanfumey L. Alcohol intake after serotonin transporter inactivation in mice. Alcohol Alcohol 2003;38:386–389.

132. Thiele TE, Miura GI, Marsh DJ, Bernstein IL, Palmiter RD. Neurobiological responses to ethanol in mutant mice lacking neuropeptide Y or the Y5 receptor. Pharmacol Biochem Behav 2000;67:683–691.

133. Homanics GE, Ferguson C, Quinlan JJ, et al. Gene knockout of the α6 subunit of the γ-aminobutyric acid type A receptor: lack of effect on responses to ethanol, pentobarbital, and general anesthetics. Mol Pharmacol 1997;51: 588–596.

134. Homanics GE, Le NQ, Kist F, Mihalek R, Hart AR, Quinlan JJ. Ethanol tolerance and withdrawal responses in GABA$_A$ receptor alpha 6 subunit null allele mice and in inbred C57BL/6J and strain 129/SvJ mice. Alcohol Clin Exp Res 1998;22:259–265.

135. Mihalek RM, Bowers BJ, Wehner JM, et al. GABA$_A$-receptor δ subunit knockout mice have multiple defects in behavioral responses to ethanol. Alcohol Clin Exp Res 2001;25:1708–1718.

136. Quinlan JJ, Homanics GE, Firestone LL. Anesthesia sensitivity in mice that lack the beta3 subunit of the gamma-aminobutyric acid type A receptor. Anesthesiology 1998;88:775–780.

137. Homanics GE, Harrison NL, Quinlan JJ, et al. Normal electrophysiological and behavioral responses to ethanol in mice lacking the long splice variant of the γ2 subunit of the γ-aminobutyric type A receptor. Neuropharmacology 1999;38:253–265.

138. Blednov YA, Jung S, Alva H, et al. Deletion of the alpha1 or beta2 subunit of GABAA receptors reduces actions of alcohol and other drugs. J Pharmacol Exp Ther 2003;304:30–36.

139. Blednov YA, Walker D, Alva H, Creech K, Findlay G, Harris RA. GABAA receptor alpha 1 and beta 2 subunit null mutant mice: behavioral responses to ethanol. J Pharmacol Exp Ther 2003;305:854–863.

140. Kralic JE, Wheeler M, Renzi K, et al. Deletion of GABAA receptor alpha 1 subunit-containing receptors alters responses to ethanol and other anesthetics. J Pharmacol Exp Ther 2003;305:600–607.

141. El-Ghundi M, George SR, Drago J, et al. Disruption of dopamine D$_1$ receptor gene expression attenuates alcohol-seeking behavior. Euro J Pharmacol 1998;353:149–158.

142. Cunningham CL, Howard MA, Gill SJ, Rubinstein M, Low MJ, Grandy DK. Ethanol-conditioned place is reduced in dopamine D2 receptor-deficient mice. Pharmacol Biochem Behav 2000;67:693–699.

143. Phillips TJ, Brown KJ, Burkhart-Kasch S, et al. Alcohol preference and sensitivity are markedly reduced in mice lacking dopamine D2 receptors. Nat Neurosci 1998;1:610–615.

144. Palmer AA, Low MJ, Grandy DK, Phillips TJ. Effects of a Drd2 deletion mutation on ethanol-induced locomotor stimulation and sensitization suggest a role for epistasis. Behav Genet 2003;33:311–324.

145. Boyce-Rustay JM, Risinger FO. Dopamine D3 receptor knockout mice and the motivational effects of ethanol. Pharmacol Biochem Behav 2003;75: 373–379.

146. Rubinstein M, Phillips TJ, Bunzow JR, et al. Mice lacking dopamine D4 receptors are supersensitive to ethanol, cocaine, and amphetamine. Cell 1997;90: 91–1001.

147. Bowers BJ, Owen EH, Collins AC, Abeliovich A, Tonegawa S, Wehner JM. Decreased ethanol sensitivity and tolerance development in γ-protein kinase c null mutant mice is dependent on genetic background. Alcohol Clin Exp Res 1999;23:387–397.

148. Harris RA, McQuilkin SJ, Paylor R, Abeliovich A, Tonegawa S, Wehner JM. Mutant mice lacking the γ isoform of protein kinase c show decreased behavioral actions of ethanol and altered function of γ-aminobutyrate type A receptors. Proc Natl Acad Sci USA 1995;92:3658–3662.

149. Bowers BJ, Wehner JM. Ethanol consumption and behavioral impulsivity are increased in protein kinase Cγ null mutant mice. J Neurosci 2001;21:RC180.

150. Bowers BJ, Elliott KJ, Wehner JM. Differential sensitivity to the anxiolytic effects of ethanol and flunitrazepam in PKCγ null mutant mice. Pharmacol Biochem Behav 2001;69:99–110.

151. Thiele TE, Willis B, Stadler J, Reynolds JG, Bernstein IL, McKnight GS. High ethanol consumption and low sensitivity to ethanol-induced sedation in protein kinase A-mutant mice. J Neurosci 2000;20:RC75.

152. Ruan Y, Tecott L, Jiang M-M, Jan LY, Jan YN. Ethanol hypersensitivity and olfactory discrimination defect in mice lacking a homolog of *Drosophila neuralized*. Proc Natl Acad Sci USA 2001;98:9907–9912.

153. Grisel JE, Mogil JS, Grahame NJ, et al. Ethanol oral self-administration is increased in mutant mice with decreased β-endorphin expression. Brain Res 1999;835:62–67.

154. Hall FS, Sora I, Uhl GR. Ethanol consumption and reward are decreased in μ-opiate receptor knockout mice. Psychopharmacology 2001;154:43–49.

155. Weinshenker D, Rust NC, Miller NS, Palmiter RD. Ethanol-associated behaviors of mice lacking norepinephrine. J Neurosci 2000;20:3157–3164.

156. Popova NK, Vishnivetskaya GB, Ivanova EA, Skrinskaya JA, Seif I. Altered behavior and alcohol tolerance in transgenic mice lacking MAO A: a comparison with effects of MAO A inhibitor clorgyline. Pharmacol Biochem Behav 2000;67:719–727.

157. Maul B, Siems W-E, Hoehe MR, Grecksch G, Bader M, Walther T. Alcohol consumption is controlled by angiotensin II. FASEB J 2001;15:1640–1642.

158. Risinger FO, Freeman PA, Greengard P, Fienberg AA. Motivational effects of ethanol in DARP-32 knock-out mice. J Neurosci 2001;21:340–348.

159. Szumlinski KK, Toda S, Middaugh LD, Worley PF, Kalivas PW. Evidence for a relationship between group1 mGluR hypofunction and ethanol sensitivity in Homer2 null mutant mice. Ann NY Acad Sci 2003;1003:468–471.

160. Cowen MS, Schumann G, Yagi T, Spanagel R. Role of Fyn tyrosine kinase in ethanol consumption by mice. Alcohol Clin Exp Res 2003;27:1213–1219.

161. Boehm SL, II, Peden L, Chang R, Harris RA, Blednov YA. Deletion of the fyn-kinase gene alters behavioral sensitivity to ethanol. Alcohol Clin Exp Res 2003;27:1033–1040.

162. Yaka R, Tang KC, Camarini R, Janak PH, Ron D. Fyn kinase and NR2B-containing NMDA receptors regulate acute ethanol sensitivity but not ethanol intake or conditioned reward. Alcohol Clin Exp Res 2003;27:1736–1742.

163. Hungund BL, Szakall I, Adam A, Basavarajappa BS, Vadasz C. Cannabinoid CB1 receptor knockout mice exhibit markedly reduced voluntary alcohol consumption and lack alcohol-induced dopamine release in the nucleus accumbens. J Neurochem 2003;84:698–704.

164. Racz I, Bilkei-Gorzo A, Toth ZE, Michel K, Palkovits M, Zimmer A. A critical role for the Cannabinoid CB1 receptors in alcohol dependence and stress stimulated ethanol drinking. J Neurosci 2003;23:2453–2458.

165. Naassila M, Pierrefiche O, Ledent C, Daoust M. Decreased alcohol self-administration and increased alcohol sensitivity and withdrawal in CB1 receptor knockout mice. Neuropharmacology 2004;46:243–253.

166. Blednov YA, Stoffel M, Alva H, Harris RA. A pervasive mechanism for analgesia: activation of GIRK2 channels. Proc Natl Acad Sci USA 2003; 100:277–282.

167. Hill KG, Alva H, Blednov YA, Cunningham CL. Reduced ethanol-induced conditioned taste aversion and conditioned place preference in GIRK2 null mutant mice. Psychopharmacology 2003;169:108–114.

168. Yang X, Oswald L, Wand G. The cyclic AMP/protein kinase A signal transduction pathway modulates tolerance to sedative and hypothermic effects of ethanol. Alcohol Clin Exp Res 2003;27:1220–1225.

169. Hall FS, Sora I, Uhl GR. Sex-dependent modulation ethanol consumption in vesicular monoamine transporter 2 (VMAT2) and dopamine transporter (DAT) knockout mice. Neuropsychopharmacology 2003;28:620–628.

170. Phillips TJ, Hen R, Crabbe JC. Complications associated with genetic background effects in research using knockout mice. Psychopharmacology 1999;147:5–7.

171. Buck KJ. New insights into the mechanisms of ethanol effects on GABAA receptor function and expression, and their relevance to behavior. Alcohol Clin Exp Res 1996;20:198A–202A.

172. Buck KJ. Molecular genetic analysis of the role of GABAergic systems in the behavioral and cellular actions of alcohol. Behav Genet 1996;26:313–323.

173. Lewandoski M. Conditional control of gene expression in the mouse. Nat Rev Genet 2001;2:743–755.

174. Jaisser F. Inducible gene expression and gene modification in transgenic mice. J Am Soc Nephrol 2000;11:S95–S100.

175. Bolivar VJ, Cook MN, Flaherty L. Mapping of quantitative trait loci with knockout/congenic strains. Genome Res 2001;11:1549–1552.

176. Wolfer DP, Crusio W, Lipp H-P. Knockout mice: simple solutions to the problems of genetic background and flanking genes. Trends Neurosci 2002; 25:336–340.

177. Long AD, Mullaney SL, Mackay TF, Langley CH. Genetic interactions between naturally occurring alleles at quantitative trait loci and mutant alleles at candidate loci affecting bristle number in *Drosophila melanogaster.* Genetics 1996;144:1497–1510.

178. Justice MJ, Noveroske JK, Weber JS, Zheng B, Bradley A. Mouse ENU mutagenesis. Hum Mol Genet 1999;8:1955–1963.

179. Belknap JK, Hitzemann R, Crabbe JC, Phillips TJ, Buck KJ, Williams RW. QTL analysis and genomewide mutagenesis in mice: complementary genetic approaches to the dissection of complex traits. Behav Genet 2001; 31:5–15.

180. Nadeau JH, Frankel WN. The roads from phenotypic variation to gene discovery: mutagenesis versus QTLs. Nat Genet 2000;25:381–384.

181. Novina D, Sharp PA. The RNAi revolution. Nature 2004;430:161–164.

182. Hommel JD, Sears RM, Georgescu D, Simmons DL, Dileone RJ. Local gene knockdown in the brain using viral-mediated RNA interference. Nat Med 2003;9:1539–1544.
183. Wall NR, Shi Y. Small RNA: can RNA interference be exploited for therapy? Lancet 2003;362:1401–1403.
184. Shirley RL, Walter NAR, Reilly MT, Fehr C, Buck KJ. *Mpdz* is a quantitative trait gene for drug withdrawal seizures. Nat Neurosci 2004;7:699–700.

III

SELECTED EXAMPLES: THE GENETIC BASIS FOR HUMAN DISEASE

10

HLA Polymorphism and Disease Susceptibility

Henry A. Erlich

1. INTRODUCTION

The human leukocyte antigen (HLA) region, on chromosome 6p21.3, contains more than 200 genes within this 3 Mb segment, many of which are involved in the function of the immune system *(1)*. The HLA class I (HLA-A, B, and C) and class II (DRB1, DQB1, DPB1, and DQA1) loci encode cell surface heterodimeric proteins that bind antigenic peptides and are the most polymorphic genes in the human genome (*see* Fig. 1 for HLA region map). Moreover, most of this extensive allelic sequence diversity (i.e., >500 alleles at the HLA-B locus and >300 at the DRB1 locus) is functional and affects peptide binding and recognition of the HLA-peptide complex by the T-cell receptor. Statistical analysis of HLA class I and class II sequences has indicated, based on the ratio of nonsynonymous to synonymous substitutions in the polymorphic sequences encoding the peptide binding cleft of all class I and class II loci, that these polymorphic sequences have been subjected to balancing selection *(2,3)*. Analyses of allele frequency distributions *(4)* in various human populations have also supported the action of balancing selection for all HLA loci, with the exception of DPB1 *(5)*. However, the Ewens–Watterson test *(4)*, examining allele frequency distributions, is a relatively insensitive test for balancing selection, and the ratio of nonsynonymous to synonymous substitutions for DPB1 is consistent with balancing selection *(6)*. Therefore, the DPB1 polymorphism is probably not neutral, but the selective pressures operating on DPB1 do appear to be different from those shaping the allele frequency distributions of the other HLA loci.

In the search for disease susceptibility genes, the high degree of functional polymorphism within the HLA loci makes them the ultimate "candidate

From: *Computational Genetics and Genomics*
Edited by: G. Peltz © Humana Press Inc., Totowa, NJ

HLA Region

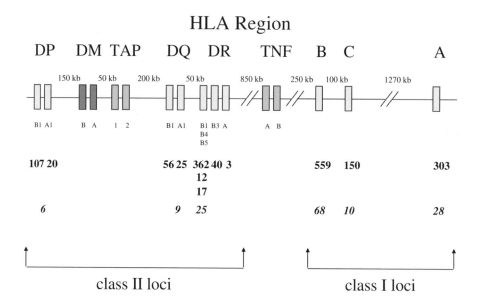

Fig. 1. Polymorphic human leukocyte antigen (HLA) and non-HLA genes in the human major histocompatibility complex (HLA Region) HLA loci are represented as teal boxes. Non-HLA loci are represented as orange boxes. Kilobase distances between loci are shown above the colored boxes. For class II HLA loci, α (A) and β (B) chain descriptors are show below the colored boxes. The number of alleles at each HLA locus is shown in bold below the α and β chain descriptors, and the number of serotypes at each locus is shown in italics.

genes." There are, in fact, more than 100 different diseases that have been associated with specific alleles of the HLA loci *(7)*. A selected subset of these HLA-associated diseases is shown in Table 1. As noted above, a variety of diseases, including autoimmune disorders, infectious diseases, cancer, adverse drug responses, and diseases of unknown etiology, like narcolepsy, have been associated with specific HLA alleles.

2. LINKAGE DISEQUILIBRIUM AND THE SEARCH FOR DISEASE-RELATED ASSOCIATIONS

In principle, the association with disease of specific HLA alleles could simply reflect linkage disequilibrium with alleles at nearby loci. This is clearly the case for the well-known association of HLA-A3 with hereditary hemochromatosis. The linkage disequilibrium between the HLA-A3 allele and the Cys282 Tyr mutation of the recently identified *HFE* locus, about 1 Mb telomeric of the

Table 1
HLA Disease Associations (Selected Examples)

Autoimmunity/Inflammation
IDDM (type 1 diabetes)
Mysenthia gravis
Inflammatory bowel disease
(UC and CD)
RA, juvenile RA
Pemphigus vulgaris
Multiple sclerosis
Ankylosing spondylitis
Psoriasis

Unknown
Narcolepsy

Cancer
Cervical carcinoma
NP carcinoma
Hodgkins disease

Infectious disease
Malaria
Tuberculosis
Leprosy
HCV
HIV

UC, ulcerative colitis; CD, Crohn's disease; HCV, hepatitis C virus; HIV, human immunodeficiency virus; NP, nasopharyngeal; IDDM, insulin-dependent diabetes mellitus; RA, rheumatoid arthritis; HLA, human leukocyte antigen.

HLA-A locus, accounts for the observed disease association *(8)*. In general, linkage disequilibrium is strong throughout the HLA region making the attribution of an observed disease association to a specific allele at a given locus difficult. However, given the remarkable extent of immunologically significant polymorphism at the HLA class I and class II loci, many, if not the vast majority, of the disease associations with alleles at these loci may well reflect functional disease determinants. The allelic products may affect differential peptide binding or differential recognition by the T-cell receptor. Additional potential mechanisms include differential activation of the T-helper cell 1 or T-helper cell 2 pathway following antigen presentation or, conceivably, differential activation of natural killer (NK) cells whose receptors (both activating and inhibitory killer immunoglobulin-like receptors) recognize HLA class I epitopes.

Arguably, the most convincing evidence that the observed disease associations reflect functional properties of specific HLA molecules comes from recent studies on celiac disease (CD). This is an inflammatory disorder involving an autoimmune attack on the intestinal mucosa that is elicited by ingestion of wheat gluten (gliadin). The strongest association with CD is with the HLA-DQ (DQ) heterodimer encoded by the DQA1*0501 and DQB1 *0201 alleles. This heterodimer is encoded in *cis* by the DR3 haplotype and in *trans* in DR5 (DQA1*0501)/DR7 (DQB1*0201) genotypes *(9)*. These genetic data argue for a direct effect of the DQ molecule rather than an association caused by linkage disequilibrium. Moreover, the peptide-binding motif for the DQ molecule encoded by DQA1*0501 and DQB1*0201 has been determined *(10)*. Native gliadin does *not* contain this peptide motif, which contains glutamic acid. However, the action of an intestinal enzyme, transglutaminase, can convert a glutamine to glutamic acid, which creates a gliadin-derived peptide capable of being bound and presented to the T-cell by the disease-associated DQ molecule. Thus, the genetics of CD can be best explained by preferential binding and presentation of a modified gliadin peptide by the DQ molecule encoded by the disease-associated alleles, DQA1*0501 and DQB1*0201 (in *cis* or in *trans*). The DQA1*03-DQB1*0302 haplotype also shows a weaker association with celiac disease. Other genes, both within and outside the HLA region, as well as environmental factors, are likely to be involved in CD, as in other HLA-associated diseases.

Another instructive example of an HLA-disease association is that of HLA-DPB1*0201 with beryllium disease *(11)*. These DPB1 associations, like the celiac disease example discussed in the previous paragraph, are consistent with the notion that the product of the disease-associated DPB1 alleles binds the disease-relevant epitope and initiates a specific disease-related immune response. HLA-associated beryllium disease represents an example of HLA "ecogenetics," i.e., a genetically determined interaction with an environmental factor, such as exposure to beryllium. HLA "pharmacogenetics," i.e., genetically determined responses to drugs, can be illustrated by the adverse hypersensitive response (experienced by around 5% of patients) to the human immunodeficiency virus antiretroviral drug, abacavir. A recent report demonstrated that this hypersensitive response to abacavir was strongly associated with the haplotype HLA-B*5701 and DRB1*0701-DQB1*-0303 *(12)*. Another example of a genetically determined adverse response to a specific drug is D-penicillamine-induced myesthenia gravis, which is also associated with specific HLA alleles. In this case, treatment of rheumatoid arthritis with D-penicillamine can induce a muscle weakness, particularly in individuals with HLA-DR1 *(13)*.

3. LINKAGE DISEQUILIBRIUM AND EXTENDED HAPLOTYPES

The strong linkage disequilibrium that characterizes the HLA region is reflected in the observation that "extended haplotypes" exist. These are specific combinations of alleles at HLA class I and class II loci that span several Mb and are found much more frequently than expected in specific populations. For example, in Chinese and some other Asian populations, the haplotype A*3303-B*5801-C*0302-DRB1*0301-DQA1*0501-DQB1*0201-DPB1*0401 is present at relatively high frequencies reflecting strong linkage disequilibrium among these many alleles *(14)*. All alleles on this haplotype are associated with nasopharyngeal carcinoma *(14)*; consequently, it is difficult (but not impossible) to sort out which allele, or combination of alleles on this haplotype is responsible for the observed disease association. For diseases, like type 1 diabetes (T1D), in which the major genetic determinants within the HLA region have been identified (DRB1, DQA1, and DQB1), other loci within the HLA region have been reported to be associated. In this case, it is critical to evaluate whether the observed associations at these loci may simply be caused by linkage disequilibrium with susceptible DRB1-DQA1-DQB1 haplotypes. In some cases, such as the association of specific DPB1 alleles *(15,16,17)*, HLA-A alleles *(18)*, or specific microsatellite markers *(19)*, the association with T1D does not appear to be caused simply by linkage disequilibrium with the high-risk DR-DQ haplotypes, implying that there are loci other than the DR and DQ loci within the HLA region that contribute to T1D risk.

4. HLA HAPLOTYPES AND DISEASE ASSOCIATIONS

As noted under Heading 3, the extensive linkage disequilibrium characteristic of the HLA loci makes it difficult, when a specific haplotype is associated with a given disease, to identify which allele or combination of alleles on that haplotype is responsible for the observed disease association. Examining disease associations in different populations, particularly those with different patterns of linkage disequilibrium, can be very instructive. For example, the DR-DQ haplotype DRB1*1501-DQB1*0602 is strongly associated with multiple sclerosis *(20)* and with narcolepsy *(21)*. Among people of European descent, these two alleles are in very strong linkage disequilibrium, and each allele is almost never observed without the other. People of African descent, however, in addition to DRB1*1501-DQB1*0602, also have haplotypes containing DRB1*1501 with other DQB1 alleles and haplotypes containing DQB1*0602 with another DRB1 allele. In the case of narcolepsy, association studies among African-American patients indicated that the DQB1*0602 allele rather than the DRB1*1501 allele was most strongly associated with disease *(21)*. In studies of multiple sclerosis among African-American patients, it was the DRB1*1501 allele that was associated with disease rather than the DQB1*0602 allele *(20)*.

In diseases like T1D, the association with DR-DQ haplotypes cannot be attributed to only one locus. The T1D association with the serological type DR4 has been known for many years. There are many different DR4 DRB1-DQB1 haplotypes, and the pattern of association for some selected haplotypes is shown in Table 2. For T1D, specific combinations of alleles at both DRB1 and DQB1 determine the extent of disease risk. A similar inference can be made from the analyses of DR-DQ haplotypes associated with inflammatory bowel disease. For both Crohn's disease and ulcerative colitis, the two clinical autoimmune disorders that comprise inflammatory bowel disease, the DRB1 allele *0103 was associated with the disease *(22)*. Typically, the DRB1*0103 allele is linked to the DQB1*0501 allele; the odds ratio for this haplotype was around 3. The disease risk was higher, however, if the DRB1*0103 allele was linked to the DQB1*0301 allele, a very rare haplotype with an odds ratio of around 8 *(22)*.

The notion that specific combinations of DRB1 and DQB1 alleles influence disease risk is consistent with a recent report of T1D associations among Filipinos *(23)*. DRB1*0405 is associated with T1D in many different populations. In several different studies, the haplotype DRB1*1401-DQB1*0503 has been associated with protection *(24)*. An unusual DR4 DR-DQ haplotype, DRB1*0405- -DQB1*0503, unique to Filipinos that carries a susceptible DRB1 and a protective DQB1 allele, was observed to have a

Table 2
Combination of HLA-DQB1 and DRB1 Alleles Confer
IDDM Susceptibility

	IDDM risk
DRB1*0401-DQA1*0301-DQB1*0302	+
DRB1*0401-DQA1*0301-DQB1*0301	−
DRB1*0405-DQA1*0301-DQB1*0302	+
DRB1*0402-DQA1*0301-DQB1*0302	+
DRB1*0403-DQA1*0301-DQB1*0302	−
DRB1*0405-DQA1*0301-DQB1*0302	+
(Japan) DRB1*0405-DQA1*0301-DQB1*0402	+
(Africa) DRB1*0405-DQA1*0301-DQB1*0201	+

IDDM, insulin-dependent diabetes mellitus; HLA, human leukocyte antigen.

neutral disease risk (odds ratio of 0.9) in this population *(23)*. This observation suggests that the susceptible DRB1*0405 allele and the protective DQB1*0503 allele may have "cancelled each other out" in terms of determining the extent of disease risk. These examples illustrate the issue of allele combinations determining disease risk for the closely linked DRB1 and DQB1 loci; there are also examples of class I (A*2402) and class II gene (DRB1(0301-DQB1(0201) combinations affecting T1D risk *(23)*.

5. HLA AND RISK ESTIMATES

For many HLA-associated diseases, e.g., T1D, there are multiple alleles at a given locus that confer susceptibility (allelic heterogeneity). Other alleles at this same locus can be negatively associated and confer protection from developing the disease, and the rest of the alleles are "neutral" in terms of disease risk. The immunological mechanisms underlying susceptibility and protection are not known. However, from a genetic perspective, protection appears to be "dominant" in the sense that individuals with a susceptible allele or haplotype (i.e., DRB1*0401-DQB1*0302) and a protective allele or haplotype (i.e., DRB1*1501-DQB1*0602) have an odds ratio significantly less than 1.0. There is a hierarchy of haplotypes and genotypes in terms of T1D risk *(25)*; the DRB1*0301-DQB1*0201-DRB1*0401-DQB1*0302 genotype has an odds ratio of around 30 in Caucasian populations.

6. ESTIMATING THE CONTRIBUTION OF THE HLA REGION TO DISEASE RISK

For some HLA-associated diseases, such as T1D, several lines of evidence suggest that the HLA region is responsible for more than 50% of the total genetic risk *(25)*. A useful measure of familial clustering, and thus, an estimate of genetic risk, is provided by the sibling risk ratio (λs) *(26)*. This is the ratio of the risk to a sibling of an affected individual relative to the population risk (prevalence). For T1D, this ratio, for Caucasian populations, is around 15. A λs value can be estimated for specific loci by linkage analysis in multiplex families. This estimate is obtained by comparing the observed proportion of affected sibling pairs that share zero haplotypes identical by descent to the proportion expected (25%) under the null hypothesis of no linkage. For a well-characterized collection of Caucasian multiplex T1D families (the Human Biological Data Interchange families), this value for the HLA region was estimated to be 4.46 *(25)*. Assuming a multiplicative model (one in which the overall genetic risk is equal to the product of the risk conferred by a specific locus, i.e., *HLA* and the risk attributed to the rest of the

HLA-A Immobilized Probe Linear Array Typing System

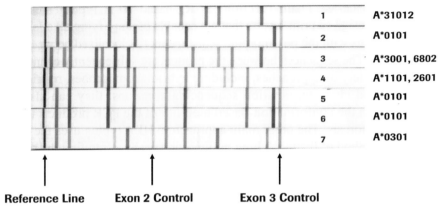

1	A*31012
2	A*0101
3	A*3001, 6802
4	A*1101, 2601
5	A*0101
6	A*0101
7	A*0301

↑ Reference Line   ↑ Exon 2 Control   ↑ Exon 3 Control

Fig. 2. Probe reactivity patterns for various HLA-A-typed cell lines are shown. The exon 2 and exon 3 control probes hybridize to all HLA-A alleles.

Another PCR-based approach, based on the specificity of primer extension rather than that of probe hybridization, has also been applied to HLA typing. This method is known variously as allele-specific amplification *(31)*, sequence-specific priming *(32)*, and the amplification refractory mutation system *(33)*. Here, a specific primer pair is designed for each polymorphic sequence motif or pair of motifs, and the presence of the targeted polymorphic sequence in a sample is detected as a positive PCR, typically identified as a band on a gel.

In general, the pattern of allelic sequence diversity at all the polymorphic HLA loci is a patchwork of discrete sequence motifs. This patchwork pattern of polymorphism is thought to reflect the operation of gene conversion-like events that have generated the extensive sequence diversity observed in human populations by recombining these short sequence motifs. One consequence of this pattern is that, in PCR-based HLA typing, a large number of different alleles can be distinguished by using a relatively modest number of oligonucleotide primers or probes that recognize these sequence motifs. On the other hand, sometimes a given pattern of sequence motifs, detected either with probes or primers or by sequencing, may be consistent with more that a single genotype, because the observed sequence motifs can be combined into more than a unique pair of alleles. This issue of "ambiguity" in DNA-based typing is discussed in Subheading 6.3.

6.3. The Problems of New Alleles and Ambiguity

As more and more PCR-based HLA typing is being carried out in more and more populations, new (previously unreported) alleles at both class I and class II loci are being detected, leading to a slow but steady increase in the number of alleles at both class I and class II loci. The vast majority of these involve new combinations of previously known sequence motifs, and thus, they can be identified without adding additional probes. Nonetheless, they can create problems for typing strategies. The identif cation of new alleles requires frequent updating of the files in the genotyping software that relate sequence motifs to alleles. The addition of these new alleles can lead to increased ambiguities in the genotype interpretation of the primary typing data, such as the SSO probe-reactivity or sequence-specific priming patterns. An additional consequence of these newly discovered alleles is to modify the interpretation of typing results obtained prior to their discovery. For example, a pattern of reactive SSO probes that was consistent with a given genotype, at one time, might, following the identification of the new allele, be consistent with additional genotypes.

Most HLA typing systems, with the exception of sequencing separated alleles, can occasionally generate an ambiguous result; here, ambiguity is defined as HLA typing data (e.g., a probe-reactivity pattern) consistent with more than one pair of alleles. In some cases, if a given probe-reactivity pattern (or other typing data) is consistent with either genotype X or Y, consideration of the genotype frequencies in the relevant populations and the likelihood that the sample is X or Y may be appropriate in interpreting the typing data. As noted in the previous paragraph allele level resolution often requires the separate amplification of the two alleles in a heterozygote. This is most commonly carried out by performing a preliminary typing (e.g., DRB1*04/DRB1*08) and then using group-specific primers for the DRB1(04 group and the DRB1*08 group, based on the sequence variation in codons 9–12 of DRB1 to amplify the alleles separately.

7. CONCLUSIONS

The HLA loci are extraordinarily polymorphic; this polymorphism affects peptide binding and presentation to T-cells and thus, influences the pattern of immune responsiveness to specific antigens and susceptibility to a wide variety of diseases. PCR-based HLA typing methods have been developed and have been applied to population genetics studies, as well as disease association studies. Many different diseases have been shown to be associated with specific alleles of the HLA class I and/or class II loci. Linkage analyses for many diseases, notably T1D, have identified the HLA region as the major disease locus. For some diseases, it appears that specific combinations of alleles determine the extent of disease risk. HLA disease associations promise to play an increasingly important clinical role in identifying individuals predisposed to specific disorders or adverse response to specific drugs or environmental agents.

REFERENCES

1. Beck S, Trowsdale J. The human major histocompatibility complex: lessons from the DNA sequence. Annu Rev Genomics Hum Genet. 2000;1:117–137.
2. Hughes AL, Nei M. Pattern of nucleotide substitution at major histocompatibility complex class I loci reveals overdominant selection. Nature 1988;335:167–170.
3. Hughes AL, Nei M. Nucleotide substitution at major histocompatibility complex class II loci: evidence for overdominant selection. Proc Natl Acad Sci USA 1989;86:958–962.
4. Ewens WJ. The sampling theory of selectively neutral alleles. Theor Popul Biol 1972;3:87–112.
5. Mack SJ, Bugawan TL, Moonsamy PV, et al. Evolution of Pacific/Asian populations inferred from HLA class II allele frequency distributions. Tissue Antigens 2000;55:383–400.
6. Gyllensten U, Bergstrom T, Josefsson A, Sundvall M, Erlich HA. Rapid allelic diversification and intensified selection at antigen recognition sites of the Mhc class II DPB1 locus during hominoid evolution. Tissue Antigens 1996;47:212–221.
7. Lechler and Warren, eds. HLA in health and disease, 2nd ed. Academic, 2000.
8. Feder JN, Gnirke A, Thomas W, et al. A novel MHC class I-like gene is mutated in patients with hereditary haemochromatosis. Nat Genet 1996 4:399–408.
9. Sollid LM, Markussen G, Ek J, Gjerde H, Vartdal F, Thorsby E. Evidence for a primary association of celiac disease to a particular HLA-DQ/heterodimer. J Exp Med 1989;169:345–350.
10. Vardal F, Johansen BH, Friede T, et al. The peptide binding motif of the disease associated HLA-DQ (alpha 1*0501, beta 1*0201) molecule. Eur J Immunol 1996;26:2764–2772.
11. Fontenot AP, Kotzin BL. Chronic beryllium disease: immune-mediated destruction with implications for organ-specific autoimmunity. Tissue Antigens 2003;62:449–458.
12. Mallal S, Nolan D, Witt C, et al. Association between presence of HLA-B*5701, HLA-DR7, and HLA-DQ3 and hypersensitivity to HIV-1 reverse-transcriptase inhibitor abacavir. Lancet 2002;359:722, 723.
13. Hill M, Moss P, Wordsworth P, Newsom-Davis J, Willcox NJ. T cell responses to D-penicillamine in drug-induced myasthenia gravis: recognition of modified DR1: peptide complexes. J Neuroimmunol 1999;97:146–153.
14. Hildesheim A, Apple RJ, Chen CJ, et al. Association of HLA class I and II alleles and extended haplotypes with nasopharyngeal carcinoma in Taiwan. J Natl Cancer Inst 2002;94:1780–1789.

15. Erlich HA, Rotter JI, Chang JD, et al. Association of HLA-DPB1*0301 with IDDM in Mexican-Americans. Diabetes 1996;45:610–614.

16. Noble JA, Valdes AM, Thomson G, Erlich HA. The HLA class II locus DPB1 can influence susceptibility to type 1 diabetes. Diabetes 2000;49:121–125.

17. Valdes AM, Noble JA, Genin E, Clerget-Darpoux F, Erlich HA, Thomson G. Modeling of HLA class II susceptibility to Type I diabetes reveals an effect associated with DPB1. Genet Epidemiol 2001;3:212–223.

18. Noble JA, Valdes AM, Bugawan TL, Apple RJ, Thomson G, Erlich HA. The HLA class I A locus affects susceptibility to type 1 diabetes. Hum Immunol 2002;63:657–664.

19. Johannsson S, Lie BA, Pociot F, et al. HLA associations in type 1 diabetes: DPB1 alleles may act as markers of other HLA-complex susceptibility genes. Tissue Antigens 2003;61:344–351.

20. Oksenberg JR, Barcellos LF, Cree BA, et al. Mapping multiple sclerosis susceptibility to the HLA-DR locus in African Americans. Am J Hum Genet 2004;74:160–167.

21. Chabas D, Taheri S, Renier C, et al. The genetics of narcolepsy. Annu Rev Genomics Hum Genet 2003;4:459–483.

22. Trachtenberg EA, Yang H, Hayes E, et al. HLA class II haplotype associations with inflammatory bowel disease in Jewish (Ashkenazi) and non-Jewish caucasian populations. Hum Immunol 2000;61:326–333.

23. Bugawan TL, Klitz W, Alejandrino M, et al. The association of specific HLA class I and II alleles with type 1 diabetes among Filipinos. Tissue Antigens 2002;59:452–469.

24. Redondo MJ, Kawasaki E, Mulgrew CL, et al. DR- and DQ-associated protection from type 1A diabetes: comparison of DRB1*1401 and DQA1(0102-DQB1*0602*. J Clin Endocrinol Metab 2000;85:3793–3797.

25. Noble JA, Valdes AM, Cook M, Klitz W, Thomson G, Erlich HA. The role of HLA class II genes in insulin dependent diabetes mellitus (IDDM): molecular analysis of 180 Caucasian, multiplex families. Am J Human Gen 1996;59:1134–1148.

26. Risch N. Assessing the role of HLA-linked and unlinked determinants of disease. Am J Hum Genet 1987;40:1–14.

27. Sokal RR, Rohlf FJ. Biometry, 3rd ed. San Francisco: W H Freeman, 1995.

28. Saiki RK, Bugawan TL, Horn GT, Mullis KB, Erlich HA. Analysis of enzymatically amplified β-globin and HLA-DQα DNA with allele-specific oligonucleotide probes. Nature 1986;324:163–166.

29. Saiki RK, Chang C-A, Levenson CH, et al. Diagnosis of sickle cell anemia and β-thalassemia with enzymatically amplified DNA and non-radioactive allele-specific oligonucleotide probes. N Engl J Med 1988;319:537.

30. Saiki R, Walsh PS, Levenson CH, Erlich HA. Genetic analysis of amplified DNA with immobilized sequence-specific oligonucleotide probes. Proc Natl Acad Sci USA 1989;86:6230–6234.

31. Wu DY, Ugozzoli L, Pal BK, Wallace RB. Allele-specific enzymatic amplification of beta-globin genomic DNA for diagnosis of sickle cell anemia. Proc Natl Acad Sci USA 1989;86:2757–2760.

32. Olerup O and Zetterquist H. HLA-DR typing by PCR amplification with sequence-specific primers (PCR-SSP) in 2 h: an alternative to serological DR typing in clinical practice including donor-recipient matching in cadaveric transplantation. Tissue Antigens 1992;39:225–235.

33. Newton CR, Graham A, Heptinstall LE, et al. Analysis of any point mutation in DNA. The amplification refractory mutation system (ARMS). Nucleic Acids Res 1989;17:2503–2516.

11

Asthma Genetics

A Case Study

William Cookson

1. INTRODUCTION

Asthma is the most common chronic disease of childhood, affecting an estimated 155 million individuals in the world. The cost of treating the disease in the United States is approx $6 billion dollars per annum *(1)*. More than half of this expense is spent on hospital care and 80% is attributable to the 20% of patients who require the most treatment *(1)*. The market to the pharmaceutical industry for asthma medication is $5.5 billion per annum *(2)*.

The diseases of asthma, eczema, and hay fever are typified by immuno-globulin E (IgE)-mediated reactions to common allergens. These allergic (atopic) diseases are increasing in prevalence and are now a major source of disability throughout the developed world. They are the result of complex interactions between genetic and environmental mechanisms.

Asthma is an inflammatory disease of the airways of the lungs. Narrowing occurs because of inflammation and mucous hypersecretion and is exacerbated as the smooth musculature in the walls of the small airways (bronchioles) becomes hyperresponsive to nonspecific stimuli. Intermittent airway constriction gives rise to the asthmatic symptoms of wheezing, coughing, chest tightness, and shortness of breath. Over time, the bronchioles may become fibrosed or scarred, and the airflow limitation may become permanent.

Eczema (atopic dermatitis [AD]) is as common as asthma, affecting between 10 and 20% of children in western populations *(3,4)*. The two diseases are strongly associated, so that 60% of children attending a clinic for eczema may also have asthma *(5)*. AD is typified by itchy, inflamed skin. The disease usually begins in infancy and early childhood, and infants with AD are prone to weeping inflammatory patches and crusted areas on the face, neck, extensor surfaces, and groin. Children and young adults tend to

From: *Computational Genetics and Genomics*
Edited by: G. Peltz © Humana Press Inc., Totowa, NJ

have dermatitis of flexural skin, particularly in the antecubital and popliteal fossae *(5)*.

Atopic mechanisms dominate current understanding of the pathogenesis of asthma *(6)* and AD *(7)*. However, approx 10% of children with either disease do not show positive skin tests to common allergens or elevations of the total serum IgE. This indicates the importance of nonatopic mechanisms in disease pathogenesis.

Both diseases show a high heritability *(h²)* (>60%) *(4,8,9)*. Identification of the genes underlying these disorders will lead to new insights into their pathogenesis and new methods of treatment. This may be accomplished by the study of candidate genes, which is unlikely to lead to new and unexpected mechanisms for disease. Novel mechanisms are more likely to be discovered through the systematic process of positional cloning.

The basic principles behind the positional cloning of single gene disorders are applicable to the cloning of genes underlying complex disorders. These principles include the demonstration of segregation within families, the use of recombination to localize disease genes to particular chromosomal segments, and the identification of the causal genes from within these segments. Each of these steps are beset by considerable uncertainties.

2. PHENOTYPE

The choice of phenotype may be critical for the success of positional cloning programs. Asthma is recognized by symptoms of intermittent wheezing, coughing, and attacks of shortness of breath. It may be accompanied by indicators of allergy, such as the total serum IgE concentration, the blood eosinophil count, and the presence of specific IgE against common allergens, detected by prick skin tests or serology. Bronchial hyperresponsiveness (BHR) to inhaled spasmogens, such as methacholine is a measure of nonspecific airway lability that accompanies asthma *(10)*. BHR is typically quantified by measuring the decline in forced expired volume in 1 s that follows increasing doses or concentrations of nebulized (inhaled) histamine or methacholine. End points may be the dose or concentration that produces a fall of 20% in forced expired volume in 1 s or the slope of the dose–response curve *(11)*.

2.1. Power

The high frequency of asthma in the population has adverse effects on the power to detect linkage. The ability to detect linkage to a particular phenotype depends on a statistic known as λs. λs is defined as the risk of disease in the siblings of an affected proband divided by the risk of the disease in the population. In general, the higher the value of λs the easier it is to detect linkage. For type 1 diabetes λs is 15, for schizophrenia λs is 8.6, but for asthma, λs is less than 2. This means that even 500 affected sibling pairs will give less than 50% power to detect linkage to a given marker *(12)*. To achieve 90% power more than 1000 sibling pairs would be required. Genetic linkage in these circumstances becomes problematic and capricious.

Quantitative intermediate phenotypes have more power to detect linkage than complex diagnostic categories, such as asthma, because they do not present difficulties with marginal cases, and because they may be more heritable than diagnostic categories. In addition, by selecting families with sibling at the extremes of trait distributions gives greatly enhanced power to detect linkage, so that the number of sibling pairs required to detect linkage with more than 90% power may drop below 100 *(13)*.

2.2. Segregation

Segregation analysis describes the study of the pattern of inheritance of disease in families. It may be used to quantify the genetic predisposition to a particular disease and its relationship to intermediate phenotypes and environmental factors. As well as a means of exploring the interrelationship between phenotypic variables, segregation analyses may also be used to measure the h^2 of various traits, with the expectation that genes underlying traits that are highly heritable may be identified more easily than those underlying weakly heritable traits. We have therefore used complex segregation analyses to explore phenotypes for subsequent linkage and association studies.

2.3. Asthma

Although it is possible to generate a brisk argument among any group of physicians about an ideal definition of asthma, most doctors in industrialized societies easily recognize the clinical presentation of an asthmatic patient. It is easier to recognize asthma in children and young adults. In older individuals, it is more difficult to distinguish asthmatic symptoms from the consequences of cigarette smoking.

Physician-diagnosed asthma reproducibly identifies disease in epidemiological surveys *(14)* and shows a high h^2 of 60–70% *(8)*. For our genetic studies, we have always defined asthma by physician diagnosis in the response to a standard (American Thoracic Society) questionnaire.

Other studies have used complex definitions of asthma *(15–17)*, usually involving the presence of absence of BHR in addition to symptoms of wheezing. Although BHR provides quantification of airway lability, it is not a completely reliable indicator of airway status. It varies with time and with treatment, and approx 5% of asymptomatic individuals will have airway hyperresponsiveness and 20–40% of asthmatics will have BHR in the normal range *(18,19)*. Clinical studies show that pronounced hyperresponsiveness does not associate well with asthma severity *(20)*. Evidence is lacking that the presence of BHR defines a more heritable trait or even a particular subtype of asthma. (This is in contrast to experimental airways hyperreactivity that is induced in murine models of asthma).

2.4. Atopy

Initially, Dr. Julian Hopkin and I observed that children within atopic families varied in the disease manifestations. Within a single family, some children might have elevated total serum IgE; whereas other children might have positive skin tests or elevated specific IgE titers against common allergens, despite having normal serum IgE concentrations. As clinicians, we felt that atopy would be recognized if any one of these traits was present. We therefore proposed a compound definition of atopy, which included one or more of positive skin tests, positive serum IgE titers against allergens, or elevations of the total serum IgE 21. Using this definition of atopy, most individuals could be classified as affected or unaffected, and borderline cases could be classified as indeterminate. Even though we were naïve to consider this trait to behave as a simple autosomal dominant *(21)*, it appears to be highly penetrant, and we have continued to use it in linkage studies *(22)*.

2.5. Quantitative Traits

We have investigated the genetic and environmental components of variance of serum total and specific IgE levels and BHR in an Australian population-based sample of 232 Caucasian nuclear families. The interrelationships of the genetic determinants of these traits were also investigated. Log_e total serum IgE levels had a h^2 of 47%. Specific serum IgE levels against house dust mite and timothy grass (added together as a radioallergosorbent test [RAST] Index), had a h^2 of 34%. BHR, quantified by the log_e dose-response slope (DRS) to methacholine, had a h^2 of 30%. We demonstrated an approx 70% overlap in the genetic determinants of total and specific serum IgE levels. However, the genetic determinants of serum IgE levels and DRS exhibited less than 30% sharing *(23)*. These data indicate that the log_e is the single most heritable intermediate trait associated with asthma and suggest that DRS and BHR are less heritable and are genetically distinct from atopy.

2.6. Genetic Linkage

Genetic linkage in humans may be assessed by parametric statistics, such as the logarithm of the odds (lod) score, or by non- or semiparametric statistics, usually based on measures of sibling pair sharing of traits and alleles. In early studies, we attempted to use lod scores *(24)*, discarding individuals with ambiguous phenotypes, but soon realized that generational effects and the decline in the prevalence of atopy and asthma symptoms with age made phenotype definition problematic in parents. Since then, we have used sibling pair methods to test for linkage to categorical phenotypes of physician-diagnosed asthma and atopy and quantitative traits of total serum IgE, skin test index, and BHR (measured as DRS).

2.7. Genotypic Ambiguity and Error

Errors in genotyping can substantially influence the power to detect linkage using affected sibling pairs. These errors may have less effect in single marker linkage analysis than in multipoint analysis, when genotyping errors can easily result in false exclusion of the true location of a disease-predisposing gene *(25)*. Simulations have shown that for loci of modest effect 5% genotyping error may eliminate all supporting evidence for linkage to a true susceptibility locus in affected pairs *(26)*. Although quantitative trait loci (QTL) association analyses of common alleles are more robust to genotyping error, power can still be affected dramatically with errors in the genotyping of rare alleles *(26)*.

Exhaustive detection of genotyping errors is therefore essential for effective linkage studies. Errors may be prevented by careful quality controls, but any large-scale pedigree collection and genotyping exercise will still result in some mistakes. Examination and correction of the genotype data should therefore precede definitive linkage or association analyses.

Standard programs, such as PedCheck, identify Mendelian errors, but these are only part of the error content of a given data set. In a large panel of families, errors may arise from misplaced samples or incorrectly classified relationships, such as half-siblings, full siblings, and identical twins. We have developed a graphical tool (GRR) for verifying assumed relationships between individuals in genetic studies *(27)*. It examines the mean and variance of the allele sharing between sibling, parent, and parent-child pairs and identifies pairs that show unexpected patterns of sharing. Its use is particularly valuable in the initial analyses of genome screen data, when errors in pedigree classification may be common *(27)*. GRR is effective with information from as few as 50 markers.

Genotyping error may also be detected by the presence of improbable recombination events, typically apparent double recombinants in a small genetic interval. The computer program MERLIN *(28)* identifies all such events within dense genetic maps. This information is output to a file. The genotypes may then be checked and corrected. As the throughput of single nucleotide polymorphism (SNP) genotyping becomes higher and more automated, it is increasingly difficult to return and regenotype individual SNPs. As an alternative, the MERLIN utility PEDWIPE may be used to produce a pedigree file, in which improbable genotypes have been scored as missing.

2.8. Parent-of-Origin Effects

The risk of transmission of atopic disease from an affected mother is approx 4 times higher than from an affected father *(29)*. Similar parent-of-origin effects have been noted in other immunological diseases, including type 1 diabetes *(30,31)*, rheumatoid arthritis *(32)*, psoriasis *(33)*, inflammatory bowel disease (IBD) *(34)*, and selective immunoglobulin-A (IgA) deficiency *(35)*.

Parent-of-origin effects seem therefore to be part of a general phenomenon affecting several immune-related loci and several diseases, and it may be assumed that this process is in some way adaptive.

Most linkage studies of asthma and related phenotypes have not explored for maternal effects. This may well be because many of the most commonly used linkage programs do not routinely give results for parents-of-origin. We have used the computer program GAS (http://users.ox.ac.uk/~ayoung/gas.html), which gives nonparametric single and multipoint linkage statistics, together with the actual allele counts from which statistics are derived. Maternal and paternal transmission equilibrium test (TDT) tests are also given by GAS, and association to quantitative traits may be investigated with quantitative trait TDT (QTDT) *(36)*.

The mechanisms for these parent-of-origin effects are unknown. They may result from immune interactions between the fetus and the mother, which are recognized to take place through the placenta, as well as through breast milk *(6)*. Alternatively, the maternal effect may be the result of genomic imprinting. Genomic imprinting is a process in which the genes from one parent are differentially expressed to the allele derived from the other parent *(37,38)*.

Several known genes show parent-of-origin effects on allergic disease. These genes include the *FcεRI-β* locus on chromosome 11q13 *(5,39)*, the *LEKTI/SPINK5* gene from chromosome 5q34 *(40)* and as yet undiscovered genes at loci on chromosomes 4 and 16 *(22)*. Parent-of-origin effects must have a physical basis, which is tractable to investigation. A first step in this might be to examine epigenetic markers of imprinting, such as the variable presence of methylation on CpG residues *(38)*, with knowledge of parental atopic status and genotype.

2.9. Genome Screens

Eleven full-genome screens have been reported for asthma and its associated phenotypes *(22,41–50)* and others have been carried out in industry. Several of these screens have been performed in distinct European populations, which are German *(43)*, French *(46)*, Finnish *(47)*, Icelandic *(48)*, Dutch *(49)*, and Danish *(50)*.

Happily, there is considerable consensus about regions of genetic linkage that are relevant to asthma. Primary linkages that have been replicated in more than one screen are to 6p24-21 (the major histocompatibility complex [MHC]) in six screens *(22,41,43,44,49,50)*, 11q13-21 (near the β chain of the high-affinity receptor for IgE [*FcεRI-β*]) in four screens *(22,41,46,50)*, 1p31-36 in three screens *(41,46,50)*, 4q13 in two screens *(22,47)*, 5q23-31 in two screens (near the interleukin [IL]-4 cytokine cluster) *(49,50)*, 7p14 in two screens *(22,47)*, 12q21-24 in two screens *(43,46)*, 13q12-14 in two screens *(22,49)*, and 16q21-23 in two screens *(22,50)*.

Four groups have shown linkage to the long arm of chromosome 2, but these are spread over some distance between 2q14 (near the IL-1 cluster) *(22)*, 2q21-23 *(44)*, 2q24-34 *(49)*, and 2q32 *(43)*. It is not yet clear whether these correspond to different genetic loci.

Three groups have found regions of linkage, which, although unreplicated, are statistically significant: these are on 3q21-22 in Danish families *(50)*, 14q24 in Icelandic families *(48)*, and 17q12-21 in French families *(46)*. A fourth group has reported a single linkage on chromosome 20p12, which was part of the results of an industrial genome screen *(17)*.

Finally, three regions of linkage have been established by studying important candidate loci: these include chromosome 14q11 and the T cell receptor (*TCR*) -α/δ genes *(51)*, chromosome 5q23 and the cytokine cluster *(52)*, and chromosome 12q12-14 and interferon (*IFN*) -γ *(53)*.

2.10. Nonreplication

Thus, 10 loci have been replicated in more than one screen, but four groups have found regions of highly significant ($p < 0.001$) but unreplicated linkage: these are on 3q21-22 *(50)*, 11p13 *(46)*, 14q24 *(48)*, 17q12-21 *(46)*, and 20p12 *(17)*.

A number of reasons may explain why linkages to these loci have not been replicated in the other studies. First, they might represent false positives. It is always difficult to judge the true meanings of the probabilities that are generated from multiple variations of phenotype and hundreds of different markers. It is therefore desirable to apply empirical statistical methods to generate global *p* values from the phenotype and marker combinations used in an individual study. These methods use simulations in which the genotypes from a study are randomly combined with the phenotypes, and the number of *p* values below various thresholds is counted. The simulations are repeated thousands of times, building up an accurate picture of the real probability of a particular *p* threshold in the data set under study *(22,47,54)*.

Second, the results may reflect population-specific differences in genetic predisposition to asthma. Differences in allele frequencies for the human leukocyte antigen *(HLA)* loci and other immune genes *(55)* show clear gradients between European countries, and the screens that have been performed in Danish *(50)*, Icelandic *(48)*, and French *(46)* families may quite plausibly be detecting regional differences in polymorphism in other immune genes.

Third, there may be methodological differences between studies. The most important of these will be differences in age distribution or disease severity.

A fourth and common reason for outlying linkage results is that replication of linkage findings in complex diseases is *a priori* expected to require a substantially larger data set than that in which the original findings were made *(56)*. This is because practicable sample sizes always represent a fraction of the ideal, and some random selection of families with linkage in a particular region is likely *(56)*.

3. INDIVIDUAL LOCI AND CANDIDATE GENES

Several of the loci found by genome screens contain important candidate genes, and three loci have been the subject of positional cloning exercises. The relevant findings for these loci are summarized under the following subheadings.

3.1. The MHC

The MHC shows the strongest evidence for linkage in most studies. It is well-known that *HLA-DR* alleles restrict the IgE response to particular allergens, usually with a relative risk less than 2 *(57–60)*. Small antigens, such as aspirin and acid anhydrides, show much stronger effects *(61,62)*. The ability

Ewart et al. identified linkage of the same SHR phenotype in an A/J and C3H/HeJ cross to murine chromosome 6, corresponding to the human IL-4 cytokine complex. This region has been identified by several human linkage studies *(52,124–126)* and may contain more than one locus influencing asthma.

Our group carried out a genome screen in a BP2 and Balb/c cross, using QTLs derived from a model of ovalbumin (OVA) induced asthma *(127)*. This identified five potential loci, two on chromosome 9, and one each on chromosomes 10, 11, and 17.

The chromosome 10 QTL to induced bronchial responsiveness (IBR) showed syntenic homology with human chromosome 12q21.1-12q24.22, which has previously been shown to be linked to human asthma-associated traits *(53,128,129)*. The region linkage of IBR to mouse chromosome 11 contains loci which contributed to survival after ozone-induced pulmonary inflammation in a AJ × C57BL/6J cross *(130)* and to ozone-induced pulmonary neutrophil infiltration in a C57BL/6J × C3H/HeJ cross *(131)*. This region shows syntenic homology to human chromosome 17, which has been implicated in previous linkage studies of asthma 17q12-21 *(46,129)* and contains numerous chemokine genes.

The suggestive linkage of IBR to mouse chromosome 17 supported the previously reported linkage to SHR *(123)*. Both the original and our studies suggest that the locus may contain more than one gene influencing airway hyperresponsiveness (AHR) *(123,127)*. This region contains the *MHC* and *TNF* genes, which may have diverse effects on antigen recognition and the promotion of airway inflammation. The *MHC* and *TNF* genes have also been implicated in gold-salt-induced IgE nephropathy in a brown Norway (BN) × Lewis (LEW) rat cross *(132)*. In human families, class II *HLA* genes are known to restrict the ability to react to particular allergens *(57–60)*, and polymorphism with *TNF* genes has been associated with asthma independently of class II effects *(64)*. The suggestion that two (or more) loci are acting within this QTL in our murine model is therefore consistent with the observations in humans.

The mouse chromosome 11 QTL influencing eosinophil infiltration into the bronchial epithelium has complex human syntenic homologies, which include the distal IL-4/IL-5 cytokine cluster on human chromosome 5. It has also been implicated by a BN × LEW cross that had been used to investigate IgE nephropathy *(132)*.

A recent comprehensive study *(133)* examined the strain distribution patterns for the asthma-related phenotypes AHR, lung eosinophils, and OVA specific serum IgE induced by allergen exposure protocols in A/J, AKR/J,

BALB/cJ, C3H/HeJ, and C57BL/6J inbred strains and in (C3H/HeJ × A/J) F1 mice. Expression of AHR differed between strains and was sometimes discordant with lung eosinophils or serum IgE. The study identified two distinct QTL for susceptibility to allergen-induced AHR, Abhr1 (allergen-induced BHR) (lod = 4.2), and Abhr2 (lod = 3.7), on chromosome 2 in backcross progeny from A/J and C3H/HeJ mice. In addition, a QTL on chromosome 7 was suggestive of linkage to this trait.

The murine chromosome 2 locus identified in this study overlaps the SHR linkage identified by De Sanctis et al. *(123)* and the human IL-1 cluster. The murine chromosome 7 locus has syntenic homology to human chromosome 19 which may contain an asthma locus *(134)*.

The NC/Nga mouse is an inbred strain established from Japanese fancy mice that spontaneously develop AD-like skin lesions and elevations of the total serum IgE concentration. These lesions are characterized by massive infiltration of $CD4^+$ T-cells which produce IL-4 and IL-5, and the degranulation of eosinophils and mast cells *(135)*. This mouse may also serve as a model for asthma *(136)*. A genetic study in these mice showed linkage to chromosome 9 *(137)*. This region is the syntenic homolog of human chromosome 11q23, which linked in some human studies to eosinophil counts and specific IgE responses 22 *(138)*.

The NOA (Naruto Research Institute Otsuka Atrichia) mouse is another model of AD. Linkage of this trait has been established to the middle of mouse chromosome 14 *(139)*, in the homologous region to the recognized human atopy locus on chromosome 13q14 *(80)*.

7. LD MAPPING

Genetic linkage studies in humans and in mice have therefore generated a substantial amount of high-quality data that has led to consensus on the number and nature of several major loci influencing asthma and its associated phenotypes. Several of these loci have been further dissected by the study of important candidate genes. For regions that do not contain candidate genes, the challenge is now to move from genetic linkage to gene identification.

LD describes the nonrandom association of deoxyribonucleic acid (DNA) variants on contiguous regions of DNA. New polymorphisms first appear on an individual chromosome and are initially coinherited with every other polymorphism on that chromosome. Polymorphisms may increase in frequency in a population either through selection or through genetic drift. Genetic recombination causes progressive dissociation between the new polymorphism and distant SNPs, until after many generations only physically close SNPs are coinherited. LD may be detected by population associations between markers or between a disease phenotype (representing a functional polymorphism) and a marker or markers.

The detection of disease-marker associations by LD mapping can precisely locate genes of small effect and could be used to identify common disease genes in genome-wide scans or to reduce the number of candidate genes in a region in which linkage has been established *(140–143)*. In the presence of common disease alleles, or when the frequency of rare alleles is increased through selection, the sample sizes required for LD studies are much smaller than for equivalently powered linkage studies *(140)*.

7.1. The Nature of LD

Simulations have suggested that LD may extend for less than 5 kb, even in relatively isolated populations, so that more than 1,000,000 equally spaced markers might be required for genome-wide LD scans *(144)*. However, reviews of published data provide examples of LD at distances greater than 100 kb *(145,146)*, and there is evidence that LD patterns vary between populations *(147,148)*. LD is detectable at 500 kb in the adenomatous polyposis coli *(APC)* gene region on chromosome 5 *(149)*, and significant LD between microsatellite loci has been shown to extend to 4 cM in some chromosomal regions *(146)*. Other studies have shown that the distribution of LD is irregular in a number of chromosomal regions *(150–153)*.

We have examined the patterns of LD for dense SNP maps in three genomic regions in a sample of 575 chromosomes from two Caucasian populations of British ancestry *(154)*. We used the D' statistic as a measure of LD because it has a simple interpretation, its scale (between 0 and 1) is independent of allele frequency and it is applicable to both SNP and microsatellite data *(155,156)*.

We found that the fine structure of LD was highly irregular. Forty-five percent of the variation in disequilibrium measures could be explained by physical distance. Additional factors, such as allele frequency, type of polymorphism, and genomic location, explained less than 5% of the variation *(154)*.

The mean D' was less than 1 even for closely linked markers, and SNPs a few base pairs apart on occasion showed no LD. The results therefore indicate that care is required when interpreting allelic association as evidence of precise localization.

The limit of detection of LD between a disease and a marker is approximately defined by a D' of 0.33 *(144,154)* and by the size of the sample studied *(157)*. We found that on average D' declined below 0.33 for distances greater than approx 35 bp *(154)*. The detection of association between a marker and disease therefore limits the location of the disease gene to within an average of 35 kb in either direction. Local differences in the extent of LD may modify this figure, which may be approximated to 100 kb (±50 kb).

7.2. Detection of Association

The key decision in moving from genetic linkage (typically 10–30 Mb) to genetic association (100 kb) is the number and density of markers to type within the limits for localization of the disease gene. This interval is typically defined by the 1 lod support unit (the region covered by the linkage curve extending 1 lod less than the maximum peak), which corresponds approximately to a 90% confidence interval. If LD were to be evenly distributed, then 30 Mb could be covered comprehensively by as few as 300 SNPs (or microsatellites or other polymorphisms). However, the universal observation is that LD is irregular. Therefore, much has been made of the presence of "haplotype blocks," which have been defined as "sizeable regions over which there is little evidence for historical recombination and within which only a few common haplotypes are observed" *(158,159)*.

It has been suggested that such blocks may be typified by a limited number of SNPs, and that these SNPs may serve to capture all relevant haplotypes and disease associations. In our data we do not find evidence of such blocks: even within regions of quite high LD, LD still declines with distance, and some markers may be out of LD with their immediate neighbors.

An empirical method of moving from linkage to association may be to type waves of markers of progressive density until association between disease and a marker is identified. The density of the first wave depends on the resources available for genotyping (budget, subjects, equipment, and workers).

The power of LD mapping depends strongly on matching marker and disease allele frequencies *(157,160,161)*. This means that SNPs with a range of gene frequencies should be tested. Microsatellites reflect LD from multiple alleles simultaneously, and as LD may extend for longer distances around microsatellites *(154)*, they may be more informative than SNPs for low density scans or when searching for mutations of recent origin. Dense panels of microsatellite markers are already in use for genetic linkage studies *(162)*, and there are 12,000 microsatellites in the public domain, so that these markers also merit consideration in LD mapping.

Association between disease and a marker may be examined in cases or controls or in families. Cases and controls may be cheaper to collect, but hidden admixture is always a possibility, particularly in country such as the United States. In the absence of admixture, the power of analysis of association in families may be increased by the inclusion of all family members, correcting for familial correlations in phenotype and genotype. Statistical methods for this type of analysis include regressive models *(163)*, as implemented in SAGE, and variance components models, as implemented in QTDT *(36)* for quantitative traits, and haplotype relative risks *(164)* for categorical data.

7.3. Association Mapping

Assuming that an association has been established between a marker and disease, the next step in localization of an assumed disease gene involves defining the limits of association and the comprehensive identification of polymorphism within those limits. Although the public SNP map is becoming more reliable and comprehensive, it is not so at the time of writing, and the identification of all SNPs in a region will still depend on systematic resequencing.

The nature of the genetic variation underlying complex traits is likely to consist of common alleles that are evolutionarily old *(165,166)*. In addition, rare alleles may require prohibitively large sample sizes to detect associations with complex traits.

Our sequencing strategy has therefore been directed at the identification of alleles with a minimum frequency of 0.15. It has been shown that sequencing 20 haploid genomes gives an approx 99.9% probability of detecting alleles with a minimal allele frequency of 0.2 and an approx 99% probability of detecting alleles with a minimum frequency of 0.1 *(167)*. We therefore have initially sequenced 10 diploid genomes (5 unrelated atopic subjects and 5 unrelated controls) together with a pool of DNA from 32 unrelated individuals. Dilution experiments with known alleles indicated that we were able to detect allele frequencies more than 0.15 with this pool. Repetitive DNA segments are very difficult to resequence, and may be screened out using REPEATMASKER (Smit, AF and Green P, http://repeatmasker. genome.washington.edu).

Once a positional candidate has been identified, we have sequenced multiple clones all exons in complementary DNA (cDNA) from 22 unrelated individuals, 12 of which were atopic and 7 of which were asthmatic. This data would have 99.9% probability of identifying SNPs greater than 0.1 frequency and 95% probability of identifying SNPs greater than 0.01 frequency *(167)*.

In general, successful LD mapping will require a systematic understanding of local patterns of LD and haplotype evolution, as exemplified by the mapping of polymorphisms in the angiotensin-converting enxyme *(ACE)* gene which control circulating ACE levels *(168)*. Haplotype-based tests may be more powerful in the presence of multiple disease alleles *(169)*, but the relationship between haplotype variation and the power of haplotype-based tests has not yet been well described. We have routinely carried out haplo-type generation in simple pedigrees by the MERLIN computer program *(28)* and more complex pedigrees by SIMWALK2 *(170)*. LD between markers may be assessed by estimation of D' from the parental haplotypes *(154)* and depicted by the GOLD program *(171)*.

8. GENE IDENTIFICATION

Once an LD and association map has been completed, then the putative gene needs to be identified from the refined genetic region. With luck, only a handful of genes will be implicated by genetic association. Gene identifica-tion depends on the examination of sequence for potential genes, the identi-fication of expressed sequences with the expressed sequence tag (EST) databases, the pattern of expression of the genes within different tissues, and the inference of gene function from homology searches and examination of domain structure. These steps are considerably facilitated by the near-completion of the human genetic sequence.

8.1. Sequence Analyses

In our studies we have analyzed genomic sequence using a modification of HPREP (G. Micklem, unpublished). We have looked for matches to human, rodent, EST, sequence tagged sites, and other DNA databases, using the SWISSPROT, TREMBL, and TREMBLNEW peptide databases. We have identified CpG islands using CPG *(172)*, transcription factor elements and putative promoter regions using PROMOTERSCAN *(173)*, and exon predictions using GRAIL *(174)*, GENSCAN *(175)*, GENEPARSER *(176)*, and MZEF *(177)*.

8.2. EST Databases

We have obtained IMAGE clones mapping to regions of interest from Research Genetics. We have aligned consensus sequences for each IMAGE clone by the Genetics Computer Group program. ESTs are by intent fragmen-tary, and even consensus sequences from multiple ESTs are likely to be incom-plete. Sequences may most easily be completed by polymerase chain reaction (PCR) of cDNA RACE libraries to extend 5' and 3' cDNA ends of the IMAGE clones. Alternatively, libraries may be screened for full-length cDNAs.

The data from all these sources needs to be integrated into a full map of the region. We have collated these annotations using ACeDB (http://www.acedb.org/) and identified known genes using BLASTN178 against the EMBL DNA database.

8.3. Domain and Homology Analyses to Infer Function

We have searched the peptide databases SWISSPROT, TREMBL, and TREMBLNEW using BLASTX *(178)* for homologs to transcripts of unknown function. We have examined putative roles for recognized protein domains within transcripts using PSI-BLAST *(178)* and SMART *(179)*.

8.4. Expression: Northerns, Multiple Tissue cDNA Panels, and Positional Arrays

The general pattern of expression of the positional candidate genes may be examined by northern blots, such as the human Multiple Tissue Northern (MTN™) Blots and Human Immune System MTN blots that may be obtained from CLONTECH. We have also found very helpful the examination of cDNA panels from multiple tissues by PCR. The use of PCR allows the examination of splice variants that may not be delineated by Northern blots.

The inclusion of all human genes on commercially available DNA microarrays adds a new dimension to this process. These arrays may be interrogated with a variety of tissues from normal and diseased individuals and information on the expression levels integrated with positional information from linkage and association studies.

8.5. The Effects of Polymorphism: Multiple Variant Alleles and Splice Variation

All of this information may be used to judge if the assumed gene has been identified. The decision is easiest if clear mutations are found in the gene, as in the case of the *NOD2* gene and Crohn's disease *(180,181)*. However, it may often be the case that the effects of polymorphism on gene function are more subtle, affecting levels of expression or splice variation. In these circumstances a definitive understanding of the mechanics of disease may take some time. Systematic examination of polymorphisms for transcription factor binding by electrophoretic mobility shift assay of footprinting experiments would seem to be a helpful first step.

8.6. Gene Function

Given that positional cloning is capable of finding new and unexpected mechanisms for disease, it is quite possible that at the end of the positional cloning process there will still be some uncertainty regarding the function of the assumed disease gene in the disease process. The downstream examination of the function of genes is likely to be highly individual and difficult to organize with high throughput. The abilities to express proteins in a variety of vectors and systems, to raise antibodies, to localize proteins within cells, to identify ligands, and to knockout in mice or knockdown in cells by ribonucleic acid interface may all be required.

9. CONCLUSIONS

The positional cloning of genes underlying asthma has proven to be highly complex and demanding of considerable resources. However, several groups now have sufficient clinical collections of families and cases and controls to be able to map disease genes with robust and replicated results. The public availability of the human and murine genome sequence and improved methods of high-throughput genotyping are hugely valuable tools in disease gene identification.

A striking feature of genetic studies of asthma has been the recognition of the considerable overlap between linkage regions from human and murine studies. This overlap extends beyond asthma to many diseases of immune and autoimmune origins. It is likely to represent the common effects of evolution on polymorphism in the same key immune genes in humans and in rodents. It strongly indicates the importance of murine studies in disease gene identification and suggests that an integrated approach to mapping encompassing both species will be the best way forward.

Despite all the difficulties, real progress has already been made and the eventual complete understanding of the genetic basis of asthma and atopic disease is now assured.

REFERENCES

1. Smith DH, Malone DC, Lawson KA, Okamoto LJ, Battista C, Saunders WB. A national estimate of the economic costs of asthma. Am J Respir Crit Care Med 1997;156:787–793.
2. Stuart M. Start-Up 1999;12–20.
3. Sampson HA. Pathogenesis of eczema. Clin Exp Allergy 1990;20:459–467.
4. Schultz Larsen F. Atopic dermatitis: a genetic-epidemiologic study in a population-based twin sample. J Am Acad Dermatol 1993;28:719–723.
5. Cox HE, Moffatt MF, Faux JA, et al. Association of atopic dermatitis to the beta subunit of the high affinity immunoglobulin E receptor. Br J Dermatol 1998;138:182–187.
6. Holt PG, Macaubas C, Stumbles PA, Sly PD. The role of allergy in the development of asthma. Nature 1999;402 (6760 Suppl):B12–B17.
7. Bos J. Immunology of atopic dermatitis. Oxford: Blackwell Science, 2000.
8. Duffy DL, Martin NG, Battistutta D, Hopper JL, Mathews JD. Genetics of asthma and hay fever in Australian twins. Am Rev Respir Dis 1990;142:1351–1358.
9. Larsen FS, Holm NV, Henningsen K. Atopic dermatitis. A genetic-epidemiologic study in a population-based twin sample. J Am Acad Dermatol 1986;15:487–494.

10. Boushey HA, Holtzman MJ, Sheller JR, Nadel JA. Bronchial hyperreactivity. Am Rev Respir Dis 1980;121:389–413.

11. O'Connor G, Sparrow D, Taylor D, Segal M, Weiss S. Analysis of dose-response curves to methacholine. An approach suitable for population studies. Am Rev Respir Dis 1987;136:1412–1417.

12. Cookson W, Palmer L. Investigating the asthma phenotype. Clin Exp Allergy 1998;28 (Suppl 1) :88–89; discussion 108–110.

13. Risch N, Zhang H. Extreme discordant sib pairs for mapping quantitative trait loci in humans. Science 1995;268:1584–1589.

14. O'Connor GT, Weiss ST. Clinical and symptom measures. Am J Respir Crit Care Med 1994;149:S21–S28.

15. Postma DS, Bleecker ER, Amelung PJ, et al. Genetic susceptibility to asthma-bronchial hyperresponsiveness coinherited with a major gene for atopy. N Engl J Med 1995;333:894–900.

16. Ober C, Cox NJ, Abney M, et al. Genome-wide search for asthma susceptibility loci in a founder population. The collaborative study on the genetics of asthma. Hum Mol Genet 1998;7:1393–1398.

17. Van Eerdewegh P, Little RD, Dupuis J, et al. Association of the ADAM33 gene with asthma and bronchial hyperresponsiveness. Nature 2002;418: 426–430.

18. Peat JK, Salome CM, Bauman A, Toelle BG, Wachinger SL, Woolcock AJ. Repeatability of histamine bronchial challenge and comparability with methacholine bronchial challenge in a population of Australian school children. Am Rev Respir Dis 1991;144:338–343.

19. Sears MR, Burrows B, Flannery EM, Herbison GP, Hewitt CJ, Holdaway MD. Relation between airway responsiveness and serum IgE in children with asthma and in apparently normal children. N Engl J Med 1991;325: 1067–1071.

20. Plaschke P, Bake B. Pronounced bronchial hyper-responsiveness and asthma severity. Clin Physiol 1994;14:197–203.

21. Cookson WO, Hopkin JM. Dominant inheritance of atopic immunoglobulin-E responsiveness. Lancet 1988;1:86–88.

22. Daniels SE, Bhattacharrya S, James A, et al. A genome-wide search for quantitative trait loci underlying asthma. Nature 1996;383:247–250.

23. Palmer LJ, Burton PR, Faux JA, James AL, Musk AW, Cookson WO. Independent inheritance of serum immunoglobulin E concentrations and airway responsiveness. Am J Respir Crit Care Med 2000;161:1836–1843.

24. Cookson WO, Sharp PA, Faux JA, Hopkin JM. Linkage between immunoglobulin E responses underlying asthma and rhinitis and chromosome 11q. Lancet 1989;1:1292–1295.

25. Goring HH, Terwilliger JD. Linkage analysis in the presence of errors II: marker-locus genotyping errors modeled with hypercomplex recombination fractions. Am J Hum Genet 2000;66:1107–1118.

26. Abecasis GR, Cherny SS, Cardon LR. The impact of genotyping error on family-based analysis of quantitative traits. Eur J Hum Genet 2001;9:130–134.

27. Abecasis GR, Cherny SS, Cookson WO, Cardon LR. GRR: graphical representation of relationship errors. Bioinformatics 2001;17:742–743.
28. Abecasis GR, Cherny SS, Cookson WO, Cardon LR. Merlin-rapid analysis of dense genetic maps using sparse gene flow trees. Nat Genet 2002;30:97–101.
29. Moffatt M, Cookson W. The genetics of asthma. Maternal effects in atopic disease. Clin Exp Allergy 1998;28(Suppl 1):56–61; discussion 65, 66.
30. Bennett S, Todd J. Human type 1 diabetes and the insulin gene: principles of mapping polygenes. Annu Rev Genet 1996;30:343–370.
31. Warram JH, Krolewski AS, Gottlieb MS, Kahn CR. Differences in risk of insulin-dependent diabetes in offspring of diabetic mothers and diabetic fathers. N Engl J Med 1984;311:149–152.
32. Koumantaki Y, Giziaki E, Linos A, et al. Family history as a risk factor for rheumatoid arthritis: a case-control study. J Rheumatol 1997;24:1522–1526.
33. Burden A, Javed S, Bailey M, Hodgins M, Connor M, Tillman D. Genetics of psoriasis: paternal inheritance and a locus on chromosome 6p [see comments]. J Invest Dermatol 1998;110:958–960.
34. Akolkar PN, Gulwani-Akolkar B, Heresbach D, et al. Differences in risk of Crohn's disease in offspring of mothers and fathers with inflammatory bowel disease. Am J Gastroenterol 1997;92:2241–2244.
35. Vorechovsky I, Webster AD, Plebani A, Hammarstrom L. Genetic linkage of IgA deficiency to the major histocompatibility complex: evidence for allele segregation distortion, parent-of-origin penetrance differences, and the role of anti-IgA antibodies in disease predisposition. Am J Hum Genet 1999;64:1096–1109.
36. Abecasis GR, Cardon LR, Cookson WO. A general test of association for quantitative traits in nuclear families. Am J Hum Genet 2000;66:279–292.
37. Hall JG. Genomic imprinting. Arch Dis Child 1990;65:1013–1016.
38. Reik W, Walter J. Genomic imprinting: parental influence on the genome. Nat Rev Genet 2001;2:21–32.
39. Cookson WO, Young RP, Sandford AJ, et al. Maternal inheritance of atopic IgE responsiveness on chromosome 11q. Lancet 1992;340:381–384.
40. Cookson WO, Ubhi B, Lawrence R, et al. Genetic linkage of childhood atopic dermatitis to psoriasis susceptibility loci. Nat Genet 2001;27:372–373.
41. Xu J, Meyers DA, Ober C, et al. Genomewide screen and identification of gene-gene interactions for asthma-susceptibility loci in three U.S. populations: collaborative study on the genetics of asthma. Am J Hum Genet 2001;68:1437–1446.
42. Ober C, Tsalenko A, Parry R, Cox NJ. A second-generation genomewide screen for asthma-susceptibility alleles in a founder population. Am J Hum Genet 2000;67:1154–1162.
43. Wjst M, Fischer G, Immervoll T, et al. A genome-wide search for linkage to asthma. German Asthma Genetics Group. Genomics 1999;58:1–8.
44. Hizawa N, Freidhoff L, Chiu Y, et al. Genetic regulation of Dermatophagoides pteronyssinus-specific IgE responsiveness: a genome-wide multipoint linkage analysis in families recruited through 2 asthmatic sibs. Collaborative study on the genetics of asthma (CSGA). J Allergy Clin Immunol 1998;102:436–442.

45. Mathias RA, Freidhoff LR, Blumenthal MN, et al. Genome-wide linkage analyses of total serum IgE using variance components analysis in asthmatic families. Genet Epidemiol 2001;20:340–355.
46. Dizier MH, Besse-Schmittler C, Guilloud-Bataille M, et al. Genome screen for asthma and related phenotypes in the French EGEA study. Am J Respir Crit Care Med 2000;162:1812–1818.
47. Laitinen T, Daly MJ, Rioux JD, et al. A susceptibility locus for asthma-related traits on chromosome 7 revealed by genome-wide scan in a founder population. Nat Genet 2001;28:87–91.
48. Hakonarson H, Bjornsdottir US, Halapi E, et al. A major susceptibility gene for asthma maps to chromosome 14q24. Am J Hum Genet 2002;71:483–491.
49. Koppelman GH, Stine OC, Xu J, et al. Genome-wide search for atopy susceptibility genes in Dutch families with asthma. J Allergy Clin Immunol 2002; 109:498–506.
50. Haagerup A, Bjerke T, Schiotz PO, Binderup HG, Dahl R, Kruse TA. Asthma and atopy-a total genome scan for susceptibility genes. Allergy 2002;57:680–686.
51. Moffatt MF, Hill MR, Cornelis F, et al. Genetic linkage of T cell receptor a/d complex to specific IgE responses. Lancet 1994;343:1597–1600.
52. Marsh DG, Neely JD, Breazeale DR, et al. Linkage analysis of IL4 and other chromosome 5q31.1 markers and total serum immunoglobulin E concentrations. Science 1994;264:1152–1156.
53. Barnes KC, Neely JD, Duffy DL, et al. Linkage of asthma and total serum IgE concentration to markers on chromosome 12q: evidence from Afro-Caribbean and Caucasian populations. Genomics 1996;37:41–50.
54. Lander E, Kruglyak L. Genetic dissection of complex traits: guidelines for interpreting and reporting linkage results. Nat Genet 1995;11:241–247.
55. Libert F, Cochaux P, Beckman G, et al. The deltaccr5 mutation conferring protection against HIV-1 in Caucasian populations has a single and recent origin in Northeastern Europe. Hum Mol Genet 1998;7:399–406.
56. Suarez BK, Hampe CL, Van Eerdewegh P. Problems of replicating linkage claims in psychiatry. In: Gershorn ES, Cloninger CR, eds. Genetic approaches to mental disorders. Washington, DC: American Psychiatric, 1994:23–46.
57. Levine BB, Stember RH, Fontino M. Ragweed hayfever: genetic control and linkage to HLA haplotyes. Science 1972;178:1201–1203.
58. Marsh DG, Meyers DA, Bias WB. The epidemiology and genetics of atopic allergy. N Engl J Med 1981;305:1551–1559.
59. Young RP, Dekker JW, Wordsworth BP, Cookson WO. HLA-DR and HLA-DP genotypes and immunoglobulin E responses to common major allergens. Clin Exp Allergy 1994;24:431–439.
60. Moffatt MF, Schou C, Faux JA, et al. Association between quantitative traits underlying asthma and the HLA- DRB1 locus in a family-based population sample. Eur J Hum Genet 2001;9:341–346.
61. Dekker JW, Nizankowska E, Schmitz-Schumann M, et al. Aspirin-induced asthma and HLA-DRB1 and HLA-DPB1 genotypes. Clin Exp Allergy 1997; 27:574–577.

62. Young RP, Barker RD, Pile KD, Cookson WO, Taylor AJ. The association of HLA-DR3 with specific IgE to inhaled acid anhydrides. Am J Respir Crit Care Med 1995;151:219–221.

63. Moffatt MF, Schou C, Faux JA, Cookson WO. Germline TCR-A restriction of immunoglobulin E responses to allergen. Immunogenetics 1997;46: 226–230.

64. Moffatt MF, Cookson WO. Tumour necrosis factor haplotypes and asthma. Hum Mol Genet 1997;6:551–554.

65. Albuquerque RV, Hayden CM, Palmer LJ, et al. Association of polymorphisms within the tumour necrosis factor (TNF) genes and childhood asthma. Clin Exp Allergy 1998;28:578–584.

66. Chagani T, Pare PD, Zhu S, et al. Prevalence of tumor necrosis factor-alpha and angiotensin converting enzyme polymorphisms in mild/moderate and fatal/near-fatal asthma. Am J Respir Crit Care Med 1999;160:278–282.

67. Li Kam Wa TC, Mansur AH, Britton J, et al. Association between-308 tumour necrosis factor promoter polymorphism and bronchial hyperreactivity in asthma. Clin Exp Allergy 1999;29:1204–1208.

68. Noguchi E, Yokouchi Y, Shibasaki M, et al. Association between TNFA polymorphism and the development of asthma in the Japanese population. Am J Respir Crit Care Med 2002;166:43–46.

69. Witte JS, Palmer LJ, O'Connor RD, Hopkins PJ, Hall JM. Relation between tumour necrosis factor polymorphism TNFalpha-308 and risk of asthma. Eur J Hum Genet 2002;10:82–85.

70. Winchester EC, Millwood IY, Rand L, Penny MA, Kessling AM. Association of the TNF-alpha-308 (G→A) polymorphism with self-reported history of childhood asthma. Hum Genet 2000;107:591–596.

71. Sandford AJ, Shirakawa T, Moffatt MF, et al. Localisation of atopy and beta subunit of high-affinity IgE receptor (Fc epsilon RI) on chromosome 11q. Lancet 1993;341:332–334.

72. Shirakawa T, Mao XQ, Sasaki S, et al. Association between atopic asthma and a coding variant of Fc epsilon RI beta in a Japanese population. Hum Mol Genet 1996;5:1129, 1130.

73. Hill MR, James AL, Faux JA, et al. Fc epsilon RI-beta polymorphism and risk of atopy in a general population sample. Br Med J 1995;311:776–779.

74. van Herwerden L, Harrap SB, Wong ZY, et al. Linkage of high-affinity IgE receptor gene with bronchial hyperreactivity, even in absence of atopy. Lancet 1995;346:1262–1265.

75. Lin S, Cicala C, Scharenberg A, Kinet J. The Fc(epsilon)RIbeta subunit functions as an amplifier of Fc(epsilon)RIgamma-mediated cell activation signals. Cell 1996;85:985–995.

76. Turner H, Kinet JP. Signalling through the high-affinity IgE receptor Fc epsilonRI. Nature 1999;402(6760 Suppl):B24–B30.

77. Donnadieu E, Cookson WO, Jouvin MH, Kinet JP. Allergy-associated polymorphisms of the Fc$\varepsilon RI\beta$ subunit do not impact its two amplification functions. J Immunol 2000;165:3917–3922.

142. Collins FS, Guyer MS, Charkravarti A. Variations on a theme: cataloging human DNA sequence variation. Science 1997;278(5343):1580, 1581.
143. Lai E, Riley J, Purvis I, Roses A. A 4-Mb high-density single nucleotide polymorphism-based map around human APOE. Genomics 1998;54:31–38.
144. Kruglyak L. Prospects for whole-genome linkage disequilibrium mapping of common disease genes. Nat Genet 1999;22:139–144.
145. Collins A, Lonjou C, Morton NE. Genetic epidemiology of single-nucleotide polymorphisms. Proc Natl Acad Sci USA 1999;96:15,173–15,177.
146. Huttley GA, Smith MW, Carrington M, O'Brien SJ. A scan for linkage disequilibrium across the human genome. Genetics 1999;152:1711–1722.
147. Kidd JR, Pakstis AJ, Zhao H, et al. Haplotypes and linkage disequilibrium at the phenylalanine hydroxylase locus, PAH, in a global representation of populations. Am J Hum Genet 2000;66:1882–1899.
148. Goddard KA, Hopkins PJ, Hall JM, Witte JS. Linkage disequilibrium and allele-frequency distributions for 114 single-nucleotide polymorphisms in five populations. Am J Hum Genet 2000;66:216–234.
149. Jorde LB, Watkins WS, Carlson M, et al. Linkage disequilibrium predicts physical distance in the adenomatous polyposis coli region [see comments]. Am J Hum Genet 1994;54:884–898.
150. Clark AG, Weiss KM, Nickerson DA, et al. Haplotype structure and population genetic inferences from nucleotide- sequence variation in human lipoprotein lipase. Am J Hum Genet 1998;63:595–612.
151. Rieder MJ, Taylor SL, Clark AG, Nickerson DA. Sequence variation in the human angiotensin converting enzyme. Nat Genet 1999;22:59–62.
152. Moffatt MF, Traherne JA, Abecasis GR, Cookson WO. Single nucleotide polymorphism and linkage disequilibrium within the TCR alpha/delta locus. Hum Mol Genet 2000;9:1011–1019.
153. Templeton AR, Clark AG, Weiss KM, Nickerson DA, Boerwinkle E, Sing CF. Recombinational and mutational hotspots within the human lipoprotein lipase gene. Am J Hum Genet 2000;66:69–83.
154. Abecasis GR, Noguchi E, Heinzmann A, et al. Extent and Distribution of Linkage disequilibrium in three genomic regions. Am J Hum Genet 2001;68: 191–197.
155. Hedrick PW. Gametic disequilibrium measures: proceed with caution. Genetics 1987;117:331–341.
156. Devlin B, Risch N. A comparison of linkage disequilibrium measures for fine-scale mapping. Genomics 1995;29:311–322.
157. Abecasis GR, Cookson WO, Cardon LR. The power to detect linkage disequilibrium with quantitative traits in selected samples. Am J Hum Genet 2001;68:1463–1474.
158. Daly MJ, Rioux JD, Schaffner SF, Hudson TJ, Lander ES. High-resolution haplotype structure in the human genome. Nat Genet 2001;29: 229–232.
159. Gabriel SB, Schaffner SF, Nguyen H, et al. The structure of haplotype blocks in the human genome. Science 2002;296:2225–2229.
160. Muller-Myhsok B, Abel L. Genetic analysis of complex diseases [letter; comment]. Science 1997;275:1328, 1329; discussion 1329, 1330.

161. Tu IP, Whittemore AS. Power of association and linkage tests when the disease alleles are unobserved. Am J Hum Genet 1999;64:641–649.

162. Weissenbach J, Gypay G, Dib C, et al. A second generation linkage map of the human genome. Nature 1992;359:794–801.

163. George VT, Elston RC. Testing the association between polymorphic markers and quantitative traits in pedigrees. Genet Epidemiol 1987;4:193–201.

164. Terwilliger JD, Ott J. A haplotype-based 'haplotype relative risk' approach to detecting allelic associations. Hum Hered 1992;42:337–346.

165. Chakravarti A. Population genetics-making sense out of sequence. Nat Genet 1999;21(1 Suppl):56–60.

166. Reich DE, Lander ES. On the allelic spectrum of human disease. Trends Genet 2001;17:502–510.

167. Kruglyak L, Nickerson DA. Variation is the spice of life. Nat Genet 2001; 27:234–246.

168. Farrall M, Keavney B, McKenzie C, Delepine M, Matsuda F, Lathrop GM. Fine-mapping of an ancestral recombination breakpoint in DCP1 [Letter]. Nat Genet 1999;23:270, 271.

169. Morris RW, Kaplan NL. On the advantage of haplotype analysis in the presence of multiple disease susceptibility alleles. Genet Epidemiol 2002;23: 221–233.

170. Sobel E, Lange K. Descent graphs in pedigree analysis: applications to haplotyping location scores, and marker-sharing statistics. Am J Hum Genet 1996; 58:1323–1337.

171. Abecasis GR, Cookson WO. GOLD-graphical overview of linkage disequilibrium. Bioinformatics 2000;16(2):182, 183.

172. Larsen F, Gundersen G, Lopez R, Prydz H. CpG islands as gene markers in the human genome. Genomics 1992;13:1095–1107.

173. Prestridge DS. Predicting Pol II promoter sequences using transcription factor binding sites. J Mol Biol 1995;249:923–932.

174. Xu Y, Mural RJ, Uberbacher EC. Constructing gene models from accurately predicted exons: an application of dynamic programming. Comput Appl Biosci 1994;10:613–623.

175. Burge C, Karlin S. Prediction of complete gene structures in human genomic DNA. J Mol Biol 1997;268:78–94.

176. Snyder EE, Stormo GD. Identification of coding regions in genomic DNA sequences: an application of dynamic programming and neural networks. Nucleic Acids Res 1993;21:607–613.

177. Zhang MQ. Identification of protein coding regions in the human genome by quadratic discriminant analysis. Proc Natl Acad Sci USA 1997;94: 565–568.

178. Altschul SF, Madden TL, Schaffer AA, et al. Gapped BLAST and PSI-BLAST: a new generation of protein database search programs. Nucleic Acids Res 1997;25:3389–3402.

179. Schultz J, Copley RR, Doerks T, Ponting CP, Bork P. SMART: a web-based tool for the study of genetically mobile domains. Nucleic Acids Res 2000; 28:231–234.

180. Hugot JP, Chamaillard M, Zouali H, et al. Association of NOD2 leucine-rich repeat variants with susceptibility to Crohn's disease. Nature 2001;411: 599–603.
181. Ogura Y, Bonen DK, Inohara N, et al. A frameshift mutation in NOD2 associated with susceptibility to Crohn's disease. Nature 2001;411:603–606.

A

Advanced intercross lines (AIL), fine-mapping of quantitative trait loci, 221, 222

Airway hyperreactivity, *see* Asthma

Alcoholism, *see* Substance dependence

Alox15, susceptibility gene identification in murine osteoporosis model, 18–20

α1-Antitrypsin deficiency, *see* Emphysema

Asthma,
  candidate loci in humans,
    chromosomal regions in other immune diseases, 279
    chromosome 13q13, 277
    chromosome 20p, 278
    FcεRI-β, 277
    human leukocyte antigens, 276, 277
    interleukin-4,
      cytokine cluster, 277, 278
      receptor polymorphisms, 278
  economic impact, 269
  eczema association, 269, 270
  epidemiology, 269
  heritability, 270
  interspecies comparison of candidate genes, 127
  pathophysiology, 116, 117
  phenotype selection for positional cloning,
    bronchial hyperresponsiveness, 270–272
    eczema, 272

    genetic linkage, 273
    genome screens, 275
    genotypic ambiguity and error, 273, 274
    nonreplicated linkage, 275, 276
    parent-of-origin effects, 274, 275
    power to detect linkage, 270, 271
    quantitative traits, 272
    segregation analysis, 271
  prospects for study, 288
  rodent models,
    airway hyperreactivity (measurement), 118–120
    genetic determinants, 120
    mouse allergen challenge models, 117, 118
    overview, 12
    quantitative trait loci analysis, 120–124
  susceptibility gene identification in murine models,
    association mapping, 284–286
    expressed sequence tag databases, 286
    expression analysis, 287
    functional analysis,
      genetic modification of mice, 287, 288
      homology searching, 287
    linkage disequilibrium mapping, 282–284
    overview, 15–18, 26, 280–282
    polymorphism analysis, 287
    sequencing, 286
    transgenic mice for functional studies, 127, 128

Atopic dermatitis, *see* Eczema